Praise for Kay Redfield Jamison's

Fires in the Dark

"The desperate, uncertain, even heroic attempt to heal is at the center of Jamison's new book. . . . It is a kaleidoscopic vision of treatment and recovery that reflects her own passionately varied intellectual life."   —*The New York Times*

"A humane, elegantly written contribution to the literature of trauma and care."   —*Kirkus Reviews* (starred review)

"Jamison . . . explores the process of prying a mind from disease or despair. Healing, she writes, depends on 'harvesting the imagination' and . . . 'the balance between remembering and forgetting.'"   —*The New Yorker*

"[Jamison makes] the case for why the humanities matter in a way that is deeper and more emotionally resonant than anything I've seen before."
—Judith Warner, *The Washington Post*

"Jamison, the exquisite chronicler of her own unquiet mind, reflects on the process—and adventure—of healing in this beautiful cultural, historical, and creative exploration of what makes us whole. . . . Jamison's elegant prose, imbued with personal warmth and deep humanity, is itself a solace, lighting the way."   —Lori Gottlieb, author of
Maybe You Should Talk to Someone

"Wonderful. . . . Should make us all think again about mental illness, the profession of psychiatry, and how we heal ourselves and others."   —John Burnside, *The Guardian*

"A profound and beautiful book. The last chapter felt like a benediction. There is so much here for the art of crafting a life of meaning. . . . A marvelously creative intelligence."
—Arthur Kleinman,
Professor of Psychiatry, Harvard University

"[*Fires in the Dark*] has a unique dramatic architecture born not just of the specific content but the remarkably creative sequencing of that content and a resulting overwhelming urgency."   —Michael Hersch, composer and pianist,
Professor of Composition, Peabody Institute

"Beautiful. . . . The reach and breadth are consoling, confirming, and vast."   —Leo Kottke, guitarist

"[A] rigorous, deeply felt meditation on psychological healing. . . . An eloquent, wide-ranging, and edifying look at healing relationships of all kinds."
—*Publishers Weekly* (starred review)

"Jamison has in her life been both the healer and the healed. . . . She is focused not only on the acute stages of mental health problems but on what comes afterwards. . . . 'How do I take on the world? How do I take some purpose from this?'"   —*The Lancet*

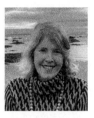

KAY REDFIELD JAMISON

Fires in the Dark

Kay Redfield Jamison is the Dalio Professor in Mood Disorders and a Professor of Psychiatry at the Johns Hopkins University School of Medicine, and an Honorary Professor of English at the University of St. Andrews in Scotland. She is the coauthor of the standard medical text on bipolar disorder and the author of the national bestsellers *An Unquiet Mind, Night Falls Fast, Exuberance*, and *Touched with Fire*. Her most recent book, *Robert Lowell, Setting the River on Fire*, was a Pulitzer Prize finalist. Dr. Jamison is a Fellow of the American Academy of Arts and Sciences and the Royal Society of Edinburgh. She is a recipient of the Lewis Thomas Prize, the Sarnat Prize from the National Academy of Medicine, and a MacArthur award.

Fires in the Dark

Fires in the Dark

Healing the Unquiet Mind

KAY REDFIELD JAMISON

VINTAGE BOOKS
A Division of Penguin Random House LLC
New York

FIRST VINTAGE BOOKS EDITION 2024

Copyright © 2023 by Kay Redfield Jamison

All rights reserved. Published in the United States by Vintage Books,
a division of Penguin Random House LLC, New York, and distributed in
Canada by Penguin Random House Canada Limited, Toronto.
Originally published in hardcover in the United States by Alfred A. Knopf,
a division of Penguin Random House LLC, New York, in 2023.

Vintage and colophon are registered trademarks of
Penguin Random House LLC.

Page 383 constitutes an extension of this copyright page.

The Library of Congress has cataloged the Knopf edition as follows:
Names: Jamison, Kay R., author.
Title: Fires in the dark : healing the unquiet mind / Kay Redfield Jamison.
Description: First edition. | New York : Alfred A. Knopf, 2023. |
Includes bibliographical references and index.
Identifiers: LCCN 2022038323.
Subjects: LCSH: Mental illness—Treatment—History. |
Psychotherapy—History—20th century. |
Rivers, W. H. R. (William Halse Rivers), 1864–1922. |
Osler, William, Sir, 1849–1919. | Jamison, Kay R.
Classification: LCC RC438 .J36 2023 | DDC 616.89/14—dc23
LC record available at https://lccn.loc.gov/2022038323

Vintage Books Trade Paperback ISBN: 978-1-9848-9820-3
eBook ISBN: 978-0-525-65718-7

Author photograph © Thomas Traill
Book design by Soonyoung Kwon

vintagebooks.com

Printed in the United States of America
10 9 8 7 6 5 4 3 2 1

For my husband,

Tom Traill

"I understood that this is what I'd been waiting for."

and
Daniel Auerbach, MD,

who built fires in the dark

Psycho-therapeutics would seem to be the oldest branch of medicine.

—W.H.R. RIVERS, MD, FRS

Fires in the dark you build; tall quivering flames
In the huge midnight forest of the unknown.
Your soul is full of cities with dead names,
And blind-faced, earth-bound gods of bronze and stone.

—SIEGFRIED SASSOON,
FOR W.H.R. RIVERS

Accompaniment. It's an elastic term: it means just what you'd imagine and more. . . . There's an element of mystery, of openness, in accompaniment: I'll go with you and support you on your journey wherever it leads. I'll keep you company and share your fate for a while. And by "a while," I don't mean a little while.

—PAUL FARMER, MD, PHD

Contents

Fires in the Dark

The Oldest Branch of Medicine

Rivers was intolerant and sympathetic. . . . He was once compared to Moses laying down the law. The comparison was an apt one, and one side of the truth. The other side was his sympathy. There is really no word for this. Sympathy is not good enough. It was a sort of power of getting into another man's life and treating it as if it were his own. And yet all the time he made you feel that your life was your own to guide, and above everything else that you could if you cared make something important of it.

—SIR FREDERIC BARTLETT, 1923

From earliest times to our own, in cave, village, or consulting room, certain individuals—healers—have stood out for being able to ease the suffering of the mourning, melancholic, or mad. Long before we could treat diseases of the brain and afflictions of the mind, priests and doctors laid on hands, listened, consoled, dispensed potions, and engaged the gods through ritual and magic. Science has progressed. Medications and psychotherapy extend hope that did not exist in earlier times, and for many, modern medicine offers cure. But to treat, even to cure, is not always to heal. This book is about the healing of psychological pain through medicine and psychotherapy, what makes a great healer, and the role of imagination and memory in the regeneration of the mind. It is about how extraordinary psychotherapy is when done well and how dispiriting it is when done badly. It is about the human and clinical reality that healing the mind is, at its heart, a journey into memory and imagination, a quest. It is a journey of accompaniment and hard work.

"The Mind at War," the first part of *Fires in the Dark*, is set in the field and shell shock hospitals of the First World War and introduces themes that are developed throughout the book. First among them, healing the mind goes back to the beginnings of medicine and religion; the need for it is as old as the needs of human nature. In recent times, healing the mind has drawn importantly upon what was learned by doctors and nurses during the First World War. They confronted unimaginable psychological pain and brought to its easing as much medical knowledge and compassion as they could. A few wrote accounts of horror and healing that are among the most powerful to come out of any war. So too did the poets who fought in the war. Doctor, nurse, and poet knew: Memory must be grappled with, death is a compelling tutor, and adversity teaches.

This book tells the story of the doctors and nurses who looked after the psychologically wounded, and the stories of those they tried to heal. It discusses two preeminent healers in depth, Sir William Osler and Dr. W.H.R. Rivers. Osler, first physician-in-chief of the Johns Hopkins Hospital and later Regius Professor of Medicine at Oxford, is considered one of the most influential physicians in history. As a doctor and teacher he was profoundly interested in healing and what makes a great healer. Osler's primary interest was in clinical practice and the scientific study of medicine, but he advised young doctors to read broadly in the humanities and taught them the judicious use of faith and suggestion in medical practice. Osler was very much engaged in the First World War, both as consultant physician to the British army hospitals and as the father of a young soldier killed on the Western Front. He came to know the limits of healing.

This first part of the book focuses particularly on the medical psychologist, physician, and anthropologist W.H.R. Rivers and on his psychotherapeutic work with Siegfried Sassoon, prominent among the war poets. To his practice, Rivers brought not only medical training but also his experience as an anthropologist who had studied cultures different from his own. He had learned from their healing rituals and ways of death, from their gods and languages and arts, and from their ways of survival.

Psychotherapy, Rivers wrote, was an attempt to check disease by measures that act through the mind, an approach based on the link that has existed throughout history "between medicine on the one hand and magic and religion on the other." The earliest ways of healing were psychotherapeutic, Rivers believed, and "if the remedies of existing peoples of rude culture provide any indication of primitive modes of thought and action, psycho-therapeutics would seem to be the oldest branch of medicine."

Siegfried Sassoon detected these ancient roots of healing in his psychotherapy with Rivers: "Your soul is full of cities with dead names," he wrote, and "earth-bound gods of bronze and stone." Rivers's understanding of him, he said, was "out beyond the boundaries of my brain." Theirs was, in Sassoon's description, an archetypal healing relationship, a profound journey. What took place in Rivers's consulting room at the Craiglockhart War Hospital for shell-shocked officers provided Sassoon with a way to approach suffering; it gave him capacity to carry forward. Rivers learned from Sassoon and his other patients, and the insight obtained from therapeutic encounters made its way not only into clinical practice but into medical and psychiatric journals as well.

It was the uses of memory—what best to remember and reconstrue, what best to forget—that engaged the imagination of many of the war poets and doctors. The poets wrote about the horror of what they had seen and done at the Western Front. They wrote to pull meaning from the acts and costs of war and to preserve the memory of those who otherwise would be forgotten. Several of the poets felt a duty to hold accountable those who were responsible for the horror, and to make the horror plain to those who had not fought. They wrote to make others see, to make it hard for them to cast off and move on. Soldier should remember soldier, Sassoon wrote:

> *Do you remember that hour of din before the attack—*
> *And the anger, the blind compassion that seized and*
> *shook you then*
> *As you peered at the doomed and haggard faces of your*
> *men?*
> *Do you remember the stretcher-cases lurching back*
> *With dying eyes and lolling heads—those ashen-grey*
> *Masks of the lads who once were keen and kind and gay?*
>
> *Have you forgotten yet? . . .*
> *Look up, and swear by the green of the spring that you'll never*
> *forget.*

To remember the dead and the maimed, to know the faces of the insane, to bear witness to the men they had commanded or served with, was to start to heal. To write about the war was to shape its terror and futility into something that could be grasped and its memory, to a point, controlled. The debt to the dead was to remember, and to carry the message forward. Nations as well as individuals grieved.

After a nation's collective horror of war, it was the duty and godsend of king and priest to tend the national grief through ritual, prayer, and music. Psychological healing was a broad necessity.

If the first part of this book is about trauma and building back from experiences of war, the second, "Healers of the Mind," centers on psychotherapy, medication, and other treatments for psychological suffering. The emphasis is on healers—priests, physicians, psychotherapists—and on psychological treatment, rather than medication. This is not because medication is less important, for it is not, but because in recent years psychotherapy has been relegated to the sidelines; this has been to the detriment of doctor and patient alike. There is no clinical or scientific reason to argue a false choice between medication and psychotherapy. Psychotherapeutics, as Rivers said, is the oldest branch of medicine; as such, it is deeply embedded in the needs of our race.

"Healers of the Mind" discusses the deep religious and magical roots of psychotherapy—funerary yarrow in Neanderthal caves, rituals of healing in the Greek temples and on Homeric battlefields, faith and suggestion, confession, redemption, and pilgrimage—and the role that psychotherapy plays in building walls to protect the mind, and in giving order to a chaotic personal universe; to exploring the roots of suffering, and in pursuing meaning and purpose in life: all of these while edging the mind toward risk and quest.

Consolation and confession—among the oldest instruments of healing—are territory shared by priest and doctor. To comfort in times of despair, to struggle with injustice, to bring peace to the troubled: These are charges of the healer. Consolation, evolved from amulet and temple ritual into eulogy, sermon, prayer book, and then the consulting room, is a critical task of priest, physician, and, more recently, psychotherapist. "I will not leave you comfortless," it says in the Gospel of John. "I will come to you." Consolation breeds hope, and hope, given fulsomely and honestly, seeds the ground for healing. In hope lies belief that we can make our way out of desolation and endure suffering long enough to make it to the far side of despair.

Great healers learn how to repair and make whole the sick mind. This book looks at what makes a healer great, and which qualities are shared by healer and priest. The doctor who ministers to the wounds of body and mind may be well-trained in clinical methods but requires as well character that lends to healing. "Often the best part of your work," William Osler told young doctors, "will have nothing to do with potions and powders, but with the exercise of an influence of the strong upon the weak." The influence must be just and well-considered. Resolution and hard work, like diagnostic and therapeutic acumen, are constitutive to a good doctor. They enable doctors to bring "comfort and help to the weak-hearted," to console not only others but themselves "in the sad hours," and to act as convoy through dangerous waters. Psychotherapy and medication underpin the modern treatment of mental suffering; thanks to science, they continue to evolve. Such treatments make healing possible; they lay the groundwork. But to heal requires more: active engagement of the imagination, learning, and seeking. Healing is a journey; it gleans from experience. Imagination, with experience, expands the territory.

Work heals. William Osler referred to work as the "true balm of hurt minds," and it is both part of the journey and, at times, the end point. Work is an active part of healing; it sustains, reaffirms, and replenishes. It gives purpose, as William James and Viktor Frankl knew well. Recovering lost dreams and passions by reengagement in work absorbs the mind, finds meaning. Writing, the poet Robert Lowell said, "takes the ache away"; it wraps frayed nerves with a "bandage of grace and ambergris." Many of the asylum doctors knew the benefit of work for their patients, and the Scottish psychiatrist A. J. Brock knew it particularly well. His psychotherapeutic treatment of the poet Wilfred Owen during the First World War, discussed toward the end of the book, was grounded in prescribed creative and physical work.

The final part of the book, "The Healing Arts," addresses the role of imagination in psychological healing and discusses the importance of art, adventure, adversity, and courage. Those who suffer—who are depressed, frightened, grieving—can learn from the heroic and the mythic; they can learn from those who have been through ordeal and suffering and who have not just survived, but prevailed. We learn from these archetypes—the explorer, the king, the poet—who make it to the distant side of ordeal: who give back what they have learned, who inspire, and who leave behind them words and deeds that can heal others. We learn that bold action can be an antidote to suffering. This is not recognized as much as it could be. We live in a time when encouraging a becalmed, quiet mental state—a focus on present and gentled sensation—is valued, taught, and trademarked. This serves many people well, but by no means everyone and certainly not at all times. Casting about in more disquieting pools may heal the mind differently and lay a groundwork for contending with future setbacks. An active approach to adversity, a swim toward dangerous waters, can help the mind regenerate. It can brace the will, get past a time of suffering, and help make sense of it. Minds are different and healing them is likewise so.

The active engagement of sufferer with healer is necessary to make sense of the experience of suffering—grief, depression, trauma, madness—by learning how to navigate hard psychological straits, to face painful memories, to gauge and harness intense or erratic moods, and to find vitality when it has been depleted. The task of a good doctor or psychotherapist is to guide the journey from suffering to health; to be, as Sassoon said of Rivers, a guide in the "devastated regions / When the brain has lost its bearings in the dark." It is a journey of accompaniment.

The book ends on the good that can come from adversity. Making it through suffering, whether patient, doctor, hero, or artist, can strengthen oneself and hearten others. It is by no means necessary for psychological healing that it come from a doctor, priest, or psychotherapist. Love can heal. Books and nature and music heal, in different ways. Music in particular is balm and blessing. It quickens and unites, arouses to common purpose. It pours blood into the heart, touches, and heals. Musicians, when themselves opened by heartbreak, can reach others through their art and lives. This is powerfully observed in the life and art of singer-activist Paul Robeson. Robeson's unassailable sense of moral purpose gave strength to tens of thousands of those less strong. He did not bend in his convictions. His singing and leadership, his social activism helped heal and give voice to the humanity he was certain binds us all. He suffered, he sang, and he spoke for those who had little cause to believe. He extended hope to those who had none. "Paul is medicine to me," said Robeson's brother, himself a minister. "The music of his soul has cured me of many maladies." Not all who heal others are doctors or priests.

There are cycles of life that tie us: the fallow seasons and the fecund; the disturbing times and the quiet ones. The mind that has suffered and has come back to health is a singular example of regeneration in nature. Healing allows this restoration; it creates capacity to move with more grace and gravity through change in circumstance. And when time demands, as it will, a "lowering of the sail and a gathering in of the sheet," healed wounds confer strength.

This book is a personal one in many ways, influenced inevitably by my experiences as a psychotherapist, professor, and patient. The hospital where I work, Johns Hopkins, has been from its beginning an exemplar of excellent clinical medicine. William Osler, whose life begins this book, was the embodiment of a great healer. My thinking about healing has been deeply shaped by my colleagues at Johns Hopkins who continue in the Oslerian tradition.

Fires in the Dark is indebted as well to my own treatment by a doctor and psychotherapist who exemplifies the art and science of healing. *What matters to you?* he asked. *How can I make a difference?* I learned from him how to plot a course through mania and depression and ways to negotiate the paths leading into the past, and find the uncertain ones that branched into the future. Although ultimately one must find one's own way. I rarely felt alone. To accompany is the gift and necessity of a healer. Over the course of a hard illness I learned to draw more deeply upon husband, family, and friends; to find in nature what only nature can give; and to experience from music and books the meaning only they can accord to grief and suffering.

As many have done, I have learned to piece together a world of sustaining things: Washington, always. The Chesapeake Bay and Big Sur, St. Andrews and London. The late works of Beethoven and Schubert. The Book of Common Prayer. William Bradford and Robert Lowell. Paul Robeson. Maria Callas. Sinatra. The Oz books and the Hornblower saga. Willa Cather. Pasternak and Hardy. The epics of Homer; the writings of the Antarctic explorers Scott and Cherry-Garrard; the pioneers of the American West. Early, lastingly, and close to the heart: the Arthurian tragedy—Malory's *Le Morte d'Arthur* and, returned to often, *The Once and Future King*. Books read for love and often to heal. Always books, places, music: islands in the mind, islands of one's own making.

This book is not about specific tenets and techniques of psychotherapy. There are good books that do this—books that describe in detail the philosophical underpinnings, methods, and outcomes of different types of treatment—but that is not my interest here. Psychotherapeutic techniques, like medications, come and go. Human nature and its needs are more constant. My book is, more than anything, a reflection on healing the mind. It is an archipelago of thoughts, experiences, and images. It is a book that looks back on the ancient, learns from the modern, and tries to discern the common threads and practices of extraordinary healing. It seeks for what Siegfried Sassoon wrote about his psychiatrist, W.H.R. Rivers: *Rivers came in and closed the door behind him. Quiet and alert, purposeful and unhesitating, he seemed to empty the room of everything that had needed exorcising.*

I

The Mind at War

Healing the Broken

CHAPTER I

The Shadow of a Great Rock

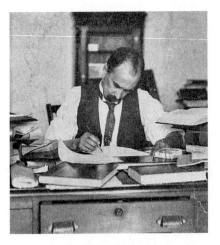

William Osler, 1891
At work on *The Principles and
Practice of Medicine*
The Johns Hopkins Hospital

*Live in the ward. Do not waste the hours of
daylight in listening to that which you may read
by night. But when you have seen, read.*

It is a hard matter and really not often necessary (since
nature usually does it quietly and in good time) to tell a
patient that he is past all hope. As Sir Thomas Browne
says: "It is the hardest stone you can throw at a man to
tell him that he is at the end of his tether"; and yet, put
in the right way to an intelligent man it is not always
cruel.

—SIR WILLIAM OSLER, 1909,
"THE TREATMENT OF DISEASE"

Theirs was, I think, the happiest household I ever knew
in those days before the Madness," remembered Sir
John Slessor. The Oxford home of Sir William and Grace
Osler seemed "always to be full of sunshine," ringing with
laughter and crammed with young doctors streaming in and
out to borrow books and talk medicine into the night. Osler,
Regius Professor of Medicine, was the preeminent physician
on either side of the Atlantic, and seen by many as the father
of modern medicine. (The esteem remains. A recent study
of American doctors, completed one hundred years after
Osler's death in 1919, found that American doctors continue
to regard him as the most influential physician in history.)
Osler was, to those he treated and taught, the embodiment
of the healer.

For young men of a particular class—those who filled
Osler's library and drawing room—Oxford was, in the years
leading up to the First World War, a world of promise and
privilege and summer days that lent themselves to nostalgia.
It was a world that cracked in August 1914. John Slessor, frequent guest in the Osler home during those years, fought

in the air in both world wars and later became Marshal of the Royal Air Force. His memories of the Great War were personal. He believed that those who survived its butchery tended to be "unduly sentimental about the friends of our distant youth, those golden young men who died in the holocausts of the 3rd Ypres and the Somme." Yet he understood that looking back made the future tenable, knew the "hell where youth and laughter go," the pain from the death of a world and of so many friends who defined that world. For him, the friend "above all to whose loss I have never been able to reconcile myself" was Edward Revere Osler, the only child of William and Grace Osler, in whose sunlit, laughter-filled house he had spent so much of his youth. Revere, named for his great-great-grandfather, the Boston silversmith and Revolutionary War hero Paul Revere, was adored by both his parents, unabashedly so by his father. From the first day, Osler was smitten with his son.

Revere and Slessor fished for trout and perch in the Oxford rivers, played cricket, exchanged books, and sketched ships and cathedral arches. They left to their separate schools and caught up at holidays. When war was declared they returned together to "a strange Oxford" already reconfiguring for action, a town soon to be overtaken by troops and hospitals. The life they had known in the town—young men in flannels, long-skirted girls, garden parties and skating on frozen ponds—faded fast and then was gone. Revere left his undergraduate studies at Oxford to serve first with a Canadian hospital unit and then, impatient to be more actively engaged, took up his commission as a second lieutenant in the Royal Field Artillery. Revere (see photo section) wrote to his father from the desolation of the Western Front in 1916. "Not an inch of earth that has not been upturned is left," he told him. "In places the shell holes are twelve feet deep, and filled with putrid mud and occasionally with a corpse at the bottom. All kinds of abandoned equipment lies everywhere, and on every sky-line rifles stick in the mud with bayonets tied across them to indicate a grave." To his mother he described the grimness of the trenches, the charred trees and the "old helmets, dead horses, and crosses." The Front inspired not so much horror as "something more than horror, more akin to a state of complete depression." He had never realized, he said, how much he missed the quiet world of Oxford, how much he loved his parents, how much he missed fishing and home.

Revere returned to Oxford on leave in May 1917. He had not slept in a bed for seven months, his father said. "His nerves are A.1. but it has been a hard experience and it is not easy to get him to talk much." Only a few months earlier Osler had written to Revere that seldom had father and son been so happy together: "No regrets cloud the clear past of 21 years—and this is a good deal to say. You have been everything that a father could wish. . . . I hope when the tyranny is overpast we may have more happy days together."

It was the unrealized hope of many fathers. The Battle of Passchendaele began within months of Revere's return to the Front. It was a slaughter. Within a day of the battle's start the field hospitals were overwhelmed. George Crile, an American surgeon, described the conditions of his hospital behind the front line: "Every bed, every aisle, every tent, every inch of floor space was occupied by stretchers—then the rows of stretchers spread out over the lawn, around the huts, flowing out toward the railway." The operating rooms ran day and night. "Each operating team did a hundred operations a day, but only one out of ten cases that should have been done. . . . Over ten thousand wounded passed through in the first forty-eight hours. I had two hundred deaths in one night in my own service." The doctors and nurses were not to take notice when shells exploded, Crile was told by his commanding officer. It was a meaningless directive: "The surgeon is barraged with fractures; shelled with broken heads; bombed with bellies; gassed with wounds."

Revere Osler's battery was shelled by the Germans during the late afternoon of August 29. Badly injured, with shrapnel in his chest, thigh, and abdomen, he was carried to a gun pit to have his wounds dressed; from there he was taken by stretcher and ambulance to the 47th Casualty Clearing Station, a medical facility just beyond enemy gunfire. By chance, four of the most skilled American surgeons were serving in field hospitals nearby; all knew Revere's father well from their years at Johns Hopkins when Osler was the first physician-in-chief: Harvey Cushing, pioneer neurosurgeon and chief neurosurgical consultant to the American Expeditionary Forces; George Crile, the first surgeon to have succeeded in performing a direct blood transfusion; George Brewer, chief consultant in surgery to the First Army; and William Darrach, a distinguished surgeon and academic.

Cushing, a close friend of the Osler family and later Osler's biographer, received a message at ten o'clock that night after a long day of operating: "Sir Wm. Osler's son seriously wounded at 47 C.C.S. Can Major Cushing come immediately?" It could not have been much worse, Cushing wrote in his journal. He cabled Osler straightaway: "Revere seriously wounded: not hopelessly: conscious: comfortable."

"Obviously all was lost," Crile wrote later. "The long marquee tent was quiet and dim; the end was fast approaching." Revere was conscious for a short time and "a faint smile illuminated his face when told that his father's American friends were there." The surgeons operated on him through the night but Revere died the next morning. The doctors, although in hourly contact with death, felt a particular pain at the death of Osler's son. Cushing cut a button from Revere's uniform to give to Osler, and Crile, who had been in Baltimore at the time of Revere's birth, recalled with sorrow, "I thought about the two times that Sir William's son had claimed my attention. Tonight and twenty years ago, the first and the last."

"We saw him buried in the early morning," Cushing wrote in his journal. "A soggy Flanders field beside a little oak grove to the rear of the Dosinghem group—an overcast, windy, autumnal day—the long rows of simple wooden crosses . . . The boy wrapped in an army blanket and covered by a weather-worn Union Jack, carried on their shoulders by four slipping stretcher-bearers. A strange scene—the great-great-grandson of Paul Revere under a British flag, and awaiting him a group of some six or eight American Army medical officers—saddened with the thoughts of his father . . . Some green branches were thrown in for him to lie on. The Padre recited the usual service—the bugler gave the 'Last Post'—and we went about our duties. Plot 4, Row F."

That evening, across the Channel, William Osler sat in his library and wrote about the death of his only child: "4:15 pm. I was sitting in my library working on the new edition of my text-book when a telegram was brought in from Harvey Cushing, at no. 41 Casualty clearing station. 'Revere dangerously wounded, comfortable & conscious, condition not hopeless.' I knew this was the end. We had expected it. The Fates do not allow the good fortune that has followed me to go with me to the grave. Call no man happy till he dies. The W. O. [War Office] telephoned in the evening that he was dead. The one consolation was that Harvey Cushing was with him & that he & Crile and Brewer also old friends died [sic] everything possible. A sweeter laddie never lived."

NAME.	Su. 26	M. 27	Tu. 28	W. 29	Th. 30	F. 31	Sa. 1
Dr Scott Holland	c				c		
Mrs Hall, sheeple Barton			c		.		c
Dr Cummings. C.a m C			c				
Mr Harrison. (Rec off			c				
Mrs Paradise. Theden					c		
Lt. Cullen. (Carter)					c		

4¹⁵ p.m.

I was sitting in my library reading recent asthma
articles for the new Edition; only left work when
a telegram was brought in from Harvey Cushing,
at No 41 Casualty clearing station. "Revere dangerously wounded, comfortable & conscious, condition
not hopeless." I knew this was the end: we
had expected it. The Fates do not allow the
good fortune that has followed me to go with
him to the grave. Call no man happy till he dies
The W.O. telephoned in the evening that he was
dead. The one consolation was that Harvey
Cushing was with him & that he & Crile and
Brewer also old friends did everything possible
a sweeter laddie never lived, with a gentle
loving nature. He had developed a rare taste
in literature, and was devoted to all my
old friends in the spirit — Plutarch, Montaigne
Browne, Fuller and above all to Isaac Walton
whose compleat angler he knew by heart &
whose "Lives" he loved. . We are heart-
broken, but thankful to have the precious
memory of his loving life.

Day book of Sir William Osler
Entry upon the death of Revere Osler
August 1917

The physician's work lies on the confines of the shadow-land, and it might be expected that, if to any, to him would come glimpses that might make us less forlorn when in the bitterness of loss.

—SIR WILLIAM OSLER, *Science and Immortality*

Death had been Osler's tutor for the shadow-land. As a young pathologist he had performed nearly a thousand autopsies; he was keenly aware of the debt owed by the living to the dead. The dead-house taught lastingly and well, he said. On the title page of the book that recorded his autopsies, Osler quoted the esteemed pathologist Sir Samuel Wilks: "Pathology is the basis of all true investigation in Practical Medicine." To study death, to handle the dead, was to study life. It was to understand not only disease and the processes of dying, but to gain some understanding of the human condition. To conduct an autopsy—the ancient examination, "to see for oneself"—forced a doctor to face the precariousness of life, not only for the body on the table so recently alive, but for the doctor. Death taught its own inevitability; it made clear the limits of healing. Not all suffering could be made better by doctor or priest. It was the charge of the healer to understand the limits of medicine and to act upon possibility, not illusion. "In seeking absolute truth we aim at the unattainable," Osler told young doctors, but "must be content with finding broken portions."

In the early 1900s, during his time as chief of medicine at Johns Hopkins, Osler expanded his interests beyond disease to what doctors might learn from the dying about suffering and healing. Doctors and nurses at the Johns Hopkins Hospital recorded their observations of nearly five hundred dying

A STUDY OF THE ACT OF DYING.

JOHNS HOPKINS HOSPITAL.

Name ____ Hosp. No. ____ Date Oct. 22nd 1902.

Age 39 Nationality American. Religion P. C. H. Roman Catholic

Nature of disease Mitral Stenosis + Insufficiency. Thrombosis. Embolism

Length of illness Three years of mo. in hospital – onset. August 1898.

The act of dying:

If sudden and very sudden – condition serious for 24 hours before.

Did respiration stop before pulse—how long? Yes – about one minute.

Coma or unconsciousness before death — how long? About three hours.

If any fear or apprehension, of what nature. See over –

    Bodily. i. e. pain. none for about twelve hours before death

    Mental. none immediately before see over

    Spiritual — remorse, etc. none –

                                J. M'Crae Over

This card is not to be filled out unless done within twenty-four hours of the death of the individual.

N. B. The object of this investigation is to ascertain the relative proportion of cases in which (1) the death is sudden; (2) accompanied by coma or unconsciousness; (3) by pain, dread or apprehension. Prof. Osler requests the intelligent co-operation of the members of the medical and nursing staff. Please note fully any other special circumstances connected with the act of dying.

"A Study of the Act of Dying"
Case note for a study by William Osler
The Johns Hopkins Hospital

Ever since admission on Jan 4th 1898 the patient has been extremely afraid of death – She has repeatedly thought herself to be dying and was always in a condition of panic regarding this – The day before her death was the anniversary of her father's death and she dwelt much on this fact during the day. The serious symptoms came on during the afternoon of Oct. 21st. At this meal she thought of dying but later on said nothing of it. About 1 pm on the day of death she asked me if her condition was serious and if the priest ought to be sent for. She was told that her condition was very grave and that the priest had better be called. She said nothing regarding this and accepted it without any comment. There was no doubt in my mind that she fully understood and knew exactly her condition. Both this she had also evidently no fear so far as one could judge. J. M'Crae patients, noting the extent of the patients' spiritual and mental fear or apprehension, their state of consciousness before death, and whether death had been sudden or prolonged.

"I have careful records of about five hundred death-beds, studied particularly with reference to the modes of death and the sensations of the dying," Osler said. "Ninety suffered bodily pain or distress of one sort or another, eleven showed mental apprehension, two positive terror, one expressed spiritual exaltation, one bitter remorse. The great majority gave no signs one way or the other; like their birth, their death was a sleep and a forgetting. The Preacher was right; in this matter, man hath no pre-eminence over the beast—'as the one dieth so dieth the other.'" It was a more sanguine summing up than perhaps was warranted.

John McCrae, whose clinical note for Osler's research study is shown on the previous page, was a house officer under William Osler and later a family friend. A pathologist and poet, McCrae served as an army doctor during the First World War. In 1915 he wrote "In Flanders Fields"—where "poppies blow / Between the crosses, row on row"—the most widely quoted poem of the war, in a field dressing station a mile from where, two years later, his friend Revere Osler was first treated for the wounds that killed him. McCrae's poem, published in England within months of his writing it, was struck through with valor, sacrifice, and duty to king and country; it had a lasting effect on the British public. Poppies remain the symbol of national cause and remembrance, worn by sovereign, soldier, and citizen to keep faith with the dead.

(William Osler, close to McCrae as he was, did not share McCrae's unwavering belief in the war. He was distraught by the killing and maiming of the thousands of young men he saw in the English war hospitals; more personally, he felt that Revere's transfer from a medical to a combat unit had been influenced by McCrae's pro-war enthusiasm. His son's "long association with Jack McCrae," Osler wrote, "made him a bit bloodthirsty.")

Poppies—sheets of them, miles and millions of them, spread across the battlefields of the Western Front. Bred up from death, given life from nutrients seeped from corpse into soil, their roots, another war poet, Isaac Rosenberg, wrote, "are in man's veins." It had been so for many wars. The summer after the Battle of Landen in 1693, the Duke of Perth remarked upon the metamorphosis of fields of death into fields of scarlet as he walked the battlefield still strewn with the heads and bones of soldiers. The poppies had sprung up everywhere, he said, "as if last year's blood had taken root and appeared this year in flowers." Two hundred years later Lord Macaulay wrote similarly that the soil "fertilised by twenty thousand corpses, broke forth into millions of poppies." It could be imagined, he said, that Isaiah had figured rightly: "The earth was disclosing her blood, and refusing to cover the slain."

When John McCrae died in France in 1918, Harvey Cushing attended his funeral. It was a large gathering and a brilliant afternoon. McCrae's horse was led by two grooms, his boots reversed in the tradition of the fallen commander. Cushing observed that soldiers were "scouring the fields this afternoon to try and find some chance winter poppies to put on his grave—to remind him of Flanders, where he would have preferred to lie." For John McCrae, life and death, like poppies arising from the blood-soaked fields, had been bound together from the beginning. His autopsy book, kept by him as a young pathologist, was testament to this. It is a fastidious record of more than four hundred postmortems he had conducted and, as he put it rather arcanely, the "diverse straunge and fearsome condicions that have ledde to ye same final ende." One studied the dead to outwit disease in the living, he said. One recognized the transience of life, the lessons learned from the deaths of others. "God have them of his grace," he wrote.

Throughout his life, McCrae's poetry and medical practice were rooted in what he had learned from the dead: how better to heal suffering, how best to comfort the dying, how better to live, how better to contend with ambiguity. This thinking he had in common with Osler. "Medicine is a science of uncertainty and an art of probability," Osler said. A physician must maintain and be able to tolerate uncertainty about things of great matter and keep close a pressing sense of

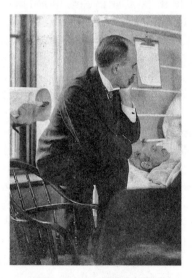

William Osler at the bedside
The Johns Hopkins Hospital

He was a keen observer, a brilliant clinician. He was a great teacher. But his main strength lay in the example he set to his fellows and his students. He was a quickening spirit.

mortality. Healing required intimate knowledge of the limits of healing.

What made Osler a great physician? Many things. He was steeped in the practice, science, and history of Medicine. Medicine was a summons, like that of priesthood: "You are in this profession as a calling, not as a business," he told medical students in 1907. Medicine "exacts from you at every turn self-sacrifice, devotion, love and tenderness to your fellow-men. Once you get down to a purely business level, your influence is gone. . . . You must work in the missionary spirit, with a breadth of charity that raises you far above the petty jealousies of life." He taught that hope should be dispensed as freely as potions, or more so. He held the doctors he trained to a high standard in science, clinical knowledge, and humanity. He saw the best in his house staff and expected them to act as he perceived them.

Osler was a legendary diagnostician, clinical teacher, and healer. "His very presence brought healing," said Clarence Farrar, who trained under Osler at Johns Hopkins and later became a psychiatrist and editor of *The American Journal of Psychiatry*. Osler at the bedside, he said, was an exercise in "immediate unplanned psychotherapy." The word "psychotherapy" would not have come easily from Osler's lips but, whatever the term, he was a healer. He spoke with a gentle voice, conveyed confidence, and gave comfort. He knew clinical medicine as well as anyone, and he knew to respect what he did not know. Patients and students instinctively trusted him. Osler's kind of healing, wrote Farrar, was "an emanation of a sensitive and fine personality that understood how to handle people. He had a remarkable gift of empathy. There was healing in his voice. The vocal tone, the facial expression, the chosen word, all united to enhance the effect of the treatment measures he might use or the advice he might give."

In a time when laboratory science was new to medicine, Osler was steeped in it—he was expert in pathology, infectious disease, and microbiology—and he insisted that his students and house staff be well-versed in these things as well. He taught them clinical medicine at the bedside rather than in the lecture hall alone. He did not brook medical or scientific ignorance, nor did he tolerate arrogance. He expected civility and was himself the model of it. He respected the uncertainty and variability of disease and human nature. "If you want a profession in which everything is certain," Osler once said, "you had better give up medicine." Variability was the law of life. "No two individuals react alike and behave alike under the abnormal conditions which we know as disease."

Osler was notably interested in the relationship between disease and the person who lives with or dies of the disease. A disease, he said time and again, is not just a constellation of symptoms with a natural course. It is something that occurs to an individual—someone who has strengths and weaknesses in the circumstances of his life, as well as drawbacks and advantages in his character. It is these that determine how the disease is perceived, fought, and handled. William Sydney Thayer, resident physician under Osler and later his successor as physician-in-chief, said that Osler "taught us that the treatment of the patient was the most important element in the treatment of disease, that the patient not the disease was the entity." Echoing the Roman playwright Terence, he added that Osler was a man and "nothing human was foreign to him."

Each year at the Johns Hopkins Hospital, and at most teaching hospitals across the country, the Hippocratic Oath is administered to graduating medical students. The oath binds them to professional and ethical standards set down more than two thousand years ago by Hippocrates and his followers. Three years after their graduation from medical school, senior residents who have completed their training as house staff on the Osler Medical Service at Johns Hopkins take another oath. Written by Thomas Traill, a professor of medicine at Johns Hopkins and longtime faculty leader on the Osler Medical Service, it is specific to the values taught by both Hippocrates and William Osler. It is a statement of calling: "I affirm my vocation to be a doctor, to practice and teach the highest standard of medicine, and to uphold the tradition of Osler's medical service. I will act only in the interest of my patients, to enhance my own judgment with the counsel of others; to assist my colleagues in every way; and to extend my professional hand to the unfortunate. I will continue to learn, to study, and to teach. I will count my success as physician and teacher by the lives that I have touched." To be a good physician, Osler taught, and still teaches, is to heal the sick, to extend hope and give comfort, and to care for those with less advantage. It is to continue to learn, teach, and read. It is to practice medicine with seriousness of purpose, consummate science, and a quickening spirit.

In a lay sermon to students at the University of Edinburgh, Osler reflected on the place of suffering in life, and how doctors must contend with the "pestilence of darkness" and the "sickness of the noon-day." He started his talk with words from Isaiah:

> *And a man shall be as an hiding*
> *place from the wind, and a covert*
> *from the tempest; as rivers of water*
> *in a dry place, as the shadow of a*
> *great rock in a weary land.*

A healer should be a refuge, Osler taught, the shadow of a great rock. These things Osler believed, and these things he was.

Osler sought to understand what the healer could and could not do for the sick and dying; how mortality and suffering registered differently, patient to patient, and doctor to doctor; and how science and faith separately and together fit into the doctor's work. It was to understand the role a doctor's temperament played in healing. How ought dispassion to weigh in with emotion? What did it mean to heal? Who were the great healers? To which of them did one turn for instruction? How did one live with uncertainty? Which books did one live by? Always, Osler asked, which books were the best guides through life; which books were the best to inspire and inform the doctor? ("It is astonishing with how little reading a doctor can practice medicine," Osler remarked, "but it is not astonishing how badly he may do it.") From which books did one draw courage? By which did one learn to die? (Osler was well-known for manifesting, as well as believing in, equanimity, although several who knew him well saw an "essential melancholy" that gave to his work "a sensitivity and a healing power that others did not have." A colleague observed, "For some 15 years I saw Osler daily. He always seemed to be essentially a melancholy man. . . . Melancholy seems to me to be his essence, almost his driving force.")

Osler read deeply and encouraged young doctors to do so. Death and melancholy, fellow travelers as they often are, were the focus of two writers he read and reread, whose books he most intimately knew. Sir Thomas Browne's *Reli-*

gio Medici, Osler's "close companion since his school days," was, he said on many occasions, his most precious book. It was surpassingly original. "We are," wrote Virginia Woolf about Thomas Browne, "in the presence of sublime imagination." "All was mystery and darkness," she added, "as the first explorer walked the catacomb swinging his lanthorn." Robert Burton's *The Anatomy of Melancholy* was another book Osler read time and again. Both Browne, a physician and naturalist, and Burton, a scholar and vicar, were fixed on man's fragile ties to existence. "I that have examined the parts of man," wrote Browne, "know upon what tender filaments that Fabrick hangs." To be a doctor was "to preserve the living, make the dead to live, to keep men out of their Urnes," he said. The "discourse of humane fragments in them, is not impertinent unto our profession; whose study is life and death, who daily behold examples of mortality, and of all men least need official *memento's*, or coffins by our bed side to minde us of our graves."

Browne and Burton had sweeping intellects, minds that dipped and flew: "As a long-winged hawk, when he is first whistled off the fist, mounts aloft," wrote Burton, "and for his pleasure fetcheth many a circuit in the Air, still soaring higher and higher till he be come to his full pitch." From their far rovings Browne and Burton gathered bits of nature, history, and psychology, and remade to themselves the doctrines of religion and science; they then wove them, with self-account, into books that, four hundred years later, continue to claim fresh space in the minds of those who read them: stunning, each sui generis. Browne's style is "a tissue of many languages," wrote Samuel Johnson of *Religio Medici*, "a mixture of heterogeneous words, brought together from distant regions." The treatise was seminal and compassionate, one that could help both healer and sufferer. "By compassion we make others' misery our own," Browne had written. "And so, by relieving them, we relieve ourselves also."

As for Robert Burton's *Anatomy of Melancholy*, Osler held that it was the greatest medical treatise written by a layman. It was "serious in purpose, and weighty beyond belief." No book in any language, Osler said in a talk to the Elizabethan Club at Yale in 1913, "presents such a stage of moving pictures—kings and queens in their greatness and in their glory, in their madness and in their despair . . . the fools who were accounted wise, and the wise who were really fools; the madmen of all history . . . the world itself, against which he brings a railing accusation." Sufferer and physician must be actively engaged in the treatment of melancholy, Burton's *Anatomy* taught. Faith and medicine must be brought to bear, minds prized open. Osler found in Burton the affirmation that work could heal when other things did not, and that writing about one's own suffering might help others also in pain.

"I was fatally driven upon this rock of melancholy," Burton wrote. "To ease my mind in writing, I writ of melancholy, by being busy to avoid melancholy." His testament, observed Osler, made "an antidote out of that which was the prime cause of his disease." He had kept Saturn as his lord: "Undertaken partly to do himself good, partly out of a fellow feeling for others, he spent his time and knowledge in laboriously collecting out of the vast chaos and confusion of books a *cento* for the consolation of the afflicted in spirit. That which others heard and read of he had felt and practiced himself." Burton had aimed to ease his mind by writing, he confessed in *The Anatomy of Melancholy*, for he had an agony of mind, a festering in his head, which he was "desirous to be unladen of."

The books that Osler had advised others to read, and

that had counseled him as a doctor, were to console him differently in the years after his son died. "If unhappy—have hope," he quoted Burton. "If happy—be cautious."

⟜

The night that Revere died, Osler wrote to a friend, "We have been preparing for the blow. I felt sure the fates would hit me through him. I have escaped all these years without a great sorrow." A few days later Grace Osler expressed their grief: "Our boy has gone—gone—buried in that dank ground in Belgium." It was heartbreaking, she said, to hear her husband "sobbing hour after hour and never to see the boy again . . . he bluffs it during the day . . . but oh—the darkness—and the thought of our dear boy . . . and we are not there."

Osler kept some saving perspective by being aware of the losses that other parents experienced during the war. He wrote to his colleague William Halsted, surgeon-in-chief at Johns Hopkins Hospital and Harvey Cushing's former chief of service. "Cushing was with him at the end which is a comfort," Osler told him. "It is a hard blow but we hope to take it bravely. Others have been hit harder. I have three friends here who have lost two boys, their all & one who has lost three." We are, he added, "utterly desolated."

Osler went back to work as consultant physician to war hospitals in England. "We are taking the only medicine for sorrow," he said: "Time & hard work." It was a prescription he had given to many: Time and hard work. "We all knew his heart was broken," Nancy Astor commented. After Osler had completed making rounds at the army hospital on her Cliveden estate, "he went through the wards in his same gay old way, but when he got to the house—for luncheon alone with me—he sobbed like a child."

Osler had made it his rule in life to maintain equanimity in the midst of setback and gift alike. But one who saw beyond the measured manner to the wound beneath was a janitor who shared small talk with Osler most days as he arrived at the Oxford physiology laboratory. Osler's face was grave, he said. His manner was dark, his banter gone. "It is Mr. Revere, sir," he said to one of the professors. "And Sir William won't get better."

Osler lived for a year after the war ended, two years after Revere's death. He kept busy. He saw patients, consulted, gave lectures, and wrote clinical papers about nervous and medical diseases of war. He and Lady Grace entertained hundreds of young doctors and recuperating soldiers in their Oxford home. He donated a collection from his library, including first editions of Donne and Milton, Keats and Whitman, to Johns Hopkins University as a memorial to Revere, but he looked to the living as well. When the city of Oxford proposed raising money for a war memorial, Osler suggested to the mayor that they instead "put every halfpenny you get into decent houses for the poor." He lived his counsel to others, that "work is the true balm of hurt minds." It was counsel that fell short. A colleague from Johns Hopkins who visited Osler in Oxford noted that "there was a subdued look" in Osler's eyes that "haunted me." He remained cordial and charming but he had lost "the real, sustained snap."

Always, Osler turned to books. He reread not only those writers he had so often read before—Browne and Burton, Plutarch, Emerson, Montaigne, Marcus Aurelius—but came around to a writer whose works had previously left him largely unmoved. Walt Whitman had been Osler's patient when Osler was a young professor and Whitman in his late sixties, by then a famous poet. At that time Whitman's poetry was not to Osler's taste. It was too radical, too raw. It was more personal than Osler found comfortable. During the war, and after Revere was killed, Osler read Whitman in a different light. Whitman had been a nurse in Washington during the Civil War; he had cared for the wounded and been with them when they died. Whitman knew gangrene, the sound of the saw, and screams in the night.

Whitman and Osler were alike in more ways than would seem evident. They knew how to tend wounds and lay on hands, how to offer hope. They knew that words give meaning to suffering; that words are a means to heal the living and to remember the dead. From Whitman's "The Dresser":

Bearing the bandages, water and sponge,
Straight and swift to my wounded I go,
Where they lie on the ground, after the battle brought in;
Where their priceless blood reddens the grass, the ground;

Or to the rows of the hospital tent, or under the roof'd
hospital;
To the long rows of cots, up and down, each side, I return;
To each and all, one after another, I draw near—not one do
I miss;
An attendant follows, holding a tray—he carries a refuse
pail,
Soon to be fill'd with clotted rags and blood, emptied, and
fill'd again.

. . . .

I dress the perforated shoulder, the foot with the bullet
wound,
Cleanse the one with a gnawing and putrid gangrene, so
sickening, so offensive,

*While the attendant stands behind aside me, holding the
tray and pail.*

. . . .

*Returning, resuming, I thread my way through the
hospitals;
The hurt and wounded I pacify with soothing hand,
I sit by the restless all the dark night.*

"Such was the War," Whitman said. "It was not a qua-
drille in a ball-room."

Osler was working on a lecture about Whitman in the
weeks before he died and increasingly he recommended
Whitman's *Memoranda During the War* to his friends. The
war hospital—the "unending, universal mourning-wail of
woman, parents, orphans"—was the untold horror.

In January 1919, Harvey Cushing dined with Osler at
Christ Church, the Oxford college of both Osler and Revere.
The dinner by candlelight was solemn and celebratory, the
first to be held in three years. "The war is surely over," Cushing wrote in his journal. "It was very fine, Wolsey's great
hall by firelight," the close surround of ages past. Afterward
Cushing and Osler walked back to the Osler home and Cushing was put to bed with "a hot water bottle at his back, a bed
lamp at his side, and Walt Whitman's *Memoranda* of another
war put in his hands to read." Whitman's writing stayed
with Cushing, himself exhausted from the years of operating
on terrible head wounds under dangerous conditions, and
drained from witnessing the deaths of so many young men.
When Cushing wrote his own account of the First World
War, *From a Surgeon's Journal*, he took his epigraph from
Whitman. "The marrow of the tragedy is concentrated in

the Hospitals," Cushing quoted: "Much of a Race depends on what it thinks of death and how it stands personal anguish and sickness." Cushing's surgical war journal was witness, like Whitman, to the anguish of war.

⌒

William Osler died in December 1919. His body was laid out on a table in his house for the postmortem examination; following medical tradition, Osler had asked his attending physician to perform the autopsy. It was for others, as it had been for himself: to look, to examine, to see for oneself.

Osler's funeral was held at Christ Church Cathedral in Oxford on a gray afternoon shot through with the "thin light of winter." His coffin, covered by a purple pall, rested on an oak stand under Christopher Wren's bell tower. "The Cathedral was packed to the doors," wrote Lady Grace. "I felt a sensation of immense pride. . . . [He was] loved and respected by the world."

The night of his funeral, Osler's coffin rested in the Lady Chapel. It lay in the oldest part of the medieval cathedral, just steps from the memorial to Robert Burton. A sheaf of lilies from Lady Grace lay on the velvet pall; so too did Osler's favorite copy of *Religio Medici*, the one he had kept by his bedside and had inscribed, in fairer days, to Revere. He was, wrote Lady Grace, lying "under the arched roof Revere always sketched, & Burton's monument at his head—It is too wonderful."

CHAPTER 2

The Night Nurse

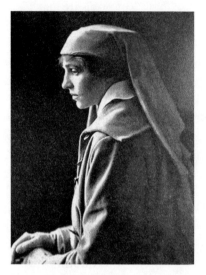

Mary Borden
Nurse on the Western Front
1914–1918

What have all these queer things to do with the dying of this man? Here are the cotton things and rubber things and steel things and things made of glass, all manner of things. What have so many things to do with the final adventure of this spirit?

He was taken to the operating room where a large piece of shell was removed and [his] wound packed; he suffered agonies and died two hours later. How useless these deaths seem to be. I watched him to the end and these hours of waiting are indeed hard to bear as everything has been done and there is nothing left for one to do but watch for the end. No matter how busy the staff may be, someone is always assigned to watch a patient who is near death, and I think it is a splendid rule.

—ALICE FITZGERALD, 1916,
"MEMOIRS OF AN AMERICAN NURSE"

In autumn of 1915, Sir William Osler spoke to a group of doctors in northern England. "The world is drunken and the nations are mad," he said, quoting Jeremiah. The madness could be seen and heard in the battlefields of Europe. There was a tract of land four miles long and just over one mile wide covered by "thick layers of the dead, heaps upon heaps, with hundreds of men standing upright, stiffened in death among the prone corpses." One could see from bluffs in France a city of British hospital tents, Osler continued, one that "spread out for miles between the dunes and the downs," with scores of British hospital wards under great tents of canvas. Innumerable "specks of white and khaki"—doctors and nurses from throughout Britain, the United States, and the Commonwealth—moved among the tents, tending and sorting the wounded. Hour after hour, the injured and dead were transferred from the ambulances and hospital trains to the wards.

Science had played its Promethean part, Osler said, and "made slaughter possible on a scale never dreamt of before . . . The shrapnel and the hand-grenade tear, bruise, and break, lacerating flesh and joints, blowing away limbs or part of the face or head, causing wounds not only terrible in themselves but certain to become infected with clothing and earth. Even the bones of a man's comrade have been blown into him." Then, Osler added, there were the insane.

Yet as Henry Adams observed about the Civil War, where there was chaos there too was opportunity. War propelled the creation of more deadly weapons but it also set the circumstances for advances in medicine and science. The overflowing war hospitals, the hundreds of thousands of wounded and dead, commanded not only urgency but improvisation. Osler's friend and colleague George Crile wrote that military surgery "has its shadows and its highlights. The highlights are romantic, for in a brief season whole areas of the body are conquered; great principles are worked out; foundation stones laid."

The war presented opportunity, number, and necessity to innovate and measure. Military doctors and scientists published their clinical findings and implemented change at an unprecedented pace. The torrent of wounded and dead made it possible for doctors to study the pathology of wounds and to have access to tissue and blood in ways not possible before the war. "If he wants post-mortem material," said Crile, "he chooses from the daily pile. If he desires transfusions he keeps a stream of blood flowing from donor to recipient, day and night." Harvey Cushing described his "incomparable opportunities" to study "every imaginable part of the brain through surgery or autopsy." Unthinkable numbers of war dead offered grim but effective teaching.

All fields of medicine and surgery advanced rapidly during the war: general, orthopedic, plastic and reconstructive surgery; neurosurgery; radiology; burn management, vaccination, and anesthesia; prosthetics, triage, treatment and prevention of contagious disease, blood transfusion, and blood storage. Healing wounds, always the particular priority in surgery, preoccupied doctors, nurses, and scientists. Wounds—lacerated, hemorrhaging, deep into the tissue— were sorted in triage and then in priority cleaned, debrided, and irrigated. Care was fastidious. Dressings were changed and tended by nurses who had learned to be adept and imperturbable. Wound healing uniquely required that the healer be hardened and gentle, both.

Ellen La Motte, a Johns Hopkins nurse working in France during the war, described caring for a patient whose wound had become infected by gas gangrene, recognizable in a moment by its "crackling and smell." The skull was fractured and a shell had lodged in the soldier's brain. But it was gas gangrene in his thigh that would kill him. "The wound stank. It was foul." The doctor "took a curette, a little scoop, and scooped away the dead flesh, the dead muscles, the dead nerves, the dead blood-vessels. And so many blood-vessels being dead, being scooped away by that sharp curette, how could the blood circulate in the top half of that flaccid thigh? It couldn't. Afterwards, into the deep, yawning wound, they put many compresses of gauze, soaked in carbolic acid, which acid burned deep into the germs of the gas gangrene, and killed them, and killed much good tissue besides. Then they covered the burning, smoking gauze with absorbent cotton, then with clean, neat bandages, after which they called the stretcher bearers, and [the patient] was carried from the operating table back to the ward."

Alexander Fleming was among the army doctors and scientists who studied the bacterial infection of gas gangrene that led rapidly to sepsis and to death. He was moved to action by what he saw: "Surrounded by all these infected wounds, by men who were suffering and dying without our being able to do anything to help them, I was consumed by a desire to discover, after all this struggling and waiting, something which would kill those microbes." His commitment to wound healing continued after the war. In 1929 he discovered penicillin in his London laboratory, the drug that revolutionized battlefield medicine, including the treatment of gas gangrene, in the Second World War. Suffering inspired doctors, scientists, and poets alike (see photo section).

Science from the battlefield brought rapid change not only to medicine and surgery but to psychiatry as well. The doctors and nurses who treated psychological damage caused by war were confronted by suffering and incapacity of a kind and magnitude without precedent. The scale on which the war produced disturbances of the mind could not be imagined, observed the British psychiatrist W.H.R. Rivers. Therapeutic pragmatism was imperative. Psychiatrists had to confront broken patients, figure ways to help them reconstruct their minds, and above all how to help them imagine a navigable future. They needed to infuse hope and nerve in order to encourage psychological recovery. War was a "vast crucible," said Rivers, an extreme trial that could rearrange or destroy the mind. Its perversities were hard to fathom, harder to deal with, and ethically intractable. Medical officers were expected to get their patients well enough to return them to the front line, an expectation counter to the practice and beliefs of physicians. It was yet more wrenching for psychiatrists, whose relationship with their patients was based on a unique trust. Therapeutic procedures, Freud said, did not aim so much at recovery as to restoring the soldier's fitness for service. The war, he stated bluntly, put doctors in the position of having "to play a role somewhat like that of a machine-gun behind the front line, that of driving back those who fled."

Many of the British and American doctors were intellectually indebted to German psychiatrists and scientists. Rivers had published with the preeminent German psychopathologist Emil Kraepelin and, like Osler, he had studied in German laboratories and hospitals. Both were admirers of the German scientific tradition and were dismayed to find themselves on the opposing side to their colleagues during the war. Nonetheless, British psychiatrists, newly exposed to the writings of Freud and Jung, adapted German psychoanalytic approaches into their work, as well as using more traditional medical treatments. Most recognized the critical role of work and physical and creative endeavors in healing. Others, unable or disinclined to distinguish psychological trauma from malingering, were more punitive. Not a few soldiers suffering from psychological trauma were shot for cowardice; often it was the job of a doctor to pin a piece of white cloth to the shirt over the condemned man's heart so that the firing squad could more accurately shoot him. No doctor had been trained to do this, to help to kill.

Nor had any nurse. War brought to nurses, as it did to doctors, protracted exposure to suffering and death. Their work was dangerous and exhausting. They were not prepared for what they saw in the field hospitals, nor for what they had to do. Their profession taught them to heal the body and treat the mind. The nurse was a link between the ancient world of healers—balm and prayer and laying on of hands—and, thousands of years later, the operating rooms, antiseptics, anesthesia, and X-ray machines of the Great War. The nurses kept some of the ways of the distant past and were proficient in modern ones. They listened to the night screams of their shell-shocked patients and controlled, as best they could, the damage from hemorrhage, gas poisoning, and sepsis. They were broadly judicious in the use of morphine.

Nurses assisted surgeons in the operating rooms as they amputated limbs and, afterward, tended the soldiers as they woke to their losses. They worked in the mud and the cold, sick or depressed; they worked while being bombed, and assisted at operations under the scream of shells. And some sat down at night, however tired, to write about what they had seen. They wrote about snapping open ampoules of morphine, knowing that some patients would be relieved of their pain and that some would die more quickly due to the kindness of strangers. They debrided wounds, sat with the dying, and wrapped the dead; they wrote about the futility of war. They wrote, too, about the wonder of life in the midst of it all.

The nurses who volunteered to serve in the war were a diverse group. For many, war nursing provided a means to escape class barriers. For others, an affluent background had given privilege but little independence or excitement. The war changed that and, as with the war poets—Siegfried Sassoon, Wilfred Owen, and Robert Graves, among others—their attitudes about the war evolved from patriotic idealism and a sense of duty to a more complicated mix of duty and world-weariness. Many of the nurses began their war years in blithe spirit. "We all met on Victoria Station," wrote one young nurse as they waited in their "flowing violet cloaks and sky blue dresses" for the train that would take them to the Front. They were high on hope and anticipation with little idea of what was ahead or how their stories would unfold. For most, a mix of belief in the national cause, youthful imagining, and commitment to nursing sped them on their way. "It is one of the most detestable things about war," observed fifty-three-year-old Edith Wharton, writing as a journalist from France in 1915, "that everything connected with it, except the death and ruin that result, is such a heightening of life."

In June 1917, the transport ship *Finland* sailed from America to France carrying the doctors, nurses, and medical students who would staff the Johns Hopkins Base Hospital No. 18 in Bazoilles-sur-Meuse. J.M.T. Finney, the director of the thousand-bed hospital and later chief surgical consultant for the Allied Expeditionary Forces, said of his Hopkins colleagues that the "suppressed excitement and expectancy" was palpable. They were embarking on a journey that would be dangerous but also exhilarating; it was one they knew would save lives and change their own. There was an "acute sense of high adventure," agreed the dean of the medical school. "A piece of the corporate body of Hopkins sailing into the unknown."

The *Finland*, escorted by a guard of destroyers, was a troop transport ship; for the doctors and nurses on board, however, the Atlantic crossing belonged more to the innocence of the world they were leaving—white-tie balls and medical studies with no mention of bullet wounds or poison gas—than the one toward which they sailed. There were formal dinners and dance cards on which to pencil the names of dance partners. These *programmes du bal* were a link to the receding world. A year later the nurses wore gas masks. The young women who had danced under the stars on the deck of the *Finland* had become unrecognizable (see photo section).

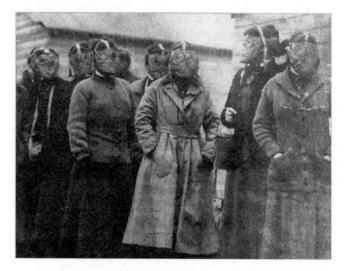

Johns Hopkins nurses wearing gas masks, 1918

They must be able to bear the gigantic waste and pity of it all, the endless killing and maiming and still keep cheerful and well-balanced and always seeing the best side of things.

—VIOLETTA THURSTAN, 1917,
A Text Book of War Nursing

Alice Fitzgerald, born into a wealthy Baltimore family, entered the Johns Hopkins School of Nursing against the advice of her parents. They were horrified that she saw any sort of work as a part of her future, and certainly not nursing. Her mother, Alice Fitzgerald said, wished her "to dance well and finally to depart from the family hearth in a cloud of tulle and orange blossoms." This was not her intention. Ten years after graduating from nursing school she was on the Western Front. "I have lived a week in 24 hours," she wrote in her memoir. "There are now 400 patients in the hospital and only 7 nurses to take care of them. We do the best we can but it can only be a minimum of care for each. In fact, the hardest lesson I have had to learn from the War is that war nursing is not seeing how much you do for each patient but how little." Baltimore society, like the dance cards on the *Finland*, was a long way from the Front.

Four months later Alice Fitzgerald described the danger and difficulty of her work. "We had a frightful night and I do not see why some of the nurses do not develop shell shock. I was awakened early in the evening by a fearful explosion, which shook my tent, and was followed by a long and loud rumble. At the same time, I saw a vivid red light through the tent walls, so I got up just as a second explosion took place." A long night of explosions followed; then the anti-aircraft guns started. Mud, thick and present much of the year, made work yet more difficult: "The patients are kept on stretchers laid on the ground and I have to kneel or crouch in the mud to nurse them, dress them and feed them. What is nursing here?" Fitzgerald found herself sympathetic to soldiers with self-inflicted wounds. "Is a man sane or insane when he attempts to wound himself in order to get away from the unutterable horrors of War?" she asked. Wounding himself could be his "only deliverance . . . the only way of escape from the hell of the trenches." How could healing take place in such conditions?

William Osler, Alice Fitzgerald's chief of medicine when she was a nursing student at Johns Hopkins, had said that doctors and nurses were "essential players at the exits and entrances of life." This was particularly so for those who went to the Front. The exits were frequent and hard, more so as the war intensified. Many nurses described the images and experiences that had fixed in their minds and stayed long after the war ended. Ellen La Motte, like Alice Fitzgerald a graduate of the Johns Hopkins School of Nursing, wrote a chilling account of her time on the Front. She did not see war as noble or heroic; she was repelled and outraged by it. Her book, *The Backwash of War*, is a bitter one, offering neither cloak against the reality of war nor tenderness toward her colleagues or readers. "This is the Backwash of War," she wrote. "It is very ugly. There are many little lives foaming up in the backwash. They are loosened by the sweeping current, and float to the surface, detached from their environment, and one glimpses them, weak, hideous, repellent."

La Motte's book opens with an unpitying account of the effect of war on the mind of a young soldier who had deserted his post: "When he could stand it no longer," she wrote, "he fired a revolver up through the roof of his mouth, but he made a mess of it. The ball tore out his left eye, and then lodged somewhere under his skull, so they bundled him into an ambulance and carried him, cursing and screaming, to the nearest field hospital. . . . He must be nursed back to health, until he was well enough to be stood up against a wall and shot. This is War. Things like this also happen in peace time, but not so obviously." Too much gauze and ether, too many bandages were used to treat him, she thought. "It was an expensive business, considering." The night nurse, as she writes of herself, was indeed "given to reflection."

Other nurses who wrote about their war experiences had a more broadly traditional and compassionate view of nursing and healing. Mary Borden was one. An Anglo-American poet and novelist, independently wealthy, she established a field hospital near the Front and was a nurse there from 1914 to 1918. Her memoir about the war, *The Forbidden Zone*, at times heart-stopping, is relentless in its portrayal of the futility of war and the limits of healing:

> Ten kilometres from here along the road is the place where men are wounded. This is the place where they are mended. We have all the things here for mending, the tables and the needles, and the thread and the knives and the scissors, and many curious things that you never use for your clothes. . . .
>
> This is the place where he is to be mended. We peel off his clothes, his coat and his shirt and his trousers and his boots. We handle his clothes that are stiff with blood. We cut off his shirt with long scissors. We stare at the obscene sight of his innocent wounds. He allows us to do this. He is helpless to stop us. We wash off the dry blood round the edges of his wounds. . . .
>
> We conspire against his right to die. We experiment with his bones, his muscles, his sinews, his blood. We dig into the yawning mouths of his wounds. . . . We lay odds on his chances of escape, and we combat with Death, his saviour.

War nurses, the personification of healers, were expected to be versed in clinical medicine, able to improvise under dangerous circumstances, and, as best they could, keep their patients alive and in comfort. They accompanied the living as they got better and stayed with them if they did not.

To stay with a patient in the presence of coming death is a type of healing, albeit a healing that cannot last. I once asked my husband, a cardiologist at Johns Hopkins, what he tells his patients when it is clear they are going to die. He said, "I tell them that we will be seeing one another more often, and that I will be adjusting their medications from time to time." His message is clear: I am not leaving you. You are not alone. We are in this together.

Nurses spoke of having life-and-death powers thought inconceivable before the war. "We could revive the cold dead," Mary Borden wrote, "snatch back the dead who were slipping over the edge; hoist them out of the dark abyss into life again." Her hands could "instantly tell the difference between the cold of the harsh bitter night and the stealthy cold of death. Then there was another thing, a small fluttering thing. I didn't think about it or count it. My fingers felt it. I was in a dream, led this way and that by my acute eyes and hands that did many things, and seemed to know what to do."

The uncanny sense of life or coming death, the reckoning that the nurse possessed an inexplicable capacity that could heal, was not uncommon. Baroness de T'Serclaes, in *Flanders and Other Fields*, described a similar quality. "I possessed a kind of power which seemed to be able to drag men back literally from the jaws of death," she wrote. "I was a fully trained nurse in the technical sense, but this was something more than technical efficiency. It was the breathing back of the Life Force, a kind of spiritual resuscitation."

To see a soldier through depression and anxiety was part of their work. "It was very frightening for young boys, eighteen and nineteen years old, to be having their leg off and all those dreadful things, terrible things, they used to have and they used to say sometimes to me, 'Will you be with me, sister,' I used to say, 'Yes, I shall be with you, I'm going with you [to the operating theatre], and I'm going to stay with you and I shall come back with you."

(Fifty years earlier, Louisa May Alcott wrote to her family in New England about her life as a nurse in Washington during the Civil War, about tending and watching, accompanying. Her work began after the amputations and other surgeries were completed, she said. "When the poor soul comes to himself, sick, faint, and wandering; full of strange pains and confused visions, of disagreeable sensations and sights. Then we must soothe and sustain, tend and watch; preaching and practicing patience, till sleep and time have restored courage and self-control.")

Mary Borden described how she, and the priest she summoned to her hospital from a near village, stayed with a twenty-year-old soldier to his death:

> He was quite conscious to the very end and he was afraid. He could not bear to be left alone. At twelve he whispered—"Je ne vois plus clair—Je ne vous vis [*sic*] presque plus—Allez cherche [*sic*] le prêtre, mais soyez la vite revenue." I ran for Guerin, an Abbé in Salle IV, and then I stood by and watched that priest do a wonderful thing. He put all his strength, all his faith, all his tenderness at the disposal of that boy— and he reached across the chasm and got to him— Guerin, by the force of his own will, changed for that wretched, terrified child, the character and quality of death. It was as if he quite simply lifted him up and carried him across the river.

Nurses were meant to ease the minds of their patients— bear witness to suffering, not flinch from it; be still with it and apprehend its meaning. Penny Starns, in *Sisters of the Somme*, writes that most of the wounded soldiers had witnessed "shocking scenes of barbarity and destruction. Tales abounded of horses being blown clean up into trees, their innards draping across withered winter branches. Patients described men for whom there had been no hope, those with completely exposed abdomens and severe head wounds, limbs blown feet away by the impact of shell explosions." The stench of burned flesh and screams of soldiers in the night stayed in the minds of nurses long after the end of the war.

Nurses knew when to fight death and when to accept that death would win. When death was unappeasable, they knew how to provide such comfort and peace as dying would allow. When medicine and surgery could do nothing more, the presence of a nurse could make the reality of medical limits more bearable. Recognizing the difference between the possibility of life and the certainty of death was everything. Morphine and clinical experience each played its role in healing, but "the gift of understanding," said English nurse Violetta Thurstan, was "the most precious a nurse can have. Imagination, tact and sympathy are other names for it." In the midst of instructions for young nurses in how to manage gas gangrene and hemorrhage, Thurstan's textbook of war nursing suggests the respite of a lime blossom tisane, a calming and sleep-inducing recipe for patients: a tonic of comfort, a sympathetic laying on of hands. A nepenthe.

⌐

"It was my business to sort out the wounded as they were brought in from the ambulances and to keep them from dying before they got to the operating rooms," wrote Mary Borden. "I was there to sort them out and tell how fast life was ebbing in them. . . . It was my business to create a counter-wave of life, to create the flow against the ebb. It was like a tug of war with the tide." The war with the tide took capacity and puissance. So too did bearing witness—listening well and compassionately—to the horror of battle and the trenches;

remorse for having killed others; dread in the wake of maiming and fear in the midst of dying. Sitting, listening, staying. Not flinching in the presence of death.

Nurses and doctors had limits. Life bled out, wrote Mary Borden. "A nurse comes along carrying a lantern. Her white figure moves silently across the ground. Her lantern glows red in the moonlight. She goes into the gangrene hut that smells of swamp gas. She won't mind. She is used to it, just as I am." Pain is everywhere, beyond the reach of her ampoule and syringe. "What can the nurse do?" she asks. "She can straighten a pillow, pour drops out of a bottle, pierce a shrunken side with a needle." It will make no difference. She is "really dead, past resurrection. Her heart is dead. She killed it. She couldn't bear to feel it jumping in her side when Life, the sick animal, choked and rattled in her arms." To resurrect the heart could be no small thing.

For many of the wartime medical staff and their patients, seasonal festivities rooted in nature and common observance gave a transient balm and relief against the dreariness of the operating rooms, dead rooms, and wards. Christmas was a time of light in a dark season. It was a reminder that hope exists in a cold time; it was a ribbon back to family and security, a tap into memory. Christmas was evocative and beautiful, an island of tradition that brought the familiar into the unpredictable. It was a healing force.

"As soon as routine is broken a new element enters," Gavin Maxwell wrote years later in *Ring of Bright Water*. What enters is fear. "After some tempest of the spirit in which the landmarks seem to have been swept away, a man will reach out tentatively in mental darkness to feel the walls, to assure himself that they still stand where they stood."

In war, Christmas was a wall that stood. It became a lull in the horror, a short-lived passage home. Beatrice Hopkinson, an English nurse who served at a casualty clearing station near the Front, described Christmas Eve as a time of fleeting beauty and solace; a place of important, if fugitive, sanctuary. The nurses and doctors gathered in the courtyard of the hospital carrying candles and lanterns and singing "While Shepherds Watched Their Flocks." The words of the carol went deep, she wrote. "Mighty dread had seized their troubled mind"; all knew. And yet it beseeched, "To the earth be peace." Perhaps. For some. For a while. They walked the wards with hymnals and lighted candles, singing the old carols. It would not last, but it was no less deeply felt for that.

It is the rare war memoir that does not describe the peace and warmth and backward glance that wartime Christmas gave to the wounded and to those who cared for them. The lighted wards, holly from the woods, fir trees cut from the forest, gifts from the medical staff for the patients—plum pudding, biscuits, cigarettes and jam, a glass of port or brandy—and the familiar carols brought contrast and respite. Nature's cycles, and the celebrations arising from them—bleak, free, and then blossoming—gave an interlude of peace to soldier and healer alike. For some. For a while. Nature reminded that life had its rhythms; intimated that the carnage might pass; or that it might pass long enough to believe in the possibility of renewal. Snow would go to snowdrops and then to wood violets: There was hope in this. Winter, like other unforgiving things, would be forced to its grave. Edward Thomas, a British poet killed in France in 1917, had taken hope from the life cycles he had observed in his English countryside: "Winter may rise up through mould alive with violets and primroses and daffodils," he wrote, "but when cowslips and bluebells have grown over his grave he cannot rise again: he is dead and rotten, and from his ashes the blossoms are springing." Winter took long in its dying but, in its own time, it would give rise to life. Nature would proliferate. Peace would come to the troubled mind. Or so one hoped.

J. M. Barrie, in his rectorial address delivered at the University of St. Andrews not long after the war, talked about spring, the war's lost season; it being lost, he said, the other seasons were unsettled, awry. "The war has done at least one big thing," the playwright told the students. "It has taken spring out of the year. And, this accomplished, our leading people are amazed to find that the other seasons are not conducting themselves as usual. The spring of the year lies buried in the fields of France and elsewhere."

Enid Bagnold, an English nurse who served in France (and who, after the war, wrote *National Velvet* and *The Chalk Garden*), wrote of her instinct that life was coming back. The soldiers in France, living so close to death, she thought, must be more aware of life than those who are not. "The crown of the hill here holds the last snows, but for all that the spring smell is steaming among the trees and up and down the bracken slopes in the garden next door. There is no moon, there are no stars, no promise to the eye." There only is promise from what one remembers, and what one imagines of the future, from one's experience that life returns each year from death. "In the dense, vapouring darkness the bulbs are moving. I can smell what is not earth or rain or bark."

Erich Maria Remarque described the quickening of nature in *All Quiet on the Western Front*, the great German novel about men who, "though they escaped shells, were destroyed by war." The narrator, a young soldier, deadened by the killing and horror that had become his life, writes about a field thick in scarlet poppies; life streams back into him. War had warped what soldiers knew. "Our knowledge of life is limited to death," he said. But occasionally nature gave them a reprieve:

These are wonderfully care-free hours. Over us is the blue sky. On the horizon float the bright yellow, sunlit observation-balloons, and the many little white clouds of the anti-aircraft shells. Often they rise in a sheaf as they follow after an airman. We hear the muffled rumble of the front only as very distant thunder, bumblebees droning by quite drown it. Around us stretches the flowery meadow. The grasses sway their tall spears; the white butterflies flutter around and float on the soft warm wind of the late summer. We read letters and newspapers and smoke. We take off our caps and lay them down beside us. The wind plays with our hair; it plays with our words and thoughts.

War remained. Healing was transitory, uncertain. *What will happen afterwards?* the soldier asks. *And what shall come out of us?* Which of us will live, and which not? Remarque ends his book:

He fell in October 1918, on a day that was so quiet and still on the whole front, that the army report confined itself to the single sentence: All quiet on the Western Front.

CHAPTER 3

Rivers

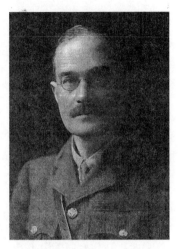

Capt. W.H.R. Rivers
Royal Army Medical Corps, 1917

The problem . . . was to find some aspect of the painful experience which would allow the patient to dwell upon it in such a way as to relieve its horrible and terrifying character.

If imagination is active and powerful, it is probably far
better to allow it to play around the trials and dangers
of warfare than to carry out a prolonged system of
repression.

—W.H.R. RIVERS, 1920,
Instinct and the Unconscious

In 1920, two years after the end of the War, Captain W.H.R.
Rivers, late of the Royal Army Medical Corps and now
praelector in natural science at Cambridge, testified before
the War Office Committee of Enquiry into Shell-Shock. He
was direct, as was his habit. When asked what he thought of
the term "shell shock," Rivers told the committee he objected
to it "root and branch." The cause of breakdown was stress,
he emphasized; concussive shock from high-explosive shells,
when it happened, was only the "last straw in a morbid process for which the mental stresses and strains of warfare [had]
long prepared the ground." The term "shell shock" had
devolved into a confusing constellation of medical, psychological, and literary concepts; by the end of the war, the word,
although widely used by the public, was in disfavor with military and civilian doctors alike. Still, it was a descriptive term
and used even by those who disliked it. Doctors and nurses
who had seen shell shock—the trembling, the stammering,
the sightless staring, the madness and quick-startle panic, the
nightmares—were familiar with the devastation it caused. By
whatever name it went, Rivers knew it well.

When asked if there was such a thing as a mental wound
arising from "shell shock," Rivers agreed that there was. He
himself referred to it as trauma, he told them, but "wound"

being the English term, he agreed with its use. Wound was a good, plain word. Mental wounds were what Rivers wrote and lectured about and they had changed him as a doctor and as a person. They were what he had treated late into the night in British war hospitals and what had established him as without peer among the war psychiatrists, a psychotherapist's psychotherapist. He had been adamant in support of soldiers being treated as ill, rather than as malingerers; he had argued vehemently against the censorious views, often expressed by the British military and elite classes, that shell shock patients were cowards.

Wounds to the mind, he told the War Commission, were beyond any usual cure; certainly they were beyond the patient's usual power of repression. Thrusting aside distressing sights and sounds from memory, ordinarily one of the more effective mechanisms of psychological survival, had been of limited avail to these patients. The war memories that soldiers tried to put out of their minds, Rivers said, were too powerful; the attempt sent doctor and patient alike on a fool's errand. The description of shell shock by Rivers and his colleagues foreshadowed much of what we now think of as post-traumatic stress disorder.

"If you think about the experience which men went through in France, seeing their friends at their side with their heads blown off," he continued, it was not surprising that the day-to-day repression that soldiers might more usually draw upon was "altogether unsuited for an experience of that scale." In the early years of the war, it was widely recommended that soldiers should cast behind them the horror of war, replace their war experiences with less morbid thoughts. Doctors and commanding officers told their soldiers, "Put it out of your mind, old fellow, and do not think about it; imagine that you are in your garden at home." This made no sense; it was destructive and at odds with human nature. To grapple best with pain, Rivers believed, the soldier must stare at it straight on until there is "familiarity which breeds indifference, if not contempt."

Many of his own patients, Rivers told the War Board, had been advised by other doctors to banish thoughts of war from their minds and to direct their thinking to gentler topics, to thoughts of forest and sea. This was understandable counsel, to a point. Direct questions about the war from family and friends often made traumatic memories worse; it was usually futile to try to convey the brutality of war to those who had not experienced it. But to repress terror in the conscious hours only encouraged its return in the night. Then the memories and images came back in recollected and hallucinated horror. There ought to be a mid-course between too active an engagement with traumatic memories and too little. The rare person who masters the balance between remembering and forgetting, Kierkegaard said, is "in a position to play at battledore and shuttlecock with the whole of existence." The doctor should temper dangerous engagement and help navigate between trying to banish traumatic thoughts altogether and dwelling upon them to a pathological degree. It was as harmful to fix upon harrowing memories, or to "brood upon feelings of regret and shame," as it was to exclude them entirely. Not that one could.

To heal, Rivers believed, one must encourage patients to engage memory: First, to remember what they have pressed out of consciousness. Then, to recollect the unbearable in a more circumspect way; to grapple with dark forces in order to obtain mastery over them. To be a healer was to make a patient's "intolerable memories tolerable," to share in the darkness of the patient's mind. It was the doctor's charge, Rivers said, to "use the controlled reflection of horror to understand what the patient has been through, to allow him to meet the horror in his own strength." In the grip of suffering the patient needed to be helped to "face the facts" and to understand the situation in all its complexity. The doctor should accompany and be as convoy in dangerous waters.

This was far from a passive process. It carried tough expectations, predicated on a moral code assumed in the officer class that Rivers treated: courage, loyalty, responsibility for the men they commanded, and control over the expression of fear. The war neuroses, Rivers wrote, stemmed in part from conflict between self-preservation and societally imposed standards of conduct. Rivers understood this but came to his clinical work with a broadly informed and sympathetic view of human behavior. His therapeutic philosophy, rooted in self-knowledge and self-reliance, was compassionate and optimistic as well as tough; it was built on ageless principles of healing. It assumed that patients will actively engage in treatment and bring to it the necessary mental and moral strength. It also assumed that the journey into the interior of the mind did not have to be made alone.

These psychotherapeutic principles were formed not only by Rivers's training as a doctor and psychologist but by years of field studies as an anthropologist. He had observed in the South Pacific, in Egypt, and among the Todas of southern India that myth and curative rites were central to healing, as was the personality of the healer-sorcerer. Power lay not only in the healer but in those seeking to be healed. Faith and suggestion were both critical. The relationship between healer and ill was subtle, potent, and very old to the race.

Siegfried Sassoon, in his memoirs, portrayed Rivers as the archetypal healer—unnervingly wise, sympathetic, and demanding—who brought Sassoon to a reckoning between his public opposition to the war and his duty to the men under his command. He depicted Rivers as doctor, Virgil, and priest, the personification of how subtle understanding and a just reading of character mended in him what the war had broken. Rivers set him toward the future, Sassoon said. "The past was still there to be used as a sedative in discreet doses—three drops in half a wine glass of water, so to speak. Looking at the future was quite a different matter." To mend, one needed to know what had broken.

~

[Rivers] was intensely occupied with the drama of human life, and this made him an interested auditor and a valuable counsellor in serious trouble. Triviality he abhorred. . . . He created an atmosphere in which the insignificant could not survive.

—SIR HENRY HEAD, 1922

William Halse Rivers Rivers was born in 1864 in Chatham, Kent, and christened there by his father, an Anglican priest. Rivers was English to the bone, bred in England's traditions, full participant in her values, and ardent lover and expresser of her language. For centuries his ancestors had been at the service of three defining institutions of England—Cambridge, the Church of England, and the Royal Navy. His birthplace, a town on the River Medway, had been home forty years earlier to the young Charles Dickens, who wrote the town and its dockyard into his novels. The Chatham Dockyard, formally established as a Royal Dockyard in 1567 by Elizabeth I, had been used earlier by the navy of her father, Henry VIII. Among the great British warships built there was HMS *Victory*, Nelson's flagship, and the ship that in 1805 bore Nelson's body back from Trafalgar to be buried in St. Paul's Cathedral.

The *Victory*'s master gunner at Trafalgar was William Rivers. He oversaw the exercising, loading, and firing of the ship's 104 cannon. His detailed account of the conflict has been indispensable to historians for their understanding of the most important sea battle of the nineteenth century. His son, also William Rivers, served on HMS *Victory* as a midshipman and aide-de-camp to Nelson. W.H.R. Rivers, the psychiatrist and anthropologist, born sixty years after Nelson's death, was keenly interested in the Rivers connection to HMS *Victory* and Nelson. Family documents relating to the role Gunner Rivers and Midshipman Rivers played at the Battle of Trafalgar were among the few personal papers found at his death. Rivers, generally acknowledged as the originator of the genealogical method used in social anthropology, kept a scholarly as well as personal interest in kinship studies throughout his life. Pedigrees are important, Rivers believed, because they allow direct as well as oblique entry into the past and make it more likely that significance will be attached to things otherwise unnoticed. His own interests in ancestry took him from his father's parish records and the Chatham Dockyard of his youth to tracking down the role of his Rivers ancestors in the sea battle that changed European history. Later his scientific interest in ancestry would lead him to unravel complicated kinships of South Pacific islanders and those of the Toda in southern India.

The line from past to present, present to past is seldom direct. The poet Robert Lowell, encouraged by his psychiatrist to examine his family history as a way to understand his life and "ancestral madness," studied his genealogy in detail and took what he had discovered into his poetry and autobio-

William Rivers
Gunnery notebook
HMS *Victory*

graphical writing. "I woke up the other morning with a curious feeling of continuity," he wrote to his cousin in the midst of his ancestral research. "Great falling festoons of loose green vines, trees and white woodwork. One thing dropping, slightly tangling and touching another indefinitely. And a feeling that as we pass through our fairly brief lives, we stay long enough to pass something on that someone else catches by his fingertips." A bit of his grandfather and an older world seemed now to touch his daughter, he said. Rivers too felt the passing on, the transfer of collective memory, the continuity.

Ancestry for Rivers, as for Lowell, was a many-sided thing: fact, social marker, definer, history, myth, and metaphor. For both, it was a portal to the history of the human race. For Rivers, kinship terms carried with them the possibility of earlier forms of social organization; these linguistic "survivals" granted a glimpse into ancestors and the world before. It had never occurred to him, Rivers wrote in *Conflict and Dream*, that a kinship term used by a people, unaware that it may reveal their history, "might be regarded as a hidden source of knowledge comparable with a piece of unconscious experience." Survivals had been likened to fossils, noted Rivers, a "preeminently 'hidden source' of knowledge," but ties to modern ideas of the unconscious—memories, thoughts, and feelings that are beyond conscious awareness, yet influence behavior—were of even more interest. Kinship language, ritual, and social institutions offered insight analogous to the access dreams gave to the unconscious. ("Also I am ancestral," wrote Siegfried Sassoon. "Aeons ahead / And ages back, both son and sire I live / Mote-like between the unquickened and the dead— / From whom I take, and unto whom I give.")

The Church, the Royal Navy, and Cambridge had molded Rivers and his ancestors. The mystery of the Church, his father's Anglican priesthood and those of his forebears, The Book of Common Prayer, with its majestic language and anciently rooted rites of baptism, burial, confession, and ministration to the sick, bore upon his thinking as a doctor, anthropologist, and psychologist. He learned from his upbringing, as well as from his field studies, that faith, magic, religion, and the rituals that defined them were common to nearly all social systems and that these human beliefs were critical to psychological healing. Rivers, baptized by his father into a Church that traced its beginnings to pagan rituals, as well as to early kings and saints, kept his mind open to the ways man worshipped his gods. When it came to his own death, he would call upon the rituals of the church of his fathers. His funeral request was notably specific, ritualistic, and Church of England, a tangled continuity of myth and Establishment.

Cambridge, where his father and so many Rivers men before him had studied, held a generous part of his affection and was the center of his intellectual world. He was elected a fellow of St. John's College and lived there most of his adult life. Rivers dedicated *The History of Melanesian Society* to "St. John's College, Cambridge, to whose fellowship this book is largely due." (For his book, he received the Royal Medal from the Royal Society, the first to be awarded for anthropology. Previous recipients had included Michael Faraday, Charles Lyell, Charles Darwin, and Joseph Lister.) Rivers's rooms at Cambridge swarmed with undergraduates, faculty, and visitors from London and abroad: novelists and poets, experimental psychologists, anthropologists, philosophers, doctors, former patients, and politicians. "His study was like a market square," observed the novelist and journalist Arnold Bennett. "Undergraduates came into it at nearly all hours." They descended upon Rivers for breakfast, tea, dinner, and all times in between. Rivers, famous for his warmth, wit, and intellectual liveliness, assumed serious conversation and work from his students. Frivolity, but not laughter, was left at the door.

"At Cambridge you knock and enter," wrote Frederic Bartlett, professor of experimental psychology at Cambridge. "The room was beautiful, with its brown panelled walls, but nothing else was. It was in an awful muddle, with books and papers and odds and ends of anthropological trophies all over the place." The room was always in chaos, Bartlett said, but when "Rivers came out of his inner study . . . somehow at once the room came alive, and the things in it were right after all. There he was, rather tall, trim, quick and light in his movements, in navy blue. You got a swift impression of straight, broad shoulders and a jutting chin, and at once of a tremendously alert mind."

Those who knew Rivers found it difficult to put into words what made him such a force. He was infectiously enthusiastic, broadly informed about human nature, and had a fast, dry wit. His sharp intelligence was almost always gentled with kindness, and acid observation was offset with eruptive exuberance. Staff notes written about him when he was a military psychiatrist at Craiglockhart War Hospital state, "Capt. Rivers when excited got explosive . . . like a soda water ciphon [*sic*] going off & puffing." Rivers had a "boundless enthusiasm for his work," said one of his students at Cambridge. He had a genuine interest in their work, too, and he took their ideas and conversation seriously. He cut lazy thinking little slack but was direct and open to criticism. He acknowledged errors freely. "When students no longer contradict me flatly to my face, I shall know that I have grown old," he once said.

The good teacher, Rivers believed, discourages imitation and adulation. He "leads his pupils to see how opinions are formed. He gives them strength and knowledge to deal with the many difficult situations by which they must sooner or later be confronted." Such a teacher puts his pupils into a position not only to understand, but to reason: not to replicate the ideas and ways of the teacher, but to create, question, set their own course. A great teacher shows how to think and how to imagine. Rivers's philosophy of teaching was cut from the same bolt as his philosophy of psychotherapy.

As a Cambridge don, Rivers won allegiance "not by asking for it, but by deserving it," a colleague said. He had dignity "because it was unconsciously there." Sympathy, enthusiasm for the ideas of others, belief in his own, a high bar of expectation, the capacity to elevate: These qualities of the great teacher were also the qualities of the great psychotherapist.

Rivers's belief in his work, and in human possibility, be it in his students or patients, was perhaps his greatest capacity. "It was his belief, in himself, in his work, in the value and

possible greatness of nearly every human life he touched,"
said Bartlett. It made him an "outstanding power to many,
and the best possible kind of friend to a few." Cambridge, and
the fellows and students whose lives he so affected there, kept
their respect and affection for him long after his death. Rivers
was brilliant; he cared; he led. He was like no other they had
known before or after.

The bond Rivers held to Cambridge was intellectual and
personal. His bond to the sea was different. As with his Royal
Navy forebears who had sailed from the Chatham Dockyard,
an irreplaceable part of Rivers's experience and work came in
long sea voyages. After graduating from St. Bartholomew's
Hospital in London in 1887, the youngest medical graduate
in its nearly eight-hundred-year history, Rivers took to sea as
ship's surgeon to Japan and North America. It was the first
of many voyages by Rivers, who, in his relatively short life,
would sail to Melanesia, New Zealand, Polynesia, the West
Indies, the Canary Islands, Madeira, Norway, the New Hebrides, and Portugal.

He traveled for scientific discovery, but he went to sea as
well to allay his chronic restlessness and a desire for change
and novelty. ("One of the strongest elements in my mental
make-up," he said about himself.) On board ship he could
read and think. Or not think. At times he went to sea to rein
in his mind, to slow the tumble of thoughts. He described
an occasion when he struggled to untangle a problem he was
working on: "I got into such a state that I hardly slept at all.
I woke so early so often that my short hours of sleep were
having a serious effect on my health. . . . Following my usual
custom of never travelling by land when it is possible to go by
sea, I went to London one evening, slept the night there and
took the river steamer. . . . The journey had the favourable
effect on me that sea or river always has in allowing me to

live without thinking and I had a quiet and more or less som-
nolent day with the minimum of mental activity of any kind.
I went to bed very early and woke the next morning with the
solution to my difficulty."

He went to sea to heal. He "always had to fight against ill-
health: heart and blood-vessels," said a colleague. Throughout his life he suffered periods of depression and nervous
exhaustion, which not uncommonly followed periods of
feverish activity. He stammered, a twist of fate as his uncle,
James Hunt, was an internationally regarded speech therapist who treated, among others, Charles Lutwidge Dodgson
(Lewis Carroll), a friend of the Rivers family. When Rivers
was a house officer at the National Hospital in Queen Square
in 1892, records indicate that he was obliged to resign due
to "nervous exhaustion." In a talk he gave later that year, he
told his audience that nervous afflictions were "more common than supposed" and that a "complete holiday" was the
best treatment. From time to time he returned to his family
home in Kent to recover from "over-work" and to rest.

Rivers's colleagues spoke of his times of "horrible weariness," spelled by periods of great activity. Frederic Bartlett
wrote: "Sometimes when I dropped in to see him I would
find him sitting still, apparently doing nothing, and looking
desperately tired. He would take off his steel rimmed spectacles and pass his hand over his eyes. And then he would jump
up and be active again. He wrote, talked, read, dashed about,
took on new things and kept on old ones all in a terrific hurry
as if he thought he wouldn't have time to finish." Exhaustion
came in the wake of "dashings about," but it was his vitality
that held sway with friends and colleagues. "A spontaneous
remembrance of Rivers would reveal him alert and earnest in
the momentum of some discussion," recalled Siegfried Sassoon. "When walking he moved very fast, talking hard, and

often seeming forgetful that he was carried along by his own legs." Because his energy and health were inconstant, Rivers learned early that if he were to be an active participant in the world he needed long periods of rest and, when he could, voyage at sea. To heal others, he began with himself.

The English institutions in which Rivers was bred—the Church, Cambridge, and the Royal Navy—strongly shaped his conduct and principles. Only later in his life, with experience and moral authority gained from his upbringing within the Establishment, did he question the preeminence of these institutions. He knew and admired the strength of traditional professional, middle-class and upper-middle-class values such as duty, restraint, bravery, loyalty, and adherence to rules. But he saw their limits, especially during war.

"Fear and its expression are especially abhorrent to the moral standards of the public [that is, private] schools at which the majority of officers have been educated," Rivers wrote, not only as a medical officer in the Royal Army Medical Corps but as someone himself who had been educated at an English public school established in the sixteenth century. For young officers, the values inculcated in public school and the expectations of their social class made it difficult to live up to their own standards in wartime. "The public school boy," continued Rivers, "enters the army with a long course of training behind him which enables him successfully to repress, not only expressions of fear, but also the emotion itself." This class-bred sense of duty, the powerful responsibility the officer felt for the men under his command, and the obligation not to break down left him vulnerable during hard times.

The junior officer, Rivers wrote, believes that it is his special duty "to set an example in this respect to his men, to encourage those who show signs of giving way." This sense of duty, bred to fullness in the more innocent days of Edwardian England, was clear: "The officer shall appear calm and unconcerned in the midst of danger." Human nature, meanwhile, argued against this. Rivers treated officers whose ideals of youth were no match for the savagery of war and who broke under its stress.

"The soldier should be encouraged boldly to face in his imagination the dangers and horrors which lie before him," Rivers said in a report to the Medical Research Committee in 1918. He should be encouraged to imagine the awful to come, to "think horribly." (Seneca had advocated visualizing terrible things that might happen, *futurorum malorum premeditatio malorum:* Rehearse in your mind all things that might befall you, he wrote: exile, torture, war, shipwreck. To imagine was to mitigate.) A few soldiers might "pass unscathed through modern warfare" because of "sluggish imagination," Rivers believed, but most had no immunity. They needed inoculating, a tinge of nightmare, a tincture of horror, to prepare against atrocity. Imagination could benefit soldiers and officers alike. "If imagination is active and powerful," Rivers suggested, "it is probably far better to allow it to play around the trials and dangers of warfare than to carry out a prolonged system of repression." Too much imagination could damage. But too much tamping down could equally damage. Mental survival lay in the consonance.

The Victorian values of Rivers's upbringing broadened when fairness and reality called for it. Harvard anthropologist and psychiatrist Arthur Kleinman has made the essential point that Rivers "perturbed and disturbed the moral ethos of his day not as a revolutionary but squarely from the center of the establishment. He liberated himself from the very cultural values that had made him and his career." Rivers, Kleinman writes, was "an exemplar of remaking moral experience by living a moral life." The shortcomings of the values bred into him were harshly exposed during and after the war. For Rivers, the social inequities in England, often perpetuated by the institutions that had shaped him, became more glaring as he grew older. Himself a Socialist and the friend of many others, he encouraged Siegfried Sassoon—who, born to privilege, acknowledged that he was seventeen before he understood that life, for most, is an "unlovely struggle against unfair odds, culminating in a cheap funeral"—to pursue Socialist politics after the war. At the time of his death, Rivers was a Labour Party candidate for Parliament. Increasingly he spent his time educating workers about their rights and speaking publicly for social reform. "To one whose life has been passed in scientific research and education the prospect of entering practical politics can be no light matter," he said. "But the times are so ominous, the outlook for our own country and the world so black," that he felt he could not refuse to stand for public office.

Rivers was open to new ideas and receptive to nonconforming views. He watched the world with curiosity more than with an inclination to judge. These characteristics contributed to his becoming a renowned psychotherapist during the war, and a revered one after. They made him, as well, an influential scholar of the theory and practice of psychotherapy. Rivers's intellectual and professional interests were wide. He was director of the first psychological laboratories in Britain, president of the British Anthropological Society, president of the Folklore Society, cofounder of the *British Journal of Psychology*, and the first president of the British Psychoanalytical Society. He studied neurology under the eminent neurologist Hughlings Jackson, assisted at history-making operations by neurosurgeon Sir Victor Horsley, and conducted nerve regeneration research with Sir Henry Head.

He published research papers with Emil Kraepelin, the most prominent psychopathologist in the world.

Even in an age that generated polymaths, Rivers stood out. He was widely recognized as an anthropologist, ethnologist, neurologist, psychologist, medical psychologist, and psychiatrist. In each field he left a mark. He studied death rituals and death houses, canoes and pottery, island names, myth, magic, and religion; sun cults and megaliths, and the religious significance of the buffalo; the naming of constellations by Pacific Islanders; navigation, possession, dreams, and the unconscious. He used indigo, violet, and bile-yellow wool samples to investigate color vision, and he studied how language categorizing and describing color had evolved among Polynesians, Inuits, and the Welsh. Rivers, as Arnold Bennett put it, had a universal knowledge and a "gift of co-ordinating apparently unrelated facts." With this facility for recognizing patterns, through persuasion and patience, he was—unlike other anthropologists before him—able to work out the complex kinship patterns of the Islanders of the Torres Strait and the Todas of southern India. He observed carefully, collected facts from across his far-ranging and brimming mind, and strung them together in new ways. He had, a colleague said, a deep love for the "beauty of organized knowledge."

Throughout Rivers's varied scientific career, his major interest was in psychology and in how man reacts to the world in which he finds himself. His anthropology fieldwork allowed him to compare beliefs and behavior across cultures and gave him a more open window into why people did what they did and why, in groups, they moved forward or fell back. "Rivers," said a colleague, "shared with Osler the power to show one half of the scientific world how and why the other half lived. He saw every problem whole."

One studied different societies, Rivers wrote, in order to

undertake "a history of the movement of thought; of the long struggle of Man with his environment; and of the countless institutions, beliefs and customs which have been the outcome of this struggle." Anthropology provided a uniquely broad perspective on the individual and, swayed by this, Rivers moved from the laboratory perspective of an experimental psychologist to a wider cultural one. "They went as physiologists," said Walter Langdon-Brown of Rivers and the other scientists who were a part of the 1898 Cambridge Torres Strait expedition. "They returned as psychologists."

A. C. Haddon, the anthropologist who headed the Cambridge Anthropological Expedition to Torres Straits, remarked that Rivers "regarded all human conditions as the appropriate study of psychology and ethnology." He would have had no argument from Rivers. Everything, he said, came back to psychology. "Every form of social activity, whether it be a marriage regulation, a religious rite, a mode of warfare, or the polishing of an implement, is in the last resort determined by psychological motives." Psychology explained human behavior and custom; it was, as well, a way to understand those who were wounded or ill in mind. It was to this that Rivers was most notably drawn.

I should go in for insanity when I return to England and work as much as possible at psychology.

—W.H.R. RIVERS, 1892

In 1892, when he was twenty-eight years old and six years out from qualifying as a doctor, Rivers began his formal psychiatric training as a clinical assistant at Bethlem Royal Hospital in London. In the interim he had been a ship's surgeon and a house officer at three London hospitals, where he had practiced general medicine, eventually specializing in neurology. He had published papers in psychiatry about delirium, neurasthenia, and hysteria.

Bethlem Hospital, which gives its name to "bedlam," the chaos of the mad, was founded during the reign of Henry III; by the mid-fifteenth century it was exclusively an institution for the insane. At the time Rivers began his clinical assistantship at Bethlem, the hospital bore few traces of its medieval past. Manacles and straitjackets were not often used and hospital activities reflected the increasingly enlightened times of late nineteenth-century asylum practice. Patients gardened, played sports, sewed, sang, and went on supervised outings to Brighton Beach and Kew Gardens. Once a month they held dances attended by "genteel" members of the neighboring community. Medicines were few and used sparingly, usually as soporifics. In the 1890s, knowledge of psychopathology included only a few major illnesses; for the most part, diagnoses were limited to mania, postnatal psychosis, melancholia, alcohol-related psychoses, and general paresis of the insane, caused by tertiary syphilis.

Rivers treated several patients who were acutely manic, others who were suicidally depressed, and a few with hallucinations and delusions associated with alcoholism. His case notes, typical of the times, were succinct. Minimally they included the patient's medical history, diagnosis, mental state, and psychiatric history. Letters, photographs, death certificates, and notes made by other doctors were often included in the charts as well. The asylum records of Alice Meek, a patient of Rivers, are typical. Miss Meek was twenty years old when she was admitted to Bethlem in April 1893 from

Medical case notes, 1893
Dr. W.H.R. Rivers
Bethlem Royal Hospital

the nearby Middlesex County Lunatic Asylum. Rivers wrote in her chart that she was moderately tall, had a pale face and light brown hair, and was deeply depressed. The patient "sits about doing nothing & looking down," he wrote, and "only occasionally brightens." She was difficult to engage and "very much frightened & thinks something is going to happen to her on account of her sins." She was psychotic, "nod[ding] assent when asked about whether she has heard voices and also whether she has seen visions."

Miss Meek showed no clinical improvement by June and in July switched into mania: She was "excited . . . gushing . . . quite happy . . . flirtatious," wrote many letters, was restless, and spent much time sketching and writing poetry. In January 1894 she had an "excess of spirits" but, if crossed, became abusive. Her clinical record documents a typical course for manic-depressive psychosis (what would now be called bipolar disorder) before the 1950s, when lithium was first available. She was discharged as "cured" in March 1894, readmitted in July, and discharged again, a year later, "uncured." Rivers's clinical notes for her are unremarkable. They show his observational ability and understanding of psychopathology but offer no hint of the extraordinary psychiatrist he would prove to be.

Rivers's clinical work at Bethlem ended when he contracted scarlet fever and was confined to a fever hospital for two months. He did not take the end of his clinical work as a great loss. He found the intellectual level of asylum psychiatry unstimulating and the attitudes of many of the asylum doctors nihilistic. In 1893 he took a position as lecturer in physiology at the University of Cambridge and four years later became the director of the first psychological laboratory in Britain. There he studied color vision, neurophysiology, and the effects of stimulant drugs, and pioneered in the development of experimental methods to study human behavior. (He was the first to conduct a study that used a "blinded" researcher, that is, where the observer of an experiment did not know which treatment was being given to which patient.)

It was to be more than twenty years before Rivers returned to clinical work in psychiatry—time he spent in the study of physiology, psychology, neurology, and anthropology. C. G. Seligman, a physician and anthropologist at the London School of Economics, remarked of Rivers that "perhaps no man has ever approached the investigation of the human mind by so many routes." These routes were to converge in the British war hospitals, first at Maghull but, more importantly, a year later at Craiglockhart War Hospital. "It was not really until the war that Rivers found himself," said his friend Walter Langdon-Brown. Rivers was fifty years old, and all who knew him would agree.

~

When war was declared in August 1914, William Rivers was in the South Pacific attending scientific meetings in Australia, revisiting Melanesia, and studying megalithic customs on a small coral island in the New Hebrides. He returned to Cambridge immediately and took on medical duties at the newly constructed army hospital built on the cricket ground of King's College. For a brief while he treated patients with neurological injuries but, at the request of a colleague, he went north to Maghull War Hospital, near Liverpool. Maghull, the first military hospital to specialize in the treatment of shell shock, was staffed by doctors and scholars from Britain's clinical and academic elite. They were in uncharted waters, improvising treatment for soldiers who had been transferred back to England from the front lines.

The staff at Maghull brought diverse backgrounds—asylum psychiatry, anthropology, psychology, neuropathology—to understanding the suffering of the shell-shocked soldiers on their wards. They all believed, as did their director, R. G. Rows, that "mental tangles ought to be straightened out by mental means." Well-read in Freud, they also immersed themselves in the writings of Jung and Janet and Dejerine. Rivers became, in the words of the neurologist Sir Henry Head, "one of that brilliant band of workers" who made Maghull and the Maudsley Hospital in London the most generative places in England for the study of the psychology of war, hypnosis, and psychotherapy.

Rivers arrived at the hospital in Maghull with "what seemed to me a jack-in-the-box leap," said his former student T. H. Pear, an authority on shell shock and later the first professor of psychology in England. "He told me that he had decided that his cloistered life at Cambridge . . . must cease." He then "paid me an honour which I shall never forget." Rivers said that he was, in effect, like a student who had been away from books. Pear went on, "Would I direct his reading for the next few weeks, and on afternoon walks—Cambridge fashion—discuss it? His first desire was to grasp what Freud meant by the Unconscious, which Rivers thought the most important contribution to psychology for a long time."

During the day, Rivers studied Freud's work on the unconscious and the meaning of dreams. In the evenings he and the anthropologist Elliot Smith talked late and with abandon about a wide sweep of other ideas. They talked "like priests, of mysteries," said Pear; their conversation flew from dragons to megaliths, mummification; ancient seats of stone; the great sea routes of the voyagers who had sailed the world to pursue "gold, pearls, and purple." (A few years later, after the war, Siegfried Sassoon wrote about a like evening of fast tumbling ideas, this time in Rivers's rooms in Cambridge. Elliot Smith and Rivers were again throwing images of ancient worlds into the air and spellbinding their listeners; their discussion flew: "five thousand years of excavated history," a "chartless Age of Ice and Stone . . . aqueducts and desiccated forests, mangled myths. Lydian coins and megaliths." They were, for Rivers, lost worlds reimagined; past worlds brought to life again.)

Although Rivers never lost his belief in the biological determinants in the onset and clinical presentation of neurosis and insanity, his interests in the psychological origins and treatment of mental disorders gradually expanded beyond purely physiological factors. He, like the other doctors at Maghull, debated diagnosis. Was the patient suffering from an anxiety neurosis (more often known as neurasthenia) or from traumatic hysteria? Were the symptoms due to regression or to repression and how did repression work? Why were dreams of war so repetitive? Could the horror of war be approached in a psychotherapeutically meaningful way? What part did faith and suggestion play in psychotherapeutic treatment?

"The war has been a vast crucible in which all our pre-conceived views concerning human nature have been tested," Rivers said not long after the war was over. "The war has shown that human behaviour in the mass is determined by sentiments resting upon instinctive trends and traditions founded upon such trends. We have learnt that reason plays a very insignificant part in determining behaviour when mankind is brought into contact with circumstances which awaken the instinct of self-preservation." The war had taught a lot and would continue to do so. Psychiatry had changed, Rivers said. There was now more "hope and promise for the future treatment of the greatest of human ills."

The war had forced psychiatrists to acknowledge the importance of unconscious factors influencing the behavior of men who engaged in killing other men or who might be killed. This led to greater acceptance of some of Freud's writings. The "uncompromising hostility," as Rivers described the attitude of English doctors toward Freud, grew less virulent. War had forced doctors to "sift the grain from the chaff and distinguish between the 'essential and the accidental.'" Clinical reality made for a more pragmatic approach. This suited Rivers well. Most important, the war had assured that psychotherapy had "taken its place among the resources of the physician."

Rivers is often referred to as "the English Freud," but it would be more accurate to say that he was a discerning, yet quite critical, expositor of some of Freud's views. He elaborated on Freud's thinking about repression and incorporated his own version into his clinical work. He was sympathetic to Freud's belief that "a thing which has not been understood inevitably reappears; like an unlaid ghost, it cannot rest until the mystery has been solved and the spell broken." To repress horror was to invite its presence later. He downplayed Freud's emphasis upon sexual experience as the "material of morbid complexes," stressing instead the instinct for self-preservation. Freud's followers, Rivers wrote, "and to a large extent Freud himself, have become so engrossed in the cruder side of sexual life that their works might often be taken for contributions to pornography rather than medicine . . . Perverse tendencies and prurient ideas are scented in every thought, waking or sleeping, of the patients who come under their care."

Rather than dismiss Freud for the caricature he had become to many English psychiatrists, Rivers took seriously, with generosity and attribution, that which he admired. Rivers thought Freud's *The Interpretation of Dreams* was a work of genius, and that Freud's writing about forgetting, specifically that it was an active, not a passive, process, was a key contribution to understanding morbid states. But he strongly disagreed with the psychoanalytic emphasis on transference— the projecting of a patient's feeling for a significant person onto the therapist—as it was antithetical to his own sense of self and to his fervid encouragement of independence in his patients. It was "a regular part of my treatment to guard against the process known to the psycho-analysts as transference," Rivers wrote. It jeopardized healing and unduly tethered the patient to his doctor; he kept watch for signs of it as it "undermined my treatment to inculcate independence."

As Rivers developed his clinical approach, he blended psychiatric theory and therapeutic pragmatism in equal measure. He kept that which worked and he modified or discarded the rest. He admired Freud as an original thinker but he maintained his distance. His respect, tempered by criticism, lent credibility to Freud's ideas. "There were enthusiastic psychotherapists before Rivers, but the orthodox [psychiatric] profession were inclined to regard them as cranks," said Walter Langdon-Brown, the Regius Professor of Physic at Cambridge. "But Rivers' position as an academic scientist was unassailable, and his adhesion to this new branch of medicine commanded respect for it."

"My own standpoint," Rivers wrote, "is that Freud's psychology of the unconscious provides a consistent working hypothesis to aid us in our attempts to discover the role of unconscious experience in the production of disease. To me it is only such an hypothesis, designed like all hypotheses, to stimulate inquiry and help us in our practice while we are groping our way towards the truth concerning the nature of mental disorder." It was only the partial truth, he said, but "it takes us some way in the direction of truth."

When Rivers was at Maghull, he reportedly found the academic study of war neurosis and psychoanalysis more interesting than actually treating patients. It was only after he was commissioned into the Royal Army Medical Corps (RAMC) and began work at Craiglockhart War Hospital in

Edinburgh that he came to be the psychiatrist of his subsequent reputation, one who delved subtly and brilliantly into shell-shocked minds. The reasons for this are not entirely clear, but one obvious difference is that, unlike his patients at Maghull, patients at Craiglockhart were officers, a class whose values and behavior he knew and understood from his upbringing. "He was wearing the King's uniform," noted T. H. Pear, "and had proud memories of many of his father's family who had been officers in the Navy." The conflict between stress and upbringing stood in clearer relief when a patient's social and educational background was similar to his own. Figure stood out better from ground when the ground was familiar.

For most of his life, Rivers had studied people who came from backgrounds dissimilar to his own; as an anthropologist, he had been wary of misinterpreting people who came from different cultures. At Craiglockhart he was close to what he knew. Personal familiarity with the world and values of his patients gave him a long lead to explore the difficult and painful. The war's requirement that he treat terrible suffering drew upon and deepened his capacity to heal. The hospital proved ideal for thinking and demanded clinical innovation. The work he did with patients who had been shattered by war "brought me into contact with the real problems of life," he said. "I felt that it was impossible for me to return to my life of detachment."

Craiglockhart itself afforded Rivers a different kind of clinical experience and a setting for reflection that served him well. The sea was near and restorative; there were acres to walk out his restlessness and to talk with other doctors. It is no coincidence that Siegfried Sassoon and Wilfred Owen, given time away from the trenches and gunfire, encouragement to write, and surrounded by the stark beauty of the

Scottish countryside, wrote many of their lasting poems at Craiglockhart; nor is it a coincidence that Rivers discovered so much that was important about the mind. This world was conducive to putting things together, repairing minds that had come apart. It was a world in which Rivers could heal, both others and himself.

It was not until the war that Rivers found himself, Langdon-Brown had said. "I think it was because he had had to heal himself that he could heal others. . . . His whole personality expanded as he grew to realize what was his true mission in life." His motivation to better understand himself, together with a particularly strong purpose to which he could commit, made him better able to study and heal the trauma of war.

The War was too big an event for one man to stand alone in.

—SIEGFRIED SASSOON,
Memoirs of an Infantry Officer

Siegfried Sassoon, who wrote at length about his wartime treatment with Rivers at Craiglockhart, was born in Kent in 1886, only a few miles from where Rivers had been born twenty years earlier. His father's family, often referred to as the Rothschilds of the East, were Baghdadi Jews who claimed direct descendancy from King David. Their roots were in Mesopotamia, Bombay, and, by the 1850s, England. Sassoon's father, Alfred Sassoon, an heir to one of the great fortunes of the nineteenth century, led a desultory life of riding, cricket, sketching, sculpting, and music. (His mother, hoping that he would become a concert violinist, bought him two Stradivariuses.) He married a non-Jew, Sassoon's Anglo-Catholic mother, Theresa Thornycroft, and was disinherited. When Sassoon was seven years old, his father left the family and returned only for brief visits. Sassoon, although he saw little of his father, remained intrigued by his paternal ancestry and believed that his poetry owed a debt to Sassoon mysticism.

Accomplishment ran throughout both sides of Sassoon's family. In addition to the success of his father's family in banking, Sassoon's paternal aunt, Rachel Beer, was editor in chief of *The Sunday Times* and *The Observer,* the first woman editor of a national newspaper (albeit newspapers owned by her family). His mother's ancestors were English farmers and artists. The farming side dated back to the thirteenth century; the artistic side, more recent, was pervasive and shot through with excellence. Sassoon's maternal grandfather, Thomas Thornycroft, and his grandmother, Mary Francis Thornycroft, were well-known sculptors. His uncle, Sir Hamo Thornycroft, created a number of the best-known public sculptures in Britain, including statues of Queen Victoria, William Gladstone, and Alfred the Great. Thornycroft's statue of Oliver Cromwell stands outside the Palace of Westminster in London; his statue of Gordon of Khartoum is in Trafalgar Square. Sassoon's aunts were also artists, as was his mother, who exhibited her paintings at the Royal Academy of Art. His mother, Sassoon believed, gave him the capacity and passion for art, a grounding sanity, and a deep connection with woods and farmland. Sassoon was born to art, privilege, and the English countryside—a land he loved, rode to the hunt, and wrote about all his life.

In 1914, two days before war was declared, Sassoon,

twenty-seven years old, enlisted in the British army. The countryside of Kent was in his thoughts then, as it was to remain while he was at the Front: "Lit by departing day was the length and breadth of the Weald," he wrote, "and the message of those friendly miles was a single chord of emotion vibrating backward across the years to my earliest rememberings." It was an unshakable love for the geography of childhood. "Beyond the night was my new beginning. The Weald had been the world of my youngness, and while I gazed across it now I felt prepared to do whatever I could to defend it."

The French countryside was different. It was stamped by death. Sassoon went to a wood following an army training session in how to use a bayonet, hoping for easement; instead, the commands of his instructor shattered the peace:

Afterwards I went up the hill to my favourite sanctuary, a wood of hazels and beeches. The evening air smelt of wet mould and wet leaves; the trees were misty-green; the church bell was tolling in the town, and smoke rose from the roofs. Peace was there in the twilight of that prophetic foreign spring. But the lecturer's voice still battered on my brain. "The bullet and the bayonet are brother and sister." "If you don't kill him, he'll kill you." "Stick him between the eyes, in the throat, in the chest." "Don't waste good steel. Six inches are enough. What's the use of a foot of steel sticking out at the back of a man's neck? Three inches will do for him; when he coughs, go and look for another."

That death was everywhere brought life into sharp focus. "There is a sense of recovered happiness in the glimpse I catch of myself coming out of my cottage door with a rifle slung on my shoulder," Sassoon wrote at the time of the bayonet lesson. "I was like a boy going to early school, except that no bell was ringing, and instead of Thucydides or Virgil, I carried a gun."

By 1917, Sassoon had fought on the Western Front, been wounded, and received the Military Cross for "conspicuous gallantry during a raid on the enemy's trenches." (Sassoon, the citation stated, had "remained for 1½ hours under rifle and bomb fire collecting and bringing in our wounded. Owing to his courage and determination all the killed and wounded were brought in.") He was admired by the men he commanded, who called him "Mad Jack" for his combination of courage and recklessness.

Sassoon became increasingly angry and bitter about the atrocity of warfare. His poetry hardened from his early heroic view of the war to being sardonic, angry, and accusatory, even as it remained compassionate when he wrote about his men. His poems spoke of maiming and death, of lost minds, and about the glorification of young soldiers' deaths by those who were older, safer, and across the Channel. It was not easy to reconcile the sensibilities and moods of a poet with the life of a soldier: "One cannot be a good soldier and a good poet at the same time." Life on the Front was in a way simpler: "Everything up there is 'soul-deadening': there is no time for emotion, no place for beauty. Only grimness and cruelty and remorse."

Sassoon's anger at the futility of the war, his rage about the death and maiming of his friends and the men he commanded, and his contempt for the "callous complacence" of those who oversaw its operation sharpened into action. In the

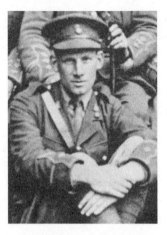

Siegfried Sassoon, 1916

Do you remember that hour of din before the attack—
And the anger, the blind compassion that seized and shook you then
As you peered at the doomed and haggard faces of your men?

summer of 1917 he wrote a declaration against the war, which was read out in the House of Commons. It began:

> I am making this statement as an act of wilful defi-
> ance of military authority, because I believe that
> the War is being deliberately prolonged by those
> who have the power to end it. I am a soldier, con-
> vinced that I am acting on behalf of soldiers. I believe
> that this War, upon which I entered as a war of
> defence and liberation, has now become a war of
> aggression and conquest. I believe that the purposes
> for which I and my fellow-soldiers entered upon this
> War should have been so clearly stated as to have
> made it impossible for them to be changed without

our knowledge, and that, had this been done, the objects which actuated us would now be attainable by negotiation.

I have seen and endured the sufferings of the troops, and I can no longer be a party to prolonging those sufferings for ends which I believe to be evil and unjust. . . .

Reaction to Sassoon's statement was, variously, that it was principled and courageous, impulsive, or muddled. For some it was treasonous. No one could seriously doubt Sassoon's courage: his Military Cross and intrepid forays against enemy troops, including single-handedly capturing a German trench and dispersing dozens of German soldiers with grenades, gave the lie to cowardice. The government faced a serious problem: They could hang a decorated officer for treason, or they could declare him mad. In this way, Sassoon came to the consulting room of Captain Rivers.

Three evenings a week I went along to Rivers' room. . . . I can visualize him, sitting at his table in the late summer twilight, with his spectacles pushed up on his forehead and his hands clasped in front of one knee; always communicating his integrity of mind; never revealing that he was weary as he must often have been after long days of exceptionally tiring work on those war neuroses which demanded such an exercise of sympathy and detachment combined.

—SIEGFRIED SASSOON,
Sherston's Progress

The Medical Board convened by the War Office to assess the fitness of Siegfried Sassoon met in July 1917. Robert Graves, a friend, fellow soldier, and poet, set on saving Sassoon's life, testified before the board that Sassoon had had a "mental collapse." He had been "beastly weak and in a rotten state of nerves." Among other things, Graves told the board, Sassoon had described his vivid hallucinations of corpses "lying about on the pavements of London." The board agreed with Graves that Sassoon was mentally disturbed. "His conversation is disconnected and somewhat irrational, his manner nervous and excitable," they concluded. "He is suffering from a nervous breakdown and we do not consider him responsible for his actions." It is unclear the extent to which Graves, in order to save Sassoon's life, convinced the board that Sassoon was mentally ill, or whether the board chose to act leniently or in a way that served the government. Either way, they decided he was suffering from shell shock and should be sent to Craiglockhart War Hospital to the care of Captain Rivers.

Thus, in July 1917, Siegfried Sassoon—second lieutenant in the Royal Welch Fusiliers, poet, fox-hunting man, and recipient of the Military Cross—sat on a train to Edinburgh. The self-dramatizing element of his mind, he wrote later, imagined a "mad-house." Less dramatically, and more hopefully, he remembered that the neurologist on his Medical Board had mentioned a doctor called Rivers. "Rivers will look after you when you get there," he had said. "I inferred, from the way he said it, that to be looked after by Rivers was a stroke of luck for me. Rivers was evidently some sort of great man; anyhow his name had obvious free associations with pleasant landscape and unruffled estuaries."

Within five minutes of arriving at Craiglockhart War Hospital, Sassoon met Rivers, now a captain in the Royal

Army Medical Corps. "There was never any doubt about my liking him," Sassoon said of their first encounter. "He made me feel safe at once, and seemed to know all about me. What he didn't know he soon found out." He was less enthusiastic about the hospital. It was a place of "wash-outs and shattered heroes." The doctors and nurses tended to the shell-shocked, but there was no escaping the faces of the 150 officers broken by war. It was "a live museum of war neuroses."

The following morning, Sassoon said, "I went to Rivers' room as one of his patients. In an hour's talk I told him as much as I could about my perplexities. Forgetting that he was a doctor and that I was an 'interesting case,' I answered his quiet impartial questions as clearly as I could, with a comfortable feeling that he understood me better than I understood myself."

Rivers filled out a medical case sheet on Sassoon, a brief account of Sassoon's military and medical history, current mental state, reasons for hospitalization at Craiglockhart, and his education at Marlborough and Cambridge. He wrote about Sassoon's poetry as well. "From childhood he has written verses at different times," he noted. During his convalescence from a riding accident early in the war—"a bad smash when schooling a horse"—he had written a poem called "The Old Huntsman," which "has recently been published with other poems under that name." Rivers encouraged Sassoon's poetry, recognizing its value in dealing with experiences during the war. Sassoon, who had, as Rivers noted, devoted his time chiefly to hunting and cricket, was a "healthy-looking man of good physique." There were "no physical signs of any disorder of the Nervous System."

Rivers did not mention Sassoon's homosexuality in his admitting note, and there is no mention of it in the other limited clinical notes available. It is unlikely that the subject was

Excerpt from Medical Case Sheet
Lieutenant Siegfried Sassoon
(Capt. W.H.R. Rivers)
Craiglockhart War Hospital

not discussed in their psychotherapy sessions; it was of central importance to Sassoon's life and writing and, although he had discussed his homosexuality with friends years before the war, it was illegal at the time he was a soldier, and for many years after. But there is no discussion of this in Rivers's notes. As was the way with Sassoon, his life was a tangle of contradiction about things most important to him: his homosexuality, love, the war, and religion. This was true of him as a soldier and remained true for the rest of his life.

Rivers's description of Sassoon's mental state at the time of his admission to Craiglockhart Hospital differed from the conclusions of the Medical Board only days earlier: "He discusses his recent actions and their motives in a perfectly intelligent and rational way," Rivers wrote about Sassoon, "and there is no evidence of any excitement or depression. He recognizes that his view of warfare is tinged by his feelings about the death of friends and of the men who were under his command in France."

Rivers was to focus on Sassoon's war-fraught nerves, his declaration against the war, and his reluctance to return to the Front. This would remain the heart of their therapeutic work. "From an early stage of his service in France," Rivers wrote in the admission note, Sassoon "had been horrified by the slaughter and had come to doubt whether the continuance of the War was justifiable." In 1916, while recuperating in England, Sassoon had been in touch with Bertrand Russell and other pacifists but "had never previously approved of pacificism and does not think that he was influenced by this communication." Nonetheless, his doubts about the war intensified. When he was fit to return to duty in July, he did not. The account of Sassoon's defiance of military authority in *The Times* is cited by Rivers in the admission note.

Sassoon met with Rivers every evening for several weeks and then three times a week after that. Rivers, recognizing that Sassoon's antiwar stance was controversial and conflicted, advised him to lie low, to "mark time" for a few weeks. The hospital authorities, he said, "would allow him all the freedom he wanted," but in the meantime he would rely on Sassoon "not to do anything imprudent." They talked about the war and his poetry, his decision about whether to return to the Front, and his feelings for the men under his command.

One evening, Sassoon recounted, "I asked him whether he thought I was suffering from shell-shock."

"Certainly not," he replied.

"What *have* I got, then?"

Rivers replied, laughing, "Well, you appear to be suffering from an anti-war complex."

In obvious ways, Craiglockhart War Hospital was far from the trenches. It was on the quiet side of the English Channel, away from the guns. Patients, protected from rain, rats, mud, and cold, ate regularly and slept in beds. They received medical and psychiatric care. The surrounding countryside and sea were luring and there were cricket fields, badminton and lawn tennis courts, golf, billiards, a beekeeping club and a poultry keeping association, a hospital magazine *Hydra*, and a model boat club. Patients went frequently into Edinburgh to shop, take tea, and visit galleries and museums.

Life in the hospital was tolerable, by day. At night, the distance from the trenches contracted. The long lawns and cricket pitches receded from the mind, displaced by nightmares, hallucinations, and emergency sessions with doctors. At night, Sassoon wrote, the men "lost control and the hospital became sepulchral and oppressive with saturations of war experience . . . One became conscious that the place was full of men whose slumbers were morbid and terrifying—men muttering uneasily or suddenly crying out in their sleep. Around me was that underworld of dreams haunted by submerged memories of warfare and its intolerable shocks and self-lacerating failures to achieve the impossible. . . . Shell-shock. How many a brief bombardment had its long-delayed after-effect in the minds of these survivors."

Craiglockhart was distant from the trenches but inseparable from what had happened there. For Siegfried Sassoon the hospital was not only a long way from the Front but yet further, impossibly far from his life before the war—an idyllic world of cricket, fox-hunting, reading, Cambridge, and writing verse. Life before the war was a world of "cloudless weather" and "hot blue skies": "It was my own countryside," he wrote in *Memoirs of a Fox-Hunting Man*. "I cannot think of it now without a sense of heartache, as if it contained something which I have never quite been able to discover." Rivers was to guide him between his irrecoverable past and difficult present, and then see him into the future.

Two issues dominated Rivers's psychotherapy with Sassoon: Sassoon's traumatic experiences during the war and his conflict about whether to return to the Front. Both required that they forge a therapeutic relationship, in order to heal Sassoon's mind, lead him to a circumspect decision about whether to rejoin his regiment, and provide him with a deeper well of understanding from which to draw after the war ended. Doctor and patient came to the relationship with different expectations, obligations, and ways of understanding experience.

Rivers, for all his empathy, was an incisive thinker. He had been attracted to science and medicine by the rigor they demanded; decades of scientific work and writing had made his mind yet more analytic. He was not only a doctor but also a medical officer whose duty was to return soldiers to the Front. Sassoon's thinking was anything but analytic; it bent toward nostalgia and dramatically drawn dichotomies. "My intellect was not an ice-cold one," Sassoon wrote in *Sherston's Progress*. "It was, so to speak, suffering from trench fever." He saw the war from the day-to-day perspective of the troops he led, less from any broader view. Feeling came more easily than reason. Rivers would encourage Sassoon to exert a tighter rein on his emotions and, in so doing, make them more effective.

Rivers and Sassoon had much in common. Both were tightly bound to symbols and language, they were bred in and drew upon the Kent countryside, and they shared a capacity to lead. Both had faith, albeit for Rivers it was not of a formally religious nature. (Sassoon, whose father was Jewish and his mother Anglican, much later in his life converted to Catholicism.) Sassoon was to say of Rivers that he had been his father-confessor and spiritual guide. His prose, letters, and poetry reflect this; Sassoon's language is shot through with demons and exorcism, benediction, faith, and guilt. Rivers was an ideal match for this. The Anglican rite of Confession had been a part of Rivers's world since his childhood in his father's parish, and it was made yet more vivid and universal through the rituals he observed as an anthropologist. He had a profound respect for the role of the spiritual, for suggestion and faith, in healing the mind; he understood the deeply human beliefs that were engrained in the origins of medicine. "Some of the modern measures of the physician," Rivers wrote, "are little more than his adoption of modes of treatment which have long been familiar, in the form of confession, to the priest."

Sin is rightly the province of priests, Rivers wrote, but there is no inconsiderable amount of confession in a patient's relationship with his doctor. It was the hope, if not the belief, of Rivers that modern medicine was "again bringing religion and medicine into that intimate relation to one another which existed in their early history." Formal religion and theology were not Rivers's interest. Rather, he recognized the power of ritual, the legacy of ancient gods, and "cities with dead names"; the force of personality of the healer and the strength of human longings, ancestral symbols, myths, and the indisputable sway of suggestion. The efficacy of healing is "largely ascribed to the personality of the sorcerer," Rivers wrote. "Some degree of confusion between personality and [healing] runs through the whole history of medicine."

Fires in the dark you build; tall quivering flames
In the huge midnight forest of the unknown.
Your soul is full of cities with dead names,
And blind-faced, earth-bound gods of bronze and stone

. . . .

You understand my thoughts; though, when *you* think,
You're out beyond the boundaries of my brain.

—SIEGFRIED SASSOON,
FOR W.H.R. RIVERS

Rivers surely held the power of priest-sorcerer for Sassoon. Such a relationship required trust and respect, and was intensified by Sassoon's vulnerability and the circumstance of war. But these are not sufficient for a strong therapeutic bond. Trust is critical, but reason is likewise essential to understanding the causes of suffering. The exercise of a patient's reason and self-observation are essential to recovery, wrote Rivers. Psychotherapy is a means to that self-discovery; through it, the patient comes to understand the cause and remedy of trauma or despair. "There is all the difference in the world between the use of reason by one who does not understand the real underlying conditions of the malady," continued Rivers, "and reason exerted when these conditions have been discovered and are themselves the material from which the reasoning starts and upon which it acts."

By exploring past thinking and behavior, and through the

retrieval of forgotten experiences, patients come to understand themselves. The recognition of motives, fears, and the context of experience was termed "autognosis" by Rivers and his colleagues. To know oneself: Without it, the ill mind was "enveloped by a sense of mystery which greatly accentuates the [negative] emotional state."

Sassoon, introspective and keenly observant by nature, energetically engaged in this analysis of self when he was at Craiglockhart and afterward. On a visit to Rivers in Cambridge after the war, he wrote in his diary: "Autognosis"— "To know Myself—this fragment of to-day— / To pluck the unconscious causes of unrest / From self-deceiving nature." He must, he wrote to himself, "behave naturally, keeping one side of my mind aloof, a watchful critic. One part of me (mostly the inherited and primitive part) is the player on the stage. But I must also be the audience, and not an indulgent one either."

Sassoon's war memories were manifestly "unconscious causes of unrest." Three months before he was admitted to Craiglockhart, he described one of his nightmares (see photo section):

> My brain is screwed up like a tight wire.... And when the lights are out, and the ward is half shadow and half glowing firelight, and the white beds are quiet with drowsy figures, huddled outstretched, then the horrors come creeping across the floor: the floor is littered with parcels of dead flesh and bones, faces glaring at the ceiling, faces turned to the floor, hands clutching neck or belly ... the hands clutching my sheets. Yet I found no bloodstains there this morning.... I wish I could sleep.

The nightmares that arise from trauma, wrote Rivers, generally manifest as a replaying of a particularly dangerous event. The content of the nightmare is true to the experience; that is, "it follows the grim reality faithfully" and is accompanied by intense emotion, "different from any known in waking life." (One of the first indications that a patient is improving, Rivers noted, is a transformation of the details of the dream; the identities of the subjects in the dream change, the circumstances begin to vary.) "The dream ends suddenly by the patient waking in a state of acute terror directly continuous with the terror of the dream and with all the physical accompaniments of extreme fear, such as profuse sweating, shaking, and violent beating of the heart." The dream tends to repeat nightly, sometimes more than once. Often the nightmare-wracked soldier will avoid sleep in "dread of its repetition."

(Walt Whitman, in his Civil War poem "The Artillery-man's Vision," wrote of the nighttime horrors and "mad joy" of war that came unbidden "through the stillness, through the dark." While his wife and infant sleep nearby, a soldier wakes to visions of battles long over: "The skirmishers begin, they crawl cautiously ahead, I hear the irregular snap! snap! / I hear the sounds of the different missiles, the short t-h-t! t-h-t! of the rifle-balls, / I see the shells exploding leaving small white clouds, / I hear the great shells shrieking as they pass." The conjured sound of cannon, "the wounded, dripping and red," the "grime, heat, rush.")

Sassoon knew that trying to block out his memories of war was futile. In June 1917, not long before he made his declaration against the war and was sent to Craiglockhart, he wrote a poem about this. It was a summer evening, he was home on leave, standing in his garden in Kent, but neither summer evening nor distance from the front line kept terror

"Repression of War Experience":

Now light the candles; one; two; there's a moth;
What silly ――― beggars they are to blunder in
And scorch their wings with glory, liquid flame—
No, no, not that,— it's bad to think of war,
When thoughts you've gagged all day come back to scare you
And it's been proved that soldiers don't go mad
Unless they lose control of ugly thoughts,
―― That drive them out to jabber among the trees.

Now light your pipe; look, what a steady hand.
Draw a deep breath; stop thinking; count fifteen,
And you're as right as rain...

Why won't it rain?
I wish there'd be a thunder-storm to-night,
With bucketsfull of water to sluice the dark,
and make the roses hang their dripping heads.

Looks; what a jolly company they are,

Siegfried Sassoon
Draft manuscript

An Address
ON
THE REPRESSION OF WAR
EXPERIENCE.

Delivered before the Section of Psychiatry, Royal Society of
Medicine, on Dec. 4th, 1917,

By W. H. R. RIVERS, M.D. Lond.,
F.R.C.P. Lond., F.R.S.,

LATE MEDICAL OFFICER, CRAIGLOCKHART WAR HOSPITAL.

MR. PRESIDENT AND GENTLEMEN,—I do not attempt to deal in this paper with the whole problem of the part taken by repression in the production and maintenance of the war neuroses. Repression is so closely bound up with the pathology and treatment of these states that the full consideration of its rôle would amount to a complete study of neurosis in relation to the war.

THE PROCESS OF REPRESSION.

It is necessary at the outset to consider an ambiguity in the term "repression," as it is now used by writers on the pathology of the mind and nervous system. The term is currently used in two senses which should be carefully distinguished from one another. It is used for the *process* whereby a person endeavours to thrust out of his memory some part of his mental content, and it is also used for the *state* which ensues when, either through this process or by some other means, part of the mental content has become

W.H.R. Rivers
The Lancet, 1918

"Repression of War Experience"

at bay. War broke through. "The garden waits for something that delays," he wrote. "There must be crowds of ghosts among the trees.":

> No, no, not that,—it's bad to think of war,
> When thoughts you've gagged all day come back to scare
>   *you;*
> And it's been proved that soldiers don't go mad
> Unless they lose control of ugly thoughts
> That drive them out to jabber among the trees.
>
> Now light your pipe; look what a steady hand.
> Draw a deep breath, stop thinking; count fifteen,
> And you're as right as rain. . . .

. . . .

You're quiet and peaceful, summering safe at home;
You'd never think there was a bloody war on! . . .
O yes, you would . . . why, you can hear the guns.
Hark! Thud, thud, thud,—quite soft . . . they never cease—
Those whispering guns—O Christ, I want to go out
And screech at them to stop—I'm going crazy;
I'm going stark, staring mad because of the guns.

Sassoon added the poem's title, "Repression of War Experience," after a talk given by Rivers to the Royal Society of Medicine in 1917 and published a few months later in *The Lancet*. Repression of painful war experience, Rivers wrote in his *Lancet* article, almost always caused more harm than good. Memory should not be corked up; it ought to be "talked over in all [its] bearings." Patients should become familiar with what caused the pain and should "dwell upon it in such a way as to relieve its horrible and terrifying character." Horror should be confronted in psychotherapy until it is replaced by the "far more bearable emotion of grief." "Remembering," Sassoon wrote in "To One Who Was with Me in the War," "we forget / Much that was monstrous, much that clogged our souls with clay."

⌒

Sassoon was sent to Craiglockhart to heal from "shell-shock" and, if it proved possible, to return to the Front. It was a strange situation for patient and doctor. Sassoon was to be brought around to returning to a war he had dramatically and very publicly denounced, and he did not have shell shock. Rivers, a doctor, was meant to heal his patient sufficiently to return him to war and likely death. Rivers, analyzing a dream he had had about pacifism and Sassoon, set out the situation: "So long as I was an officer of the R.A.M.C.," he wrote. "So long as I was in uniform I was not a free agent, and though no one can be a free agent during a war, it was a definite element in my situation at the time that my official position might be influencing the genuineness of the views I was expressing in my conversations with [Sassoon]." Rivers was expected to carry out the business of the army. In order to do that he was required to listen to, understand, and help resolve the anti-war conflicts of Sassoon. All patients knew their doctors were required to act as army officers, to return soldiers to the war, and to maintain an anti-pacifist stance.

"Life, with an ironic gesture, had contrived that the man who had lit up my future with a new eagerness to do well in it should now be instrumental in sending me back to an even-money chance of being killed," Sassoon wrote about Rivers. "As an R.A.M.C. officer he was bound to oppose my 'pacifist tendency,' but his arguments were always indirect. Sometimes he gently indicated inconsistencies in my impulsively expressed opinions, but he never contradicted me."

Soldier and doctor talked night after night about Sassoon's experience in the war, the cost of going back to it—the betrayal of principle, the risk of death—and the cost of not going back. Rivers did not put pressure on Sassoon. It was not in his nature to do so and he knew that Sassoon would put pressure upon himself. Sassoon had excelled at being a commander; he missed the men he had led and looked after, the men for whom he felt responsibility. He missed the courage and human spirit of the soldiers who "had inspired me to be at my best when things were very bad." More and more he felt guilt about his own safety and comfort at Craiglockhart, playing golf, taking tea in Edinburgh, and writing poetry.

"Autumn was asserting itself, and a gale got up that night,"
he wrote. "The longer I lay awake the more I was reminded
of the troops in the line. There they were, stoically endur-
ing their roofless discomfort while I was safe and warm."
He wrote "Sick Leave" during this time, a self-accusatory
poem berating himself for his absence from the war and from
his men:

When I'm asleep, dreaming and lulled and warm,—
They come, the homeless ones, the noiseless dead.
While the dim charging breakers of the storm
Bellow and drone and rumble overhead,
Out of the gloom they gather about my bed.
　　　They whisper to my heart; their thoughts are mine.
　　　"Why are you here with all your watches ended?
　　　From Ypres to Frise we sought you in the Line."
In bitter safety I awake, unfriended;
And while the dawn begins with slashing rain
I think of the Battalion in the mud.
"When are you going out to them again?
Are they not still your brothers through our blood?"

It became increasingly clear to Sassoon that "going back
was the only way out of an impossible situation. At the front
I should at least find forgetfulness . . . and be in the trenches
with those whose experience I had shared and understood."
Rivers, he said, had let him "drift on for twelve weeks without
the slightest pressure." He came to his decision: "When the
windows were dark and I could see the stars, I still sat there
with my golf bag between my knees, alone with what now
seemed an irrefutable assurance that going back to the War as
soon as possible was my only chance of peace." "Love drove
me to rebel," he wrote of his soldiers while in Craiglockhart.

"Love drives me back to grope with them through hell; / And in their tortured eyes I stand forgiven."

⌁

"I had said good-bye to Rivers," Sassoon wrote years later about leaving Craiglockhart in November 1917. "Shutting the door of his room for the last time, I left behind me someone who had helped and understood me more than anyone I had ever known. Much as he disliked speeding me back to the trenches, he realized that it was my only way out. And the longer I live the more right I know him to have been." Although Rivers had given both Sassoon and the Medical Board the option for Sassoon to return to England rather than going back to the Front, Sassoon turned it down. He maintained then, as he did for the rest of his life, that the only decision possible was to return to the war and his men. He felt a debt to his doctor for the rest of his life. "I must never forget Rivers," Sassoon wrote in his diary. "He is the only man who can save me if I break down again. If I am able to keep going it will be through him."

Sassoon returned to the war, posted first to Ireland and then to Palestine. (Rivers had told the Medical Board that Sassoon's nerves were not yet strong enough to fight at the Front.) In May 1918 he returned to France. A British soldier, mistaking him for a German, shot him in the head and Sassoon returned to London to convalesce. He was safe from the guns and in a hospital room filled with sunlight overlooking Hyde Park, yet he was distraught, without peace. It was not possible to be more comfortable, he wrote later, even though he had a bullet wound in his head. Still, "I was restless and overwrought. . . . The white-walled room seemed to imprison me, and my thoughts couldn't escape from themselves." He felt little desire to stay alive and an "angry feeling of wanting to be killed came over me." He was bitter and found the future unimaginable. "Everything had fallen to pieces and one's mind was in a muddle, and one's nerves were all on edge," Sassoon wrote:

> And then, unexpected and unannounced, Rivers came in and closed the door behind him. Quiet and alert, purposeful and unhesitating, he seemed to empty the room of everything that had needed exorcising.
>
> My futile demons fled him—for his presence was a refutation of wrong-headedness. I knew then that I had been very lonely while I was at the War; I knew that I had a lot to learn, and that he was the only man who could help me.
>
> Without a word he sat down by the bed; and his smile was benediction enough for all I'd been through. "Oh, Rivers, I've had such a funny time since I saw you last!" I exclaimed. And I understood that this was what I'd been waiting for.
>
> He did not tell me that I had done my best to justify his belief in me. He merely made me feel that he took all that for granted, and now we must go on to something better still. And this was the beginning of the new life toward which he had shown me the way.

II

Healers of the Mind

Priest, Physician, and Psychotherapist

CHAPTER 4

And the God Left

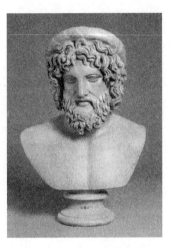

Asclepius, God of Medicine

O Lord Asclepius . . . it was you who granted us the opportunity of reaching a calm haven from the vast sea and utter dejection, and allowed us to offer our greetings to the common hearth of mankind.

He stretches out his hand and shows me a certain spot
in the sky, and while pointing at it he said: "This is the
one that Plato calls the soul of the universe." I look
and I see enthroned in the sky Asclepius of Pergamum.

—AELIUS ARISTIDES, *Orations*

Amid the Aesculapian cult, the most elaborate and
beautiful system of faith healing the world has seen,
scientific medicine took its rise.

—SIR WILLIAM OSLER,
The Principles and Practice of Medicine

In 1968, an archaeologist in Paris looked through her
microscope at a sample of ancient pollen grains excavated
from a cave in Iraqi Kurdistan. What she saw was "remarkable," Arlette Leroi-Gourhan wrote later in *Science*. The
specimen, taken from beneath the skeleton of a Neanderthal
man, contained clusters of pollen grains from at least seven
species of flowers, including yarrow, cornflower, and holly-
hock. Several clusters still retained the form of the original
anther. Tucked in as a grace note among the grains was a scale
from the wing of a butterfly that, the scientist suggested, had
probably flown in on one of the flowers. Most of the clusters
of pollen, she speculated, had been introduced into the cave
as complete flowers and at the same time; that is, the flowers
had been brought in deliberately. Based on the seasonal pattern of flowering in the region, she concluded that the corpse

of the Neanderthal man had been laid on a bed of branch and flower "more than 50,000 years ago between the end of May and the beginning of July." Her vivid account, tantalizingly specific and published in a prestigious scientific journal, provoked widespread interest and discussion.

Had the Neanderthals buried their dead with flowers, in a deliberate mourning ritual? The archaeologist who first excavated the site at Shanidar Cave, and who sent the soil samples to Leroi-Gourhan's laboratory, thought they had. He described someone in the last Ice Age "rang[ing] the mountainside in the mournful task of collecting flowers." Early Stone Age man had had a "soul," he wrote in *Science*. He had had a spiritual sense. Did Neanderthal also leave remnants of ritual healing or medicinal herbs?

Imagination is set traveling at the thought of Neanderthal mourners gathering cornflowers and yarrow, carrying their flowers to a grave within a cave, and strewing them in a pattern determined by ritual or aesthetic. But science demands evidence, more than just conjuring, and it was never possible that the idea of flowers and mourning rituals in Shanidar Cave would go unchallenged. The notion of such purposeful behavior in the Neanderthal, as evidence of early religious practice, was met with broad skepticism. Some critics were maliciously tart, others more measured. Hundreds of prehistoric burials had been uncovered, some archaeologists pointed out, but never one with flowers. Other explanations were possible.

Flowers might have been brought into the cave by rodents. The Shanidar Neanderthals may or may not have engaged in mortuary rituals, but rodents, many of whom build their nests of plants and grasses, were suggested as a more likely source of the yarrow, grape hyacinth, and other flowers in the burial earth. Or perhaps the wind had carried flowers into the cave. Scientists who studied cave structure and sediment wrote blistering critiques of scientists who studied bones and culture. Some argued that the burial sites were intentional, others that they were not. Even had there been a burial, some held, it need not have been a sentient, sacred event.

Recent science suggests another possibility, of relevance here, that the grains of pollen in the Neanderthal cave may have come from flowers collected for their healing properties rather than for burial and mourning. Penny Spikins, an archaeologist at the University of York, argues that the healing skills of the Neanderthal were sophisticated enough to include early forms of fever control, wound dressing, and use of medicinal herbs. Plaque on Neanderthal teeth has been found to have chemical remnants of yarrow, whose bitter taste, Spikins points out, made it more likely to have been used as a medicine than for food. No one knows for sure.

❧

In the Bruniquel Cave in southwest France, one thousand feet beyond the entrance, archaeologist Jacques Jaubert and his colleagues discovered circular and semicircular arrangements of intentionally marked stalagmite tips, burnt bones, and fire tracings. The reddening, blackening, and cracking of stalagmites suggested to the scientists that the structures had been heated by fire. Uranium-series dating, reported in their 2016 article in *Nature*, estimated the age of the structures to be 175,000 years. The Neanderthals who had constructed the elaborate groupings of stalagmites, Jaubert concluded, had a level of social organization that was "more complex than previously thought." There seemed no likely functional purpose for these structures, nor for lighting a fire on them, instead of on the cave floor, unless it was for a sacred ritual to give thanks, or to create awe. The scientists concluded that the altar-like arrangement likely had been part of symbolic or ritual behavior, part of the Neanderthal spiritual life. And possibly a part of the healing life as well.

We know little about what Neanderthals thought or created (see photo section). Caves collapse, bones return to dust. But what they left behind gives a surprising glimpse into prehistoric healing and ritual, enough to wonder about their notions of death, belief in the gods, and what they knew about healing. Shanidar Neanderthals may have gathered flowers to mourn their dead or to heal their sick, or for something else beyond our grasping. Surely there were shared elements—flowers, herbs, incantations, a healer—between the rituals of mourning and healing. We do not know the why of fire pits or the intention that led to regular geometric arrays of stalagmites. These discoveries offer only a hint of the psychological and spiritual life of an extinct species of human, a distant kin who shared our fears and pleasure in the world.

Who healed the sick and tended their wounds? Who sat with the dying? Were their healers as our own? How did they heal the mind?

⌒

Like Neanderthal, we turn to the natural world for healing. Nature gave us choice and opportunity to experiment with her trees and plants and rivers; they are what we live with and among, what we see and know. They tug, frighten, and provision us. Our ancestors drew upon nature's cycles and bounty for their rituals of religion and healing. We are interested in what they did before us because we, as they, are bound to nature and need it to survive.

It could not have been a long walk from using plants and trees for food and shelter to trying them for their healing prospects. Priests, healers, and others, curious or impetuous, ingested, or gave to others to ingest, a bit of bark, a flower, or a berry. Some plants killed or sickened and others healed. A few are used even now for healing. Willow bark, for one, was inscribed as a remedy on Sumerian clay tablets dating to 3000 B.C. and described in hieroglyphics in the medical papyri of the ancient Egyptian physicians. Hippocrates prescribed it to bring down fever in his patients. By the end of the nineteenth century, the active compound in willow bark had been identified as aspirin, synthesized, and used widely, to fight inflammation and fever. Like digitalis from foxglove and quinine from cinchona bark, it is among several thousand plant-based medicines in our modern pharmacopoeia. Yarrow, for one, has been used for healing from the Stone Age until more recent times. In the *Iliad*, Achilles used yarrow to heal wounds during the Battle of Troy (hence the flower's genus name, *Achillea*). Yarrow would be used later by Native American healers to bring down fever, and by both traditional Chinese doctors and Anglo-Saxon healers to stanch the flow of blood from wounds. For thousands of years, from the Aegean Sea to the islands of Scotland, man's needs and beliefs have turned to the healing power of plants.

Most cultures have discovered plants that heal the body and mind. The use of herbal medicine in China dates to the Bronze Age; *Huangdi Neijing*, a fundamental Chinese medical text and one of the earliest in medicine, has been used since the second century B.C. Centuries later, Li Shizhen, the great sixteenth-century Chinese physician, herbalist, and acupuncturist, compiled a comprehensive text of nearly two thousand drugs, *Compendium of Materia Medica*. It included physical properties of the drugs, their origins—rock, earth, water—healing uses to which they could be put, and directions for how best to prescribe them.

In time, treatments specific for disorders of the mind were added to the growing list of medicinal herbs prescribed for physical illnesses. Five hundred years before Christ, Hippocrates prescribed extracts of plants, including laurel, lotus, and myrtle, for the depressed and deranged. Pimpernel, known in its scarlet variety for ties to revolution and high adventure, was used for more than two thousand years to treat depression and other mental illnesses. Doctors in ancient Greece, and many since, believed pimpernel cured melancholy and restored joy (its Latin name, *Anagallis*, comes from the Greek words for "laughter," and "to delight again"). Doggerel suggests that it was widely used and appreciated: "No heart can think," the old rhyme goes, "no tongue can tell, the virtues of the pimpernel" (see photo section).

Persian doctors recommended damask rose and lavender for mania; to the depressed, they gave pomegranate, honey, pear juice, and white lily. The Anglo-Saxons prescribed peony and periwinkle to be drunk out of church bells. Later, in *The Anatomy of Melancholy*, Robert Burton described the many healing herbs that "purge all the melancholy vapours from the spirits." Ginger and nutmeg would soothe those in despair, he wrote. So too would dandelion, marigold, willow, roses, and sassafras, broth of violets, sweet apples, and syrup of poppy. To rectify the air, to clear it against all manner of melancholy, he and others before him suggested peels of citron, water lilies, and cloves. Native Americans used a wide variety of herbs for healing, including yarrow, honeysuckle, cattails, and lavender for depression and anxiety. Wherever in place, and whenever in time, healers discovered plants to calm the mind or to enliven it.

Egypt's "teeming soil," Homer says in the *Odyssey*, "bears the richest yield of herbs in all the world / . . . Every man is a healer there, more skilled / than any other men on earth— Egyptians born / of the healing god himself." It was an Egyptian who gave Helen of Troy the magical potion nepenthe to quell sorrow, drive off dullness, and banish grief, to escape pain. Dioscorides, the Greek physician and botanist whose herbal was used for more than fifteen hundred years, and Roman naturalist Pliny the Elder, believed that nepenthe was a potion brewed from the herb borage; when added to wine, they claimed, it promoted "mirth and hilarity." It was used for thousands of years to elevate mood and dampen agitation, to comfort, and to keep melancholy at bay. Borage, or nepenthe, Robert Burton wrote in 1620, "challenge[s] for the chiefest place" among cures for melancholy (see photo section).

The desire for a nepenthe to quell sorrow and forget pain is an original and lasting part of who we are. In Big Sur on the California coast—built, it seems, of fog, stone, and sea—is the restaurant Nepenthe. It is named for the drug of old, its founders say, an "isle of no-care." Nepenthe is a place, a state of mind, "a drug, heart's ease, dissolving anger, / magic to make us all forget our pains." Our desires are now as they were in the time of Homer and before: to heal, to gain heart's ease.

Stone-from-the-Meeting-of-the-Waters. Honeycomb.
Mint-from-the-Mountains and Peppermint Blossoms.
Date Palm, Blue Lotus, and Bark of-the-Pomegranate.
Acanthus. Film-of-Dampness-Which-is-Found-on-
the-Wood-of-Ships. Hemlock and Squill.

—EGYPTIAN MEDICAL REMEDIES,
EBERS PAPYRUS, C. 1500 B.C.

"Sixty centuries ago," William Osler wrote, "after mil-
lenniums of a gradual upward progress" and yet seemingly
"out of the ocean of oblivion," civilization—and a highly
evolved practice of medicine—came out of the fertile land of
the Nile valley. Osler said of Imhotep, the Egyptian architect
and physician of the late twenty-seventh century B.C., that
he was "the first figure of a physician to stand out clearly
from the mists of antiquity." Imhotep, Isaac Asimov added,
was also the first scientist, one who was unique, "for no other
scientist since has been made into a god."

Imhotep built for eternity. He is remembered for design-
ing and constructing the first pyramid, built forty-seven
hundred years ago. The Step Pyramid, revolutionary and
ambitious, was part of a thirty-seven-acre complex that
included the pharaoh's burial chamber, temples, pavilions,
and courtyards; living areas for priests; and great, high steps
to make ready the pharaoh's ascent into the afterlife.

Imhotep is a critical figure in the history of medicine as
well. Two thousand years before Hippocrates, he laid down a
foundation for its principles and practice. Like other Egyptian healers, his healing art was rooted in prayer, magic, and
herbs, as well as in meticulous observations of the body and
its diseases. These observations existed alongside supernatu-

ral forces, which were assumed in illness, just as they were assumed to underlie the life-giving cycles of flooding of the Nile. Imhotep, at ease with both natural and supernatural, is the first physician known to have extracted medicines from plants—the same is said of Asclepius, the Greek god of medicine—and he is the likely author of the Edwin Smith Papyrus, the oldest known surgical treatise. He described two hundred diseases. He healed the sick and made better the journeys of the dying. His temples were used as healing places long after his death and, in time, he was deified as the god of medicine and healing. The Greeks, in ultimate tribute, held him with Asclepius, their own god of medicine.

In those early years, medicine and the priesthood were linked in preparation and practice. Later, magic and the gods existed on intimate terms with emerging science as well. Magic and religion controlled the "uncharted spheres," Osler said, but science set its sights on controlling the natural world, first by understanding it and then by acting upon it.

Incantation shared a healing role with medicinal herbs. Even as Egyptian physicians advanced the science of disease and treatment, they held on to their primitive powers of suggestion, so often essential to healing. They chanted against occupying spirits and demons and invoked magic spells to make their medicines more powerful. The scientific among them studied bones and body organs and made close note of what they saw; they described symptoms and the natural course of diseases and observed which remedies cured and which did not. It was a time of generative and pragmatic medical practice. They, like the Greeks, were aware of psychological influences on illness and healing. Egyptian sleep temples, forerunners of those of the Greeks, served as hospitals, sanctuaries, and centers for purification, healing of body and mind, analysis of dreams, and meditation. Healers induced trancelike states and interpreted dreams as ways to determine the correct treatment for illness and the most auspicious path through life. Music, painting, and nature were used to calm the agitated, tend the grieving, and heal the melancholic. Egyptian doctors, and after them the Greeks, grew skilled in describing and prescribing for brain fevers, mania, and other mental disorders. As they did, they laid down the elements of medical psychology and psychiatry. They studied and tended the hurt mind.

❧

Asclepius did not appear, as the statues of him are wont to do, gentle and calm, but in a lively posture and rather frightening to behold. Serpents followed him, enormous sorts of reptiles, they too hurrying on, with their tremendous train of coils, making a whistling noise as in the wilderness and woodland glens. His associates followed him carrying boxes of drugs, tightly bound. Then the god stretched forth his hand to me.

—HIPPOCRATES, *Epistolae*

To all who approached Asclepius, Pindar said, whether stricken with the plague or wounded by a "far-flung stone," the Greek god of medicine gave deliverance from suffering. The god appeared, "stretched forth his hand," and listened. His was a god's deliverance, one that healed and gave wisdom. He created order from the chaos of his supplicants' dreams and looked into their minds as well as their bodies. To many Asclepius touched, he granted psychological relief.

He offered a bond to humanity, extended "greetings to the common hearth of mankind." Asclepius healed with his presence and his drugs and the suggestive powers used in his temples. He prescribed paradoxical remedies such as hemlock, or tasks impossible to complete. Aristides, the Greek writer and orator, was treated for years at the Aesculapian temple in Pergamon. "When the harbor waves were swollen by the south wind and ships were in distress," he said, "I had to sail across to the opposite side, eating honey and acorns from an oak tree." Asclepius demanded it of him. The god's expectation made probable that Aristides would make the demand of himself and succeed (see photo section).

To many who came to him, Asclepius taught ways to navigate not only what lay near but uncertain straits farther out. Hardship led to good. "I myself am one of those who have lived not twice but many varied lives through the power of the god," Aristides said of his healing days in the temple of Asclepius. His sickness and what he learned from Asclepius gave him courage, tenacity, and knowledge. He had acquired "precious gems in return for which I would not accept all that which is considered happiness among men . . . These regions have no harbor, but most correctly and justly is it said that this is the most secure and steadfast of all ports." One learned from suffering, one discovered new paths, new ways to survive. One was tougher, more flexible. Asclepius was rock and wayfinder, teacher and healer. He was the "stern-cable of salvation." Asclepius laid the grounds for introspection and healed the mind; he made the "harsh in illnesses mild."

Asclepius also brought the mind back from darkness and death, the Greek dramatist Menander wrote: "I had been dead during all the years of life that I was alive. The beautiful, the good, the holy, the evil were all the same to me; such, it seems, was the darkness that formerly enveloped my understanding and concealed and hid from me all these things. But now that I have come here, I have become alive again for all the rest of my life, as if I had lain down in the temple of Asclepius and had been saved. I walk, I talk, I think." Many philosophers and writers came to Asclepius temples to be treated, including Socrates, Sophocles, and Marcus Aurelius.

The mythic Asclepius, son of Apollo, himself the son of Zeus, was born near Epidaurus in ancient Greece. The Sanctuary of Asclepius at Epidaurus, one of three hundred temples built in his name, dates to the fourth century B.C. It was, in every way, designed for psychological as well as physical healing. Set among the hills and trees, away from the

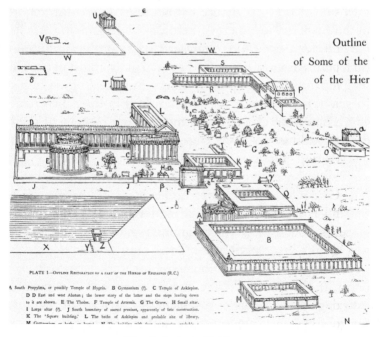

The Asclepion at Epidaurus

interferences of the world, it defined arcadia. It was beautiful and restful; the air was pure, the diet simple; there were fresh springs in which to bathe, and a theater and library for arts and learning. Pilgrims sailed to Epidaurus from cities across the ancient world to be touched by the god or his priests, and to be healed by magic, art, peaceful circumstances, suggestion, and medicine. They came to a world perfectly cast for mending minds.

Temple priests drew upon magic, religion, drama and music, suggestion, surgery, drugs, and herbs. Some of their methods—suggestion and interpretation of dreams—seem ahead of their time. They were, but the psychological underpinnings of temple healing had evolved over centuries. The priests of Asclepius had learned from their ancestors, and they understood the nature of suffering. The construction of their sanctuaries emerged from this understanding. Meditative peace came more easily in a quiet and beautiful setting, faith was more powerfully evoked in the midst of marble temples and altars and sacred waters. Still, healing was not a passive thing. Supplicants were involved in their own remedy. They were expected to articulate the content of their dreams and to be actively engaged in treatments prescribed by the priest-physicians.

Before beginning treatment, supplicants purified themselves and offered sacrifices to Asclepius—song, money, olive shoots—and proffered figs and honey cakes to the temple serpents. Blood of sacrificial animals—sheep, cattle, pigs—was caught in a vessel and poured onto the altar; entrails were cooked and feasted upon. Hymns were sung to Asclepius, the "healer of all," the god who softened "the painful sufferings of man's diseases." Sacred lights were lit. Supplicants bathed in healing waters—mineral springs, the river, the sea—meditated in a sacred grove, fed on a cleansing diet, and prayed.

The priests laid on hands and applied ash; at times, they ordered delicacies such as partridge with frankincense. Only then came incubation, during which the supplicants slept in special areas within the sanctuary. There, lulled by suggestion, and with their moods perhaps enhanced by drugs, they slept in expectation that Asclepius, or another god, or a temple priest would visit and tell them the things to be done to cure their sickness. Persians, in another time, made the distinction between "knife doctors," "wound doctors," and "herb doctors." The priest-doctors of the Asclepieia were all of these.

The suggestive powers of the temple setting and its rituals were strong. The sick in mind were cured by hypnotic power of place, and their dreams were given a healing meaning by god or priest. The infusion of hope gave rise to a greater faith in a healing god. Therapeutic order emerged from the interpretation of a supplicant's dreams, and its effect made more powerful by the drugs, surgery, and herbs that followed. One of the remedies, "Unguent Asclepius," was a particularly complicated one, worthy of the medicinal preparations of the Egyptian physicians and commensurate with those of the god for whom it had been named, the "Master of Herbs." Some of the potency of the god's remedy stemmed from its Daedalean formula and the challenge of procuring ingredients from Egypt and Asia Minor: "Common salts, rock salts, Cappadocian salts roasted, pumice-stone, white coarse soda (potass), laurel berries, at the rate of 1 pound; white hellebore, soapwort, wild raisin, Alexandrian mustard, unburnt brimstone, feverfew, salt of tartar, mastich tree blossoms, marsh-plant, at the rate of 6 ounces."

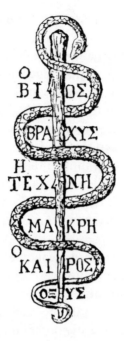

Staff of Asclepius

Life is short, the Art long, opportunity fleeting.
—HIPPOCRATES

Snakes roved freely throughout the temples, for Asclepius took pleasure in their company. Serpents, it was said, had a way with herbs. Asclepius, deft with herbs, had witnessed this. He had seen a serpent approach another of its kind, lifeless, and place herbs from inside its mouth onto the dead reptile's head. In a heartbeat, life changed place with death. Serpents could heal. They shed age and infirmity as they did their skin. They were vigilant and quick. They could change identity to survive or deceive. Long before Asclepius, serpents were associated with deities and magical powers. But it was Asclepius who brought them to the eternal. Nothing so embodies healing, from ancient temple to modern medical guild, as Asclepius and the serpent wound around his staff.

The Aesculapian cult, as Osler observed, had a psychologically sophisticated understanding of human behavior and helped lay the groundwork for modern scientific medicine. Generation after generation of physicians owed the fundamentals of their medical education to it. Hippocrates, the "Father of Medicine," who was born twenty-five centuries ago on the Aegean island of Kos, was one. He is thought to have trained at the Aesculapian temple on Kos but broke from the priest-healers there when he came to believe that disease was the result of rational causes, not religious or magical ones. There was nothing divine or sacred about disease, Hippocrates and his followers taught; physicians ought not to invoke magic or the gods. With the practice of Hippocrates, Osler wrote, "Medicine broke its leading strings to religion and philosophy."

Hippocrates, an astute clinical observer, carefully described symptoms and courses of disease in works variously written by him, his students, or his followers. Importantly, Hippocrates recognized the ascendancy of the brain in behavior. "From the brain, and from the brain only, arise our pleasures, joys, laughter, and jests, as well as our sorrows, pains, griefs and tears," he wrote. Within its confines, we learn to distinguish the "ugly from the beautiful and the bad from the good." It is the brain "which makes us mad or delirious, inspires us with dread and fear." Hippocrates had a particular interest in human nature, temperament, and madness. His clinical descriptions of melancholia and mania still ring true, and his case studies are striking for their detail. In a letter attributed to him—part of the diffuse and disputed body of Hippocratic texts—he, or one of his followers, writes to Greek physician and herbalist Crateuas about the mental turmoil of the philosopher Democritus. "They say that he is sick and needs a purge because he is in the midst of madness." Democritus was awake night and day, laughing at all things "great and small." He heard the voices of birds and traveled "into the boundlessness." It was hoped Democritus would not need drugs, but perhaps the leaves, blossoms, and roots of plants would help, "bound tightly so they will not be open to the winds and lose their concentration of pharmaceutical virtue . . . Know well we would purge the sick minds of men along with their bodies. But that is a prayer. For the present, gather especially the plants from mountains and high ridges. . . . Try to gather blossoms from marsh flowers by the ponds, river flowers, and fountain flowers."

Time was of the essence. "Send these things to us immediately. The time of year is fitting and the constraints of the so-called madness press." (Democritus, believed deranged by some, was thought a genius, or both, by others.) In all things, Hippocrates and his followers urged the awareness of time and opportunity, the obligation to closely observe, to extend compassion, and to pass on to other physicians and students that which had been learned. It was important to maintain skepticism and an open mind. That which seemed to be madness might not be so. It might be eccentricity, or wisdom of an unusual kind. The letter, though likely apocryphal, gives a glimpse into Hippocratic thought and practice.

In addition to his scientific observation of diseases and their progression, Hippocrates made explicit how a physician should conduct himself, as well as his moral and ethical obligations toward his patients. A doctor must be proficient in medical knowledge, he said, but he must have "natural" talent and disposition as well. He must work hard, be persistent, and stay conscious of the limits of his knowledge. He must be elegant, but show no signs of luxury. He must be a "gentleman in character" and, being so, "grave and kind to all." He must be serious, quick-witted, silent in the face of disturbance, gracious in disposition, and "turn to the truth when a thing has been shown to be true." Above all, a physician's priority must be to act in all ways to benefit his patient.

Hippocrates never entirely forsook the art of medicine as practiced by the gods, or at least he continued to acknowledge the gods as a kind of exemplar. "A physician who is a lover of wisdom is the equal of a god," he said. "The gods are the 'real physicians.'" Like the gods, doctors should choose the higher ground. The ideal practice of medicine should be kept at the front of one's thinking: godlike, perhaps unobtainable, but sought.

Nowhere do the moral qualities of the physician and the high ground of medical practice make themselves more clear than in the Hippocratic Oath. It begins with a bow to the gods—"I swear by Apollo Physician, by Asclepius, by Health, by Panacea and by all the gods and goddesses"—and continues on to obligate the doctor to venerate teacher, patient, and a sacred calling: "To hold my teacher in this art equal to my own parents . . . to help the sick according to my ability . . . [to] keep pure and holy my life and art." Revenants of an ancient priesthood seep into the Hippocratic pledge of purity and holiness of the physician-confessor: "Whatsoever I shall see or hear in the course of my profession . . . if it be what should not be published abroad, I will never divulge, holding such things to be holy secrets." To this day, with rare exception, the Hippocratic Oath holds the physician to the same confessional duty as that of the priest. (The "sacramental seal is inviolable," Roman Catholic canon law decrees. "It is absolutely forbidden for a confessor to betray in any way a penitent in words or in any manner and for any reason." The Anglican Book of Common Prayer says likewise. The secrecy of a confession is "morally absolute.")

The human qualities that characterize the mythic healers remain the same today. The psychological needs and desires of our ancestors and modern man are not so different. Psychotherapy, a powerful journey undertaken by healer and patient, is beholden to these same needs and desires. It is to that relationship, that kind of healing, we turn next.

"Then the god stretched forth his hand to me," Hippocrates said. "And taking it gladly I begged him to join me and not to be too late to aid me in my treatment. He replied: 'At the moment you have no need of me at all, but this goddess here [Truth], who holds sway over mortals and immortals alike, for the present will herself guide you' . . . And the god left."

CHAPTER 5

Bearings in the Dark

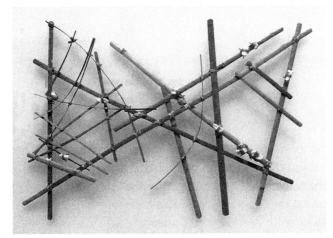

Micronesian stick chart
Islands and ocean swells

Some may not have performed their journey exclusively, or even mainly, by sailing, but may have covered large distances by paddling, passing from point to point of coasts and keeping in relation with land as constantly as possible. In such a case wind and current would have little influence except as causes of delay, though such delay may have the most important effect.

—W.H.R. Rivers

To sit quietly in a consulting room and talk to someone
would not appear to the general public as a heroic or
dramatic thing to do. In medicine there are many
different ways of saving lives. This is one of them.

—MORAG COATE,
Beyond All Reason

The bourne of healing has remained much the same as
in the days of Asclepius and Hippocrates: to treat disease as best as science allows, to console, to accompany and
bear witness, to give hope, and to make whole again. As in
antiquity, the healer is minister to the soul, however secularly
imagined that soul may be. "It is the physician's order," Maimonides said, "to keep in sight the movements of the soul,
to study them constantly." It is the healer's order to restore
the mind to soundness: to repair and mend it, to pry it from
disease, to reassemble. He asked of his doctor, wrote French
poet Antonin Artaud, that he "uplift my abasement, balance
what is crumbling, reunite what is separated, recompose what
is destroyed."

W.H.R. Rivers and William Osler knew this. Both physicians were sons of Anglican (Church of England) priests,
and both were baptized by their fathers. Rivers and Osler
spent much of their youth listening to their fathers' sermons
and prayers and observing them tend their parishioners. As
young men they were immersed in parish life, a life that
assumed faith as it assumed the air. Both observed the suffering of their fathers' parishioners and saw what their fathers
did and could not do to alleviate it. They learned the limits
of faith and of their fathers. Both held the hymns and the

language of the Bible and the Book of Common Prayer close to them and drew upon them throughout their lives. They knew better than most the words of solace, the obligation of healing: "Keep watch, dear Lord, with those who work, or watch, with those who weep this night," it says in the Book of Common Prayer. "Tend the sick . . . give rest to the weary, bless the dying, soothe the suffering, pity the afflicted."

If Rivers and Osler grew to have their doubts about the teachings of their church, and they did; if they had an uncertain faith in God, they kept a debt to the words, rituals, and

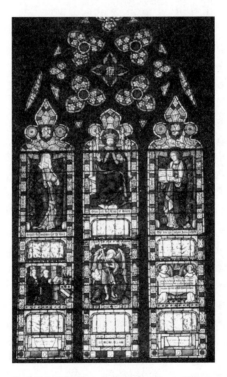

St. Michael's Church in Kent, where Henry
Rivers served as priest

music of the Anglican Church. They believed in the power of faith and ritual, and used it in their work as doctors and teachers.

The Church of England, indebted as it is to ancient worship and music, retains a primitive power to suggest, to console, and to heal. The Church carries the history of its penitents and celebrants; it keeps a keen understanding of the human need for solace and communion, a desire for the sacred, and places that evoke wonder. Rivers's sister remembered the enchantment of her father's church and the rectory where they lived. There was a large garden, tennis lawns, and a cricket pitch. The church, whose tower dates to the Normans, "had a low 'leper' window through which the pilgrim lepers had been able to look in the direction of the altar." On the far side of the church, she continued, "ran the old Roman road, along which the Canterbury Pilgrims used to take their way." Lepers, a Roman road, Canterbury pilgrims: near-perfect building blocks for a child's imagination. The combination of pagan, faith, and suffering was one to which Rivers would be drawn for life.

William Osler's upbringing was different from that of Rivers. His father, ordained by the archbishop of Canterbury, was ordered to "cure the souls in His Majesty's Foreign Possession"; that is, he was ordered to establish a church in the backwater of the Canadian frontier. Featherstone and Ellen Osler left England in 1837 to find themselves among a "wild people." Their church was a ministry of two thousand settlers living in towns scattered across more than two hundred square miles. The Devil ran rampant, the newly ordained Osler wrote. "Drunkenness, blasphemy, and several species of vice were common." Bears and wolves lived in the woods; the winters were fierce. Primitive, Osler said, did not begin to describe it (see photo section).

Osler's church was more than an Atlantic crossing away from the stained glass antiquity of Henry Rivers's church and the rectory's rolled lawns and cricket pitch. Yet for both young Rivers and Osler, the Church kept partial hold through the sacraments of baptism and burial and ministry to the sick. They watched their fathers heal parishioners through word, ritual, consolation, and force of personality. It left a lasting mark. Osler, it was said later, was more than a doctor; he was a priest as well. On the fever wards, a young doctor observed, Osler laid on hands, gave hope, and consoled the dying. He ministered to the sick. Faith—"the one great moving force which we can neither weigh in the balance nor test in the crucible," said Osler—was a determining part of who they were as doctors. Faith was indeed a "great moving force" in human life; it had found its way from desert and cave into the teaching amphitheaters of modern medicine. It was a force in the lives of doctors and their patients, be they believers or not. Faith had limits, Osler made clear. It could not knit a bone, cure cancer, or raise the dead. But God was there, worshipped or not. Hope and faith were essential forces.

Hope, wrote John Steinbeck, cushions the shock of experience:

> Probably when our species developed the trick of memory and with it the counterbalancing projection called "the future," this shock-absorber, hope, had to be included in the series, else the species would have destroyed itself in despair. For if ever any man were deeply and unconsciously sure that his future would be no better than his past, he might deeply wish to cease to live. And out of this therapeutic poultice we build our iron teleologies and twist the tide pools and the stars into the pattern.

Hope provides time, energy, and a shore toward which to swim. "In the treatment of nervous diseases," said Coleridge, "he is the best physician who is the most ingenious inspirer of hope." Hopelessness is the dark heart of depression; hope must be infused into those without it. It must be given, even knowing that it is likely to be spurned. There is consolation in words of hope, and even more consolation in the persistent extension of hope, of reiteration. I remember what one of my colleagues at Johns Hopkins said to a deeply depressed patient: "I will never, ever, ever give up on you." It was an affirmation of hope and promise of convoy, a covenant. Faith, the Bible had taught, was the substance of things hoped for, the evidence of things not seen. My colleague dealt in faith.

The Swiss psychoanalyst Carl Jung was, like Rivers and Osler, the son of a Protestant minister. Although he moved away from the beliefs of his father, Jung believed that walking the road to God, searching for God, the quest for the spiritual, was the heart of life's journey. Among his patients older than thirty-five, he wrote in "Psychotherapists or the Clergy," there was not one "whose problem in the last resort was not that of finding a religious outlook on life." By "religious outlook," he made clear, he was speaking in the broad sense of spiritual quest. It had "nothing whatsoever to do with a particular creed or membership of a church" (see photo section).

Healing was a religious problem, but only in the more general meaning of the word "religious." Religion and psychology and medicine were woven as one, but their individual strands meant different things to different people. Modern man, Jung wrote, "has heard enough about guilt and sin." He needed to understand himself in psychological ways, not only in religious ones. Man has a dark side and, as he comes to understand this, he must "reconcile himself with his own nature—how he is to love the enemy in his own heart and call the wolf his brother." One must be on good terms with one's darker side, Yeats said.

The idea that one could learn from the dark is territory well-mapped by religion. Religious and healing rituals of confession bear witness to the existence of the dark. The Babylonians and Assyrians practiced an early form of psychotherapy, based in religion and magic, which relied upon confession, suggestion, and exorcism. Confession, in a secular or religious sense, is important in many forms of psychotherapy. It is usual for the psychotherapist, wrote Jung, "to begin by eliciting from the patient a more or less voluntary confession of things he dislikes, is ashamed of, or fears. This is like the much older confessional in the Church, which in many ways anticipated modern psychotherapeutic techniques." He and Freud, Jung wrote, practiced as Confessors; in time, they traded confessional for couch. "My method, like Freud's," wrote Jung, "is built up on the practice of confession." (Confession was an integral part of many therapeutic relationships, Rivers observed. It is of no surprise that Sassoon described Rivers as his "father-confessor.")

Since the early days of Christianity, in both the Catholic and Anglican Churches—the latter of which includes the Episcopal Church in the United States—healing has been preceded by the Act of Confession, an articulation of the penitent's sins and shortcomings. "We have erred and strayed from thy ways like lost sheep," one prays from The Book of Common Prayer: "We have left undone those things which we ought to have done, and we have done those things which we ought not to have done. . . . Spare thou those who confess their faults." William James, who lamented the decline in the practice of confession, spoke to its benefits: "Shams are over and realities have begun," he said. The interior "rottenness" is taken outward; the "shell of secrecy" is forced open, the "pent-in abscess" bursts open and "gains relief."

To confess, to put into words in the presence of another, to acknowledge where one has fallen short, is to begin to comprehend the wayward and damaging, to see a pattern, thence to extend observation beyond the confessional. Redemption requires not only confession but atonement and accountability. This is critical to many different therapeutic and self-help traditions. The fourth step in Alcoholics Anonymous, for example, is to make "a searching and fearless moral inventory of ourselves"; the fifth is to "admit to God, to ourselves, and to another human being the exact nature of our wrongs." Confession teaches; it brings knowledge from shame. The catharsis that may follow—a loosening of suppressed emotions, the cleansing of wrongdoing, the reimagining of failure or inadequacy—is part of healing. It is the "most important psychotherapeutic agent in the process of confession," observed W.H.R. Rivers, "whether this form part of a religious rite or of a manifestly medical procedure." Repressed grief, anxiety, and shame, brought to consciousness, gives relief. Examining shortfalls in the self and committing to remedy thought and actions can lead to amendment, grace, and consolation. Repentance heals. It amends and makes renewal possible.

"I am ill because of wounds to the soul, to the deep emotional self," wrote D. H. Lawrence. "And the wounds to the soul take a long, long time, only time can help / and patience, and a certain difficult repentance."

◦———

In 1952, John Custance, who served as a Royal Navy officer during the First World War and as an intelligence officer in the Second, wrote *Wisdom, Madness, and Folly*. It is an extraordinary book, written under pseudonym, about his manic-depressive psychosis, an illness that brought him, as it does to many, dramatic religious experiences, including ecstatic states, delusions, and hallucinations. He argued the futility of any treatment that did not address religion in a serious way. Psychological treatment "cannot afford to ignore the religious aspect," Custance wrote. "It demands the parson as well as the psychologist. With all due respect to the very kind and well-meaning doctor who treated me, he was not much use as a father-confessor. I needed absolution, and he had none to give. It was not much use telling me to pull myself together and forget my sins." Sin was too deep in him, too real, to be dismissed as merely a product of madness.

The doctor need not be a believer in order to deal with issues of faith and confession. Many people have neither need nor interest in matters of religion, and discussing such things will not heal their minds. Morag Coate, whose *Beyond All Reason* is a meditation on the importance of psychotherapy in healing psychotic illness, spoke to the importance of the psychotherapist addressing religious belief: The question is not "Can it be proved?" but rather, "What does it do?" The doctor who grapples with faith and God and sin of all dimensions, she wrote, "does not have to be a believer. What he requires is honesty, a capacity to be concerned in other people's spiritual struggles, and a realisation that, however certain his own belief or disbelief may seem to be, he cannot himself claim to know all the answers. . . . The test of his skill in personal relationships is that, having used to the full the positive influence of his personality, he can in the end leave his patients free."

Doctors must have a "shared humanity" with their patients, in addition to knowing the limits of their knowledge. They must respect the independence of the patients they treat; that is, give them room to make mistakes and to find paths of their own; they must "leave their patients free to get well each in his or her separate individual way." If a patient believes in God, Coate argues, God is then "a real person to the patient and to be discussed as such." Most important, doctors must know enough about themselves and the world to "step across into the other's territory." They must be able to look at the world through the eyes of someone who is suffering onto madness, be able to enter another's world of confusion and ambiguities. Doctors must, as William Osler said, be able to tolerate the uncertainty that comes with human nature, disease, and treating the sick.

Morag Coate dedicated *Beyond All Reason* to "A.S.," Anthony Storr, an English psychiatrist and writer, and one of the preeminent psychotherapists in Britain. I knew Anthony first during a year's sabbatical leave in Oxford, where he practiced psychiatry and taught young doctors. We became close friends and colleagues and, when he died in 2001, I was honored to give his eulogy. I learned immeasurably from Anthony about psychotherapy, about how easy it is to do poorly and how difficult it is to do well. He was a compassionate doctor, in part because he had known depression and anxiety himself, and he brought rare understanding to the suffering of his patients. He believed that human imperfection is part of who we are and part of what the psychotherapist must hear out, take in, and take on. All of us are complex and ambivalent, which causes pain to us and to those we care about. But suffering also causes us to discover and invent, and to look intently into dark corners of memory and action. Dark can come to good. "It's not psychopathology that counts," he once said. "It's what you do with it."

Storr's father, an Anglican priest, was a canon and the

archdeacon of Westminster Abbey. When Anthony was a
child, his father would give him the keys to the abbey so that
he could take his gramophone into the sanctuary and listen
to Handel and Bach. "It was glorious," he said. "Glorious."
He learned young that religion was essential to the lives and
healing of many, but he learned with equal conviction that
music, in its sublimity, could heal and transport. Many things
could heal, or help to heal, he believed: faith, music and literature, medication, love and friendship, solitude. Psychotherapy healed in part by bringing to light what could best reach
a particular patient. Like Rivers, Osler, and Jung, Storr shed
many of the beliefs of his father's church, but he kept his love
for the ritual, the language, and the music. Faith was important to him. He knew its power and its limits, and assumed its
presence in his work as a psychotherapist.

Music was Anthony Storr's lifelong interest and passion.
In *Music and the Mind*, he discussed his belief that religion
and music alike serve to order the emotions. Religions, he
wrote, provide "a hierarchy culminating in a deity . . . They
all seem to be attempts of the human mind to impose some
kind of order on the chaos of existence." Music was not a
belief system, but "its importance and its appeal also depend
upon its being a way of ordering human existence." Music
is a "source of reconciliation, exhilaration, and hope," a gift
of purpose. It is, as Anthony ends his book, "an irreplaceable, undeserved, transcendental blessing." Art deepens and
uplifts, lends to reflection, and gives meaning. It heals.

Although he trained as a Jungian, and wrote extensively
about both Jung and Freud, Storr was skeptical about orthodox psychoanalysis. His theoretical perspective, like that
of many psychotherapists, became more eclectic and pragmatic as he grew older. He extracted what he found useful
from psychoanalysis but took as well from other forms of

psychotherapy and psychology. His writing reflects his broad interests in psychology, medicine, creativity, aggression, literature, and music, and the porous border between normal and abnormal behavior.

Anthony wrote well about psychotherapy. Like Rivers and Osler, he was curious, deeply read, open to dissenting views, and sensitive to the importance of his own role in healing patients. He was tough, kind, widely educated, and an astonishingly good listener. He was adept at making sense of jumbled thinking and chaotic lives. He had all the attributes of a healer, and this fills his writing.

He was a thoughtful teacher as well. One day, when I was expressing my difficulty in imagining Freud as an empathetic psychotherapist, Anthony suggested I visit the Freud Museum in Hampstead. He said he thought I would be surprised by the warmth and humanity of Freud's study. I was (see photo section).

Anthony did not confuse empathy with competence, and was acutely aware of the misguided temptation of psychotherapists to impress patients with their empathy. The therapist "has to be affected without acting upon his own feelings," he wrote. "To use his own feelings in the service of the patient, as a guide to understanding, not as a way of demonstrating how kind, how loving, how sympathetic he himself is." Someone had described two British prime ministers, he said: "One possessed no antennae, while the other possessed nothing else." Lack of antennae was disqualifying for anyone who wished to be a psychotherapist. But so too was an excess. Being a good therapist demanded more than being warm and "entering into another's distress." It demanded a sympathetic and intelligent understanding of the twists of temperament and the vagaries of dreams, the determining drives of fear and longing, and the desperation of hope lost.

It demanded that one learn from patients who they were and how they came to be that way. It demanded distance:

> The thing about being associated with a hawk is that one cannot be slipshod about it. No hawk can be a pet. There is no sentimentality. In a way, it is a psychiatrist's art. One is matching one's mind against another with deadly reason and interest. One desires no transference of affection, demands no ignoble homage or gratitude. It is a tonic for the less forthright savagery of the human heart.
>
> —T. H. WHITE, *The Goshawk*

In 1772, John Gregory, physician to George III and professor of medicine at the University of Edinburgh, wrote in *Duties and Qualifications of a Physician* that physicians must be conversant with human misery and of open heart, but they must not blend their own sympathies with those of their patients: "A physician of too much sensibility may be rendered incapable of doing his duty," John Gregory wrote. If there is an excess of sympathy, it will "depress his spirit and prevent him from acting with that steadiness and vigour, upon which perhaps the life of his patient in a great measure depends." Like writers, doctors ought to keep a sliver of ice in their souls. But just a sliver.

~

Afterwards he would talk in general terms about the theory of analysis, about the mortmain of the past which holds us in thrall. Sometimes, as the analysis progressed, he would show little hints of excitement—as though he scented something for which he had been waiting for a long while. . . . He patiently waited for me to discover the long road back for myself. I too began to feel the excitement of the search.

—GRAHAM GREENE,
A Sort of Life

We sought to heal the mind long before we could treat diseases of the brain. Magicians and priests healed their supplicants as much through suggestion and tincture of time as by science. The past 150 years have seen this change markedly. In the early twentieth century, psychoanalysis and electroconvulsive therapy came into their own and, in the years following the Second World War, antidepressant, antipsychotic, and anticonvulsant medications, lithium, and structured psychotherapies came into use. Treatments continue to improve, new ones are developed—mood stabilizers and antidepressants, medications for anxiety and schizophrenia, brain stimulation techniques, ketamine, psilocybin, virtual reality therapies, and others—remedies that help millions of individuals. Less beneficial, however, has been the concurrent decrease in the time given over to psychotherapy.

Medication and other non-psychotherapeutic treatments save lives, ameliorate suffering, make meaningful work possible, and allow relationships to mend. For many, medication does these things more quickly, better, and less expensively than psychotherapy. If medication is imperfect, and if medication has allowed a drift away from the use of psychotherapy, still no one who treats, studies, or suffers from mental illness, and no one who is familiar with the underlying clinical science, would return to the days before such treatment was available.

Medication restores mood, thinking, and energy well enough to reclaim much of what is lost during illness. Yet this often falls short of healing the mind. Many, their suffering improved by treatment, remain raw and fragile: They cling close to shore, avoid risk, and fear returning to the fray of life. They do not expand the territory of their beliefs or curiosities, nor do they learn as much as they might from their suffering.

Others, differently wrought, intuit what they must do in order to heal and they do it in their own way and in their own time. They draw solace from their friends and family, meditate, engage in spiritual and physical activities that bring them peace, and actively engage in treating their illness. They survey their losses and rebuild; they hold close what they value and jettison the rest. They learn. They learn from observing the journeys of others, they take note of those who have lived lives of originality and courage. They turn to music or books, immerse themselves in their work, and start on a path toward purpose and meaning. As they expand their imaginative and moral worlds they heal and, in doing so, they enlarge the worlds of those around them. Some do these things alone, without counsel. For others, psychotherapy is an irreplaceable part of the process, marking the channel for the way home.

⌒

"Psycho-therapy is rather amazing," Robert Lowell wrote to Elizabeth Bishop in 1949. "Something like stirring up the bottom of an aquarium—chunks of the past coming

up at unfamiliar angles, distinct and then indistinct." Psychotherapy is indeed a strange and amazing thing, a mix of prehistory, medicine, philosophy, religion, and, more recently,
the science of psychology. It is well-studied, widely used,
nebulous, and as frustratingly and importantly various as the
individuals who engage in it. Yet the many schools of psychotherapy have common elements in how they are practiced.

Daniel Hack Tuke, a physician and member of the
Quaker family that reformed treatment for the insane in
England, noted in his 1892 *Dictionary of Psychological Medicine* that "psychotherapy" derives from the Greek words for
"mind," "breath," and "spirit," and meant, as well, "I attend
the sick." In Tuke's time, psychotherapy was broadly defined
as treatment of disease by the influence of the mind (a working definition used by W.H.R. Rivers twenty-five years later).
Psychotherapy was restorative and the personality of the
physician or psychotherapist was critical to the restoration.

Psychotherapy, Rivers had written, is the oldest branch
of medicine. It is rooted in myth, religion, magic, and science and goes back farther than we can date or imagine it.
The Greek and Egyptian gods of medicine had practiced
psychotherapy in their own way; they had used persuasion,
distraction, art, and consolation to heal minds darkened
by melancholy or circumstance. They had interpreted the
dreams of the sick who came to them. Leopold Löwenfeld,
an Austrian physician, wrote in 1897: "Psychotherapy is no
achievement of the modern age. If we look in history towards
the first beginnings of our art, it is clear as an unmistakable
fact that among the different methods of healing which were
used at that time, psychotherapy is the oldest, and that it rep-
resents the first and original form in which the practical art
of healing was exercised." Ways to heal the mind go back
unimaginably far in human history.

Over the years, definitions of psychotherapy gained in precision what they lost in clarity. A British definition of psychotherapy from the 1970s is straightforward: psychotherapy is "a method of treating illness based on the use of psychological rather than physical techniques." The American Psychological Association defines psychotherapy in a more precise, albeit rather lifeless way, as the "informed and intentional application of clinical methods and interpersonal stances derived from established psychological principles for the purpose of assisting people to modify their behaviors, cognitions, emotions, and/or other personal characteristics in directions that the participants deem desirable." This is a utilitarian definition for clinical science, but it scarcely calls up what happens in the consulting room.

Between the vague, if intriguing, nineteenth-century definitions of psychotherapy, and the precise but sterile definitions of the twentieth and twenty-first, lies a broad array of meanings and practices. More than four hundred types of psychotherapy have been described, many based on written guidelines for how to conduct treatment. Some keep the language and methods of early psychological treatments such as psychoanalysis. Others are based on existential, self-actualization, or personal growth philosophies. The most widely used psychotherapies now are structured cognitive and behavioral methods that prescribe ways to modify behavior and patterns of thinking. These psychotherapies are practical and generally deal with issues of an immediate concern. They are less ambitious than traditional psychodynamic therapies in addressing issues of the laying down of memory, of personality, and the causes of distress. They are more amenable to systematic study, less focused on understanding the self.

At the intersection of ancient healing practices and current approaches to psychotherapy are treatments, now under study, which combine psychotherapy and psychedelic drugs for depression, trauma, alcohol and drug dependence, and intense fear of dying. Psilocybin, derived from mushrooms that have been used for centuries in indigenous religious ceremonies to induce mystical and transcendent states and to alter mood and consciousness, is the most systematically studied of the psychedelic agents. Psychotherapy has proved vital to guide and facilitate psychedelic-induced experiences. Treatment results are encouraging. If the findings hold, psilocybin-assisted psychotherapy will link current clinical practice to the use of psychedelic substances in prehistoric religious ceremonies, magical-religious practices recorded nearly four thousand years ago in Egyptian papyri, shamanistic curing rituals, and the healing rites—suggestion, dream interpretation, sacred waters, and potions—used by priests in the Aesculapian temples. Psychotherapeutics, drugs, and the sacramental—ancient and modern—converge to heal the mind.

The practice of psychotherapy varies in many ways: the degree to which psychotherapeutic sessions are structured by the therapist; the clinical training of the therapist; the frequency of visits; the relative amount of focus upon the past, present, and future; the extent to which behavior is attributed to unconscious influences, or to hereditary ones; and the degree to which the exploration of mood, experience, and memory is initiated by the therapist, by the patient, or by both. This scramble of methods, definitions, and vocabulary is confusing; it is small wonder that the wide range of philosophies and techniques makes the field vulnerable to charges of cloudy inscrutability. Inexactitude is not incompatible with clinical benefit, but it lends to doubt.

Jerome Frank, a psychiatrist and psychologist at Johns Hopkins during the second half of the twentieth century, spent most of his clinical and scientific career trying to determine which qualities of therapists and methods of treatment are shared by different psychotherapeutic philosophies. The healing power of psychotherapy, Frank came to believe, lies in several general features: its ability to increase the patient's mastery of a world experienced as chaotic and beyond control; its capacity to instill hope, to contend with demoralization, and to lessen suffering; and to provide a confessing or confiding relationship.

Frank reasoned that if different types of treatment led to similar results, as seemed to be the case from his research and that of others, there must be elements in common across quite different psychotherapeutic approaches. His book *Persuasion and Healing*, based on many years of studying psychotherapists and psychotherapy, was published in 1961 and remains one of the more influential books about psychotherapy and psychological healing. Psychotherapy, he wrote and taught, involves at its core three things: a healing agent (typically a person trained in a "socially sanctioned method of healing believed to be effective by the sufferer"); a sufferer who seeks relief; and a healing relationship that is "a circumscribed, more or less structured series of contacts between the healer and the sufferer in which the healer . . . tries to bring about relief of symptoms."

Psychotherapy works if it relieves distress and improves the ability of patients to work, to have meaningful relationships, and to better master the inconstancies of life. For this to happen, patients must learn about themselves, and then use that knowledge to become more self-reliant and to gain insight that can be used in the future. Psychotherapy, like mortar and pestle, breaks down psychological suffering into finer elements of memory, cause, defense, aspiration, and apprehension; it then reconstitutes them into new and stron-

ger arrangements of mind. A deeper knowledge of self is critical to understanding the world as it is, not as one desires it to
be. Such knowledge, well-utilized, frees up energy to explore
new things, to master, and to mend.

Exploration of the self encourages exploration not only
of mind but of life. It should be a difficult but fascinating
venture; too often it is not. Adolf Meyer, one of the foremost
psychiatrists of the first half of the twentieth century and the
first psychiatrist-in-chief at the Johns Hopkins Hospital, was
described by one of his house staff as someone who stimu-
lated the desire to explore and who had a "knack for posing questions that provoked curiosity in the patient, leading
him or her to continue the search for further reasons for the
behavior." (He would show "hints of excitement," Graham
Greene had said about his psychoanalyst. Then, "I too began
to feel the excitement of the search.")

To be demoralized is to feel overwhelmed and chartless,
disheartened by circumstances of life. This is the common
end point of many psychological and medical conditions,
including depression, trauma, grief, and physical illness. Psychotherapy seeks to address this. "The mastery of life's direction is the aim of psychotherapy," Paul McHugh and Phillip
Slavney write in *The Perspectives of Psychiatry*, a book that
has shaped the clinical practice and intellectual lives of several generations of psychiatrists. "It is facilitated by learning
how events of the past and aspects of one's own character
have conspired to produce prior frustrations and recurrent
demoralization."

Constructing life stories is critical to psychotherapeutic
work. I asked my psychiatrist once what went into laying the
groundwork of a good alliance with patients. How does he
come to know them, how do they come to trust him? He

answered with questions that he asks: "What is your story?" "What questions bring you to see me?" "What matters to you?" "What do you experience?" "What can I do to make a difference?" "How do I understand you?" Psychotherapy is a quest to find out who the patient is and how he or she came to be that way. It is a journey to find out what adds to the person's enjoyments and strengths in life; fresh ways to grapple with the past, present, and future; and how to discover innovative ways to ameliorate pain and amass joy. The therapist's understanding of the patient needs to remain open and fluid; it cannot solidify. It must be free "to organize and grow," as Adolf Meyer put it. Brought to light and into words, depression, grief, anxiety, madness, and trauma can be better grasped, better put to use to change suffering into something more endurable, serviceable. As Anthony Storr said, what matters with psychopathology is what one does with it.

⌀

Throughout the whole history of medicine from the stage of its close association with magic or religion to its full emergence as an independent social institution, the personality of the healer has been of predominant importance.

—W.H.R. RIVERS, 1918,
PSYCHO-THERAPEUTICS

Many who adhere to particular forms of psychotherapy find it counterintuitive that the relationship between therapist and patient determines the outcome of treatment more than the particular school of psychotherapy. Certain targeted methods, those based on behavioral techniques such as cognitive behavioral therapy and dialectical behavior therapy, may be particularly effective in treating specific symptoms and conditions that serve the individual poorly but, Frank concluded, the success of all techniques "depends on the patient's sense of alliance with an actual or symbolic healer." This is born out by a broad body of studies done over many years. In psychotherapy research, the therapeutic alliance—based on trust, expectation, competence, and collaborative purpose—is a consistent predictor of outcome. A recent analysis of two hundred studies, involving more than fourteen thousand patients, found that therapeutic alliance, more than anything else, predicted good treatment results.

Traits of the therapist powerfully affect the strength and constancy of this alliance. These qualities—some vague, others specific—have defined good doctors for years. "The chief of these is humanity," John Gregory told students studying medicine at the University of Edinburgh in 1772. To heal others requires a "sensibility of heart which makes us feel for the distresses of our fellow-creatures, and which of consequence incites us the most powerful manner to help them." The nineteenth-century alienists J. C. Bucknill and D. H. Tuke wrote in 1879 that physicians treating mentally distressed patients should possess "a faculty of seeing that which is passing in the minds of men . . . a firm will, the faculty of self-control, a sympathising distress at moral pain, a strong desire to remove it . . . [and the power] which enables men to domineer for good purposes over the minds of others." *A sympathising distress at moral pain, a strong desire to remove it:* True now, as then.

Therapists require also to be competent (an obvious, if not sufficiently emphasized quality). This means, among other things, to be well-versed in psychology and psychopathology, diagnosis, current in relevant clinical science, adept in the use of medical and psychological treatments, knowledgeable about the clinical course of mental diseases, and skilled in recognizing the context and diverse manifestations of psychopathology; to know when medication and hospitalization are advisable; and to freely consult books and colleagues.

Clinical research shows that in order to form a strong therapeutic alliance with a patient, psychotherapists must be discernibly engaged in the treatment process, empathetic, engendering of trust, enthusiastic, confident, open to exploring new ideas, and clear in how they communicate. These attributes of a good therapist seem scarcely surprising, but their presence in the consulting room is less common than one might hope. Critically, as psychiatrist and philosopher Karl Jaspers wrote, the psychotherapist also must be aware of "human limits and one's own limitations." They must be self-aware.

Patients, too, have traits that influence the therapeutic alliance. Disease is important, so too is the person who has it. "We do not all start off in life with the same amount of nerve capital," wrote William Osler. Were patients always "cast in the same mould," he said, "we should ere this have reached some settled principles in our art." Sara Coleridge, the daughter of Samuel Taylor Coleridge, heir to his nervous afflictions, wrote in similar vein: "Diseases are like tulips & auriculas which vary without limit according to unknown differences of soil & situation."

We share much but differ importantly. We vary in temperament, intelligence, vitality, race, religion, and class; in courage and curiosity; in our ability to rebound from suffering, and to make and keep relationships. Differences exist, they always have. Healers must acknowledge and make the best of these differences. Two ears of seed-corn grew side by side, Willa Cather wrote in *O Pioneers!* "The grains of one shot up joyfully into the light, projecting themselves into the future, and the grains from the other lay still in the earth and rotted; and nobody knew why."

⌒

Sometimes I think that the search for suffering and the remembrance of suffering are the only means we have to put ourselves in touch with the whole human condition.

—GRAHAM GREENE,
A Burnt-Out Case

Viktor Frankl, the Austrian neurologist and psychiatrist, wrote that life is marked, if not defined, by suffering and our response to it. If life is to have meaning, he said, then suffering must have meaning. He wrote from the experience of incomprehensible pain. His wife, his brother, and his parents died in German concentration camps and he himself spent three years in Auschwitz, Theresienstadt, Kaufering III, and Türkheim. In those years, he found purpose as a doctor and healer; called by that purpose, he would help to heal tens of thousands of others. Out of atrocity, he wrote *Man's Search for Meaning*, his book about survival and the surpassing human need for meaning.

In 1945, a few months after he was liberated from the camps, Viktor Frankl wrote to friends: "I am unspeakably tired, unspeakably sad, unspeakably lonely. . . . In the camp, you really believed you had reached the low point of life—

and then, when you came back, you were forced to see that things had not lasted, everything that had sustained you had been destroyed, that at the time when you had become human again, you could sink even deeper into an even more bottomless suffering." Yet, he wrote, "I take back nothing of my old affirmation of life." Without it, he continued, he did not know that he could have survived the camps. "Life is so infinitely meaningful that even in suffering and even in failure there still has to be a meaning." He told another friend that purpose would come from the suffering. "When all this happens to someone, to be tested in such a way . . . it must have some meaning." He was, he said, "destined for something."

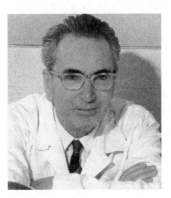

Viktor Frankl in 1965

Everything can be taken from a man but one thing: the last of the human freedoms—to choose one's attitude in any given set of circumstances, to choose one's own way.

Man's Search for Meaning, first published in Austria in 1946 and in the United States in 1959, has commanded a wide following. It is direct, compassionate, and tough; it extends hope, but not naïve hope. Or not entirely naïve hope.

Frankl believed that the primary motivating force in life is to find meaning, whether through work, art, or nature; dedication to a uniting or higher cause; or love. Rather than to ask, "What can I expect from life?" one should ask, "What does life expect of me?" We hold an obligation to life; we have an obligation to contend with suffering in such a way as to make it give meaning to our life. We hold a like obligation to remember. "Remembering is a noble and necessary act," Elie Wiesel said. "Because I remember, I despair. Because I remember, I have the duty to reject despair."

The essential thing, Frankl said, is to "transform a personal tragedy into a triumph, to turn one's predicament into a human achievement." If the circumstance cannot change, the person must. Purpose pulls us into the future, psychotherapy pulls purpose from the past. Psychotherapists must take into account not only a patient's weakness and reluctance to change, but their strengths, hopes, dreams, and human connections as well. Therapists should help the patient build upon successes shown in previous dealings with adversity by "widening and broadening the visual field," hence making purpose and meaning discernible and attainable.

Psychotherapy is not expected to be easy. Meaningful change requires effort and discomfort. "If architects want to strengthen a decrepit arch," Frankl pointed out, "they *increase* the load which is laid upon it, for thereby the parts are joined more firmly together. So if therapists wish to foster their patients' mental health, they should not be afraid to create a sound amount of tension through a reorientation toward the meaning of one's life."

It is as Siegfried Sassoon wrote about his psychotherapy with W.H.R. Rivers. Rivers, he said, had taught him that "a strenuous effort must be made to take some small share in the real work of the world." Frankl and Rivers offered hope to their patients that they would be able to achieve a life of greater purpose and meaning; both made clear that much effort would be required.

⌒

Without your wound where would your power be? . . .
Angels themselves cannot persuade the wretched and
blundering children on earth as can one human being
broken on the wheels of living.

—THORNTON WILDER,
The Angel That Troubled the Waters

"The most skilful physicians," Plato says in *The Republic*, "are those who, from their youth upwards, have combined with the knowledge of their art the greatest experience of disease." These most skillful healers, he specified, "should have had all manner of diseases in their own person." These physicians can then cure the body with the mind, but the mind itself must be well; it must have rid itself of sickness. The experience of past illness, not its present state, may give a healing advantage and confer purpose. More than two thousand years later, Jung wrote much the same. The doctor must continue to examine himself; learning from this becomes the special strength of the physician who has himself known suffering, one described by Jung and others as the wounded healer. It is the doctor's own hurt, Jung believed, "that gives the measure of his power to heal." His observation, that the wounded healer is uniquely able to heal others, is one that traces its way through the history of psychological healing, a history that is particularly well-written by the late

Stanley Jackson, distinguished professor of medical history at Yale. Jackson traced the concept of the wounded healer to the mythic Greek centaur, Chiron, who had been abandoned by his mother when he was young and who was later wounded by a poisoned arrow. Chiron's own suffering gave him not only deeper understanding of how to heal those who sought him out, but greater insight into teaching his students how to heal others with persuasion, plants, and the art of medicine. He was tutor to Achilles, Dionysus, Odysseus, and Asclepius, the Greek god of medicine, all of whom learned well and lastingly from their wounded healer.

In the sanctuary of Asclepius, on the slope of the Acropolis, there is a monument that dates from 220 A.D. The first of the "duties of a physician," it reads, is to "heal his mind." The healer must heal himself before he can begin his work with patients. Priests and physicians, if they themselves have been healed—through prayer, spiritual consolation, herbs, confession, the laying on of hands—can console by like means their supplicants. Their counterparts included shamans who, healed of their own wounds, heal others through their special abilities to induce trances and ecstatic states, acquired while they themselves were in the grip of disease or madness.

Jackson describes Jung and Freud as modern examples of the wounded healer who, having gone through times of deep emotional distress, developed new methods of psychological healing. At a broader level, he included self-help groups as wounded healing communities, such as Alcoholics Anonymous, in which members engage in mutual healing by sharing experiences of drinking beyond control. "No one escapes being wounded," wrote Catholic priest and theologian Henri Nouwen. As Anthony Storr said, it is what one does with the wound that matters. Jung advised that a critical part of what psychotherapists must do is to study their own experience and pain. Treatment of others is predicated on the doctor's sorting out in himself that which he might be expected to sort out in a patient. This capacity to transform suffering into a healing gift, exemplified in Viktor Frankl's life and work, is what gives the wounded healer power and purpose.

Some physicians and priests who themselves have suffered go on to teach from it. Nearly three hundred years ago George Cheyne (1671–1743), a Scottish physician, philosopher, and mathematician, included his own experience of melancholy as a case history in his influential 1733 medical text, *The English Malady: Or, a Treatise of Nervous Diseases of all Kinds, as Spleen, Vapours, Lowness of Spirits, Hypochondriacal, and Hysterical Distempers*. (He chose the title, he said, because the "English Malady" was a "Reproach universally thrown on this Island by Foreigners, and all our Neighbours on the Continent.") In his book, written for physicians, Cheyne described his own debilitating depression and suggested to his colleagues more humane ways to treat nervous diseases of all kinds.

No one, Cheyne stressed, could understand the pain of mental suffering except those who had known it personally. "Of all the Miseries that afflict Human Life . . . in [this] Valley of Tears," he wrote, "nervous Disorders, in their extream and Last Degrees, are the most deplorable, and beyond all comparison the worst." It was not possible, he continued, to convey to those not afflicted, the "Horror . . . [the] perpetual Anxiety and Inquietude . . . [the] melancholy Fright and Pannick, where . . . Reason was of no Use." Cheyne described the desperate solitude that depression imposes on its sufferers. Fellow physicians and friends found it difficult to be in his company. They "dropt off like autumnal Leaves," he recounted. "They could not bear, it seems, to see their Companion in such Misery and Distress, but retired to comfort themselves with a cheer-upping Cup, leaving me to pass the melancholy Moments with my own Apprehensions and Remorse."

Physicians who had been through this "Fright and Pannick," and had recovered, could help others by sharing their experiences, and by describing the toll that melancholy had taken on their professional and personal relationships. From his own experience, Cheyne suggested ways for other doctors to better treat melancholy and other nervous diseases. They should encourage compassion and patience from family and friends; prescribe milk and seed, strenuous exercise, and medicines of a wide variety, including sassafras, flowers of chamomile, winter bark, and syrup of mulberry; they should learn from others who had known despair or madness. He was aware that colleagues would criticize, even ridicule him for publicly disclosing his "Misery and Distress," but he was adamant that it was important to teach other doctors from not only a clinical but a personal perspective. "It will be a great Satisfaction to me," he wrote, "if I can at least alleviate and mitigate the Sorrows and Miseries of my Fellow-Sufferers, by the Experience I have so dearly bought."

Timothy Rogers (1658–1728), a nonconformist minister in London, was another wounded healer. He had had a severe breakdown in his twenties—"deep and settled melancholy"—that lasted for two years. When he recovered, Rogers used his experience and newfound sense of purpose to teach other ministers, physicians, and the public about depression. In his *A Discourse Concerning Trouble of Mind, and the Disease of Melancholly*, published in 1691, he wrote that it was of first importance, and indispensable, to understand the experience of those who were melancholy or mad. "Look upon your distressed Friends," he wrote, "as under one of the worst Distempers to which this Miserable Life is [subject]."

Recognize that Will is paralyzed; do not expect otherwise: "Melancholly seizes on the Brain and Spirits, and incapacitates them for thought or Action; it confounds and disturbs all their thoughts, and unavoidably fills them with anguish and vexation." Do not ask depressed friends and colleagues to do what they cannot do. It is bitterly demoralizing, a fool's errand. Show pity and compassion. Be aware that soul and body dwell together; know when to call in the skills of both minister and doctor.

If possible, Rogers continued, encourage those who are suffering to seek help from physicians who also have suffered. Take "recourse to such Doctors as have themselves felt [melancholy] for it is impossible fully to understand the nature of it any other way than by Experience." Extend hope—the first casualty of despair—to those who have lost it: "Tell them of others who have been in such Anguish, and under such a terrible Distemper, and yet have been delivered . . . those [who have been] long afflicted with Trouble of Mind, and Melancholly." The minister offered himself as a case in point: It had been hard to come to health again, he said, and hard to put himself into the public view. But hope was carried by purpose and had a particular legitimacy when it came from a wounded healer.

CHAPTER 6

Big Sur

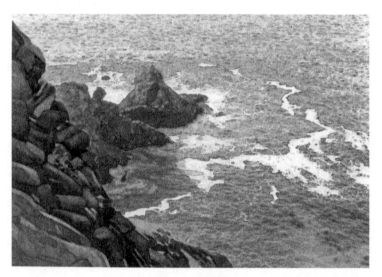

Big Sur, California

He was at ease with ambiguity, comfortable with complexity, and decisive in the midst of chaos and uncertainty. He treated me with respect and an unshakable belief in my ability to get well, compete, and make a difference. It was the task and gift of a great doctor. It was the task and gift of psychotherapy.

"These years were painful, then?" "I hardly know.
Something lies gently over them, like snow,
A sort of numbing white forgetfulness . . ."

—G. S. FRASER,
"CHRISTMAS LETTER HOME"

I had no intention of becoming a psychotherapist when I
began graduate school in psychology at the University of
California, Los Angeles. Clinical psychology seemed a foreign endeavor, very much across the aisle from those of us
interested in neurophysiology, psychopharmacology, and
experimental psychology. To become a psychotherapist was
thought to be "soft," speculative, and a waste of academic
training. Psychoanalysis cast a long shadow in those days.
Beverly Hills, which neighbors UCLA, was home-country
to psychoanalysts in Los Angeles and known as Couch Canyon. What one heard practiced there did little to improve the
image of psychotherapy.

This changed. It was the 1970s, a time not too distant
from the headier and more complicated sixties. The sixties
had been a decade of antiwar protests, nationally gutting
assassinations, indelible music festivals—Monterey, Big Sur,
Woodstock—and addled brains. Herb tea was served up with
morning glory muffins; LSD found its way into art, music,
and the psychiatric hospital. It was a time of white heat and
questioning; restlessness, love beads, and music: Nina Simone
and Joni Mitchell, John Coltrane. Etta James and Otis Red-
ding; Leonard Cohen, Simon and Garfunkel, and Phil Ochs.
Mickey Newbury. Jefferson Airplane. Leo Kottke and Kris
Kristofferson. It was a remarkable time, but it lent itself to a

kind of haziness. I participated and took in its contradictions. One was young, alive, and had assent to skirmish and dream. The sixties and seventies opened more minds and senses than they closed.

Occasionally minds cracked. Certainly mine did, although it would have cracked anyway on account of my ungovernable genes. In the mid-seventies, long after it would have been wise to do so, I got help for my troubles. By then the times were more sympathetic to psychotherapy and to minds that had frayed or fried. The decade had given energy and blessing to those seeking new ways to think about the mind. California drew in these searchers, who were scattered up and down the Pacific Coast from Berkeley and San Francisco to Southern California.

No place drew more mind-questers than Esalen in Big Sur. Encounter groups, Eastern mysticism, and the human potential movement flourished there; impassioned debate moved from lecture rooms to the hot baths built on cliffs between sea and sky. Big Sur, wild and beautiful, on the edge of the continent is, many say, where the West ends. Esalen and Big Sur, six hours north of Los Angeles, attracted musicians, artists and writers, psychologists and scientists during the sixties and seventies. Aldous Huxley, Timothy Leary, Joseph Campbell, R. D. Laing, Linus Pauling, Richard Feynman, B. F. Skinner, Jack Kerouac, Henry Miller, and Ansel Adams spoke or lived there. Discussions focused on human consciousness and newly evolving forms of psychotherapy. Along the way, psychotherapy came out of its privileged and private closet. I spent much time in Big Sur during the seventies, hiking through the redwoods and on the river trails, going to folk and jazz concerts, and listening to animated discussions about altered states of consciousness and psychotherapy. Abnormal psychology became more intellectually interesting to me, and more personally relevant. White rats rooting about in their mazes, nonparametric statistics, and principal component analysis lost their luster when set against trying to understand the aberrant and creating mind.

After two years in graduate school I spent a long summer and autumn in London to consider my academic future. Ostensibly I was at the Maudsley, a psychiatric hospital in South London affiliated with the University of London, but in fact I spent most mornings walking and reading in Hyde Park. In the afternoons I sat next to the yellowing polar bear in the Natural History Museum and worked on a play about a woolly mammoth who had amnesia and wandered the steppes. Aimless mulling is a good way to make a decision. I switched my PhD field to clinical psychology, with a specialization in psychopharmacology, and began the formal study of psychopathology. I also began to see patients.

For the first years of my training, each psychotherapy session with a patient was observed by a clinical supervisor behind a one-way mirror; after the session, there was an extended debriefing of things learned and things that ought to have been learned. It was an intense training, if obsessive and stifling at times, and a good grounding in the theory and practice of how minds evolve, unravel, become fearful, anxious, or depressed. The training was meant to teach young psychotherapists how to diagnose, treat, and heal patients of their suffering. This was an aspiration no one could question, but it was a dubious enterprise in the hands of graduate students.

I liked doing psychotherapy but felt uncertain that I was making much of a difference. People are complicated and making inroads into long-standing ways of behaving was more complicated still. When I was assigned to the inpatient service at the UCLA Neuropsychiatric Institute, I treated more severely ill patients and, strangely, I felt on stronger ground. The chief resident in psychiatry at UCLA, Dr. Daniel Auerbach, supervised my work on the ward. I learned not only from his observations of my clinical work, but by watching him treat patients directly. He was empathetic, but not in an exuding way, and he was straightforward. He did not condescend or ingratiate; he encouraged questioning. His understanding of human nature was nuanced, fed by many springs, as was his knowledge of medicine and psychopathology. He didn't pretend to know what he didn't know.

Less than a year later, a few months after I started as an assistant professor in psychiatry at UCLA, I became acutely manic—hallucinating, delusional, at one with the universe—in a worsening of the illness I had suffered from since I was seventeen. Dr. Auerbach, my former clinical supervisor, was the only one I trusted to treat me. I was only just beginning to recover from my first attack of psychotic mania and I assumed my professional life was over. My personal life was a shambles. With dread, I made an appointment to see him and drove to his office, about twenty minutes from mine at UCLA. It was an early evening in Southern California, the time of day when the light is quiet on the nerves and the hills are beautiful. I drove, unsettled and confused, up Coldwater Canyon, which was parallel to the canyon I meant to take. It was the first wrong turn of many. Even by the driving standards of Los Angeles, I should not have been driving. How many times had I driven Laurel Canyon, and Benedict and Coldwater Canyons? It didn't matter. I was lost. And I was terrified.

All of my assumptions about a blithe future were on the cutting-room floor. I was frightened I would get sick again, go mad again, and I was mortified by the things I had done when I was manic. I was bone-tired from depression. I needed psychotherapy, unimaginable to me unless on the listening side of the desk, and I had little hope that it or anything would work.

My doctor, and until only a few months earlier my clinical teacher, made it clear during our first meeting that I had manic-depressive illness (as bipolar illness was known then), that lithium was necessary, and that lithium was only a part of what I would need to get well. I was put on a course to heal and psychotherapy was a part of that course; it proved essential.

The most important thing my psychiatrist did during that first meeting was to give me hope that I would get better. I didn't believe this at the time, all seemed futile, but his belief that I would get well, and stay well, continued throughout my treatment. It was undeviating, even during my darkest depressions. Slowly, some of his faith got through. His was not a naïve or perfunctorily offered hope; it was clinically informed and seemed unassailable. His faith was persuasive enough to ferry me to the other side. He acted on the belief, with Osler and Rivers, that the power of faith is one that a good doctor uses as a matter of course. And he used it well. He made it clear that what I had to deal with now, and into the uncertain future, would be hard. I would have to go through the pain of the past, reexperience it, not circumvent it. This was not what I wanted to hear, but it is obvious now that the examination of truth, the knotty quest for it, made truth easier to take on. Cloaking pain can do no favors. It is difficult to accept, but pain is essential to healing. Things change with suffering: Some strengths and dreams erode; others emerge to take their place. Trust in a psychotherapist is predicated on hard truths, on seeing the world as it is, not as one remembers or hopes it to be.

At some point, early in treatment, I was feeling very much

alone with my illness. I did not know anyone who had been so sick and made it back. I wrote to two men who had written about their own experiences of manic-depressive illness: Joshua Logan, the director of *South Pacific*, *Mister Roberts*, *Annie Get Your Gun*, and *Picnic*; and Sloan Wilson, author of *The Man in the Gray Flannel Suit*. Both were kind enough to write back. I had asked, How do you survive your illness? How do you endure, make it through? Both said what my psychiatrist had said: It is hard. It is really hard. There is no easy way. But it is possible, you can do it, life comes back again. Neither said simply, You will be fine. They said, You will be fine, but then there was the sting, the truth, the chaser: It is really, really hard.

Now, when I talk with students who have been manic or severely depressed and they ask me how I made it through, I start with the words of Josh Logan, Sloan Wilson, and my psychiatrist: It is hard. You can do it. It is really hard.

It took a long time to heal my mind. My psychiatrist saved my life and those things and relationships most meaningful in it; he made the future bearable, and then, with work and time, my future became a quite wonderful thing. He accompanied me on a long journey that gave much and taught more. It is a hard thing to capture in words, the work of a masterful healer, but I tried to do it in this passage from a book I wrote much later about my illness, *An Unquiet Mind*:

> My psychiatrist saw me through madness, despair, wonderful and terrible love affairs, disillusionments and triumphs, recurrence of illness, an almost fatal suicide attempt, the death of a man I very much loved,

and the pleasures and aggravations of my professional life—in short, he saw me through the beginnings and endings of virtually every aspect of my life. He was tough, as well as kind, and even though he understood more than anyone how much I felt I was losing in vivacity by taking medication—lithium then, as now—he never was seduced into losing sight of the overall perspective of how costly, damaging, and life threatening my illness was. Lithium was necessary, I would have to deal with it. He was at ease with ambiguity, had a comfort with complexity, and was able to be decisive in the midst of chaos and uncertainty. He treated me with respect, a decisive professionalism, wit, and an unshakable belief in my ability to get well, compete, and make a difference.

I remember sitting in his office a hundred times during long, grim, suicidal months and each time thinking, What can he say that will make me feel better or keep me alive? Well, there never was anything he could say. It was all the desperately optimistic, condescending things he *didn't* say that kept me alive; all the compassion and warmth I felt from him that could not have been said; all the intelligence, clinical competence, and time he put into it; and his granite belief that mine was a life worth living. He taught me that the road from suicide to life is cold and colder and colder still, but—with steely effort, the grace of God, and an inevitable break in the weather—that I could make it.

Ineffably, psychotherapy heals. It makes some sense of the confusion, reins in the terrifying thoughts and feelings, returns some control and hope and possibility of learning from it all. I cannot live or stay

sane without lithium, but psychotherapy is a sanctuary. Psychotherapy is a battleground; it is a place I
have been psychotic, neurotic, elated, confused, and
despairing beyond belief. But, always, it is where I
have believed—or have learned to believe—that I
might someday be able to contend with all of this.
It is an odd thing, owing life to lithium, one's own
quirks and tenacities, and this unique, strange, and
profound relationship called psychotherapy.

The sea encourages my melancholy,
And then helps me forget it.

—DOUGLAS DUNN, "WISHFUL THINKING"

Sycamore Canyon Road in Big Sur follows the redwood
and buckeye trees lining the banks of Sycamore Creek and
ends two miles later at Pfeiffer Beach, known for its cliffs and
waves that pound hard through rock arches in the sea. Kelp
is thick in the water and there is a strange, lovely sand on the
north beach, purple from manganese garnet washed down
from the hills. The coastal plants are odd but alluring—black
evening primrose, dune buckwheat—and seasons change in
ways you will always remember. I have never known Big Sur
to be anything but moody and breathtaking. If you have to
lose your mind, as I apparently had to, Pfeiffer Beach in Big
Sur is as good a place as any to do it.

One evening as I lay on my back on Pfeiffer Beach, the
stars fell down on the ocean and sand, and then on me. It
was numinous, and as real as stars falling into the sea can be.

It rained stars. That night I flew in my mind, upward, past the stars, across fields of ice crystals, to the rings of Saturn. I didn't really, of course. It was madness, mania sprung loose in all ecstasy. But it did not seem mad at the time. That night on Pfeiffer Beach, with its falling stars, was glorious, achingly so. I would try later to recapture the wonder of that night, but it is in the nature of such experience that it is unrepeatable. In time, the images from Pfeiffer Beach were laid down in a new place, in the back of my mind, together with other incandescent, ardent memories from mania and love. There they lay quiet, for the years necessary to keep them from seducing me to harm. Later, they could be prized loose and used in safety.

I kept these memories of Big Sur to myself for many years, and measured the drabness of medicated life and depression against them. I had to reconcile the glory of having reached for the stars with a more anchored, less splendid world. It was hard to do, leaving behind star fields at my feet and rings of Saturn through my hands, but the stars and planet had no place in life other than in imagination. Psychotherapy gave me the means to sort through and rearrange such intensely seductive memories. To heal is to understand what has been lost, whether it is innocence or sanity. To heal is to reshape the experience of loss into good. Intolerable memories, Rivers said of war, should be made tolerable. Ecstatic ones, so different, yet capable of damage, should be kept on a tight rein. They should come to joy, not madness.

I returned often to Big Sur after the night on Pfeiffer Beach. The stars no longer rained down on me nor swept across the cliffs and sea. I turned to life instead: differently beautiful, intense, and wonderfully strange. I started to write at Big Sur: that love and work and a great doctor heal; that grief teaches; and that nostalgia gives comfort and some meaning but it seldom leads to much. I wrote about how the mind uses its moods of passion and grief to create, and how much one learns from the courage of explorers, artists, and pioneers. I have begun most of my books in Big Sur, including this one; it owes everything to a doctor who made grief bearable and mania replaceable.

Waves take a hard toll on the tidal invertebrates of Big Sur. Some survive by burrowing into the sand or wrapping themselves in kelp. Others—limpets, barnacles, and starfish—glue their bodies to the rocks and take nourishment from the waves, even as they are pummeled by them. "The force of the great surf . . . has much to do with the tenacity of the animals," wrote John Steinbeck. "Rather than deserting such beaten shores for the safe cove and protected pools, [they] simply increase their toughness and fight back at the sea with a kind of joyful survival."

One holds tight to a rock during danger, then breaks loose to take on the sea.

CHAPTER 7

Sowings

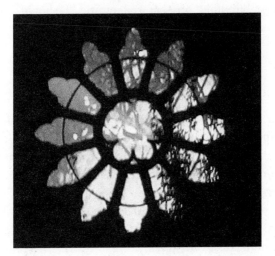

Notre-Dame in flames
Paris, 2019

*Notre-Dame de Paris is our history, our literature,
our collective imagination. . . . We will rebuild
because that is what our history deserves.*

—Emmanuel Macron,
President of France

When spring came, after that hard winter, one could not get enough of the nimble air. . . . There was only— spring itself; the throb of it, the light restlessness, the vital essence of it everywhere. . . . If I had been tossed down blindfold on that red prairie, I should have known that it was spring.

—WILLA CATHER, *My Ántonia*

On a mid-April night in 2019 the Cathedral of Notre-Dame burned. A thousand beams were on fire, the three-hundred-foot oak and lead spire had collapsed into itself, and flames were shooting through the roof. No one knew what would be the fate of the wood, stone, and the stained glass. The president of France, Emmanuel Macron, stood in front of the medieval cathedral and spoke to his countrymen. "Cette histoire, c'est la nôtre," he said. "Alors elle brûle." This is our history. And it's burning.

He spoke about Paris, the French people and their culture, and how all came together in Notre-Dame. "Notre-Dame de Paris is our history," he said. "It is our literature, our collective imagination, the place of our great moments, our epidemics, our wars, our liberations." It is "the base from which we evaluate our distances, and from which we measure ourselves." The cathedral is our story, the president continued. It is burning—We will rebuild it—It is our destiny (see photo section).

Questions filled the night: What could be saved? Could any of "the forest"—the roof made from a thousand great oaks cut down nearly nine hundred years ago—withstand the fire? Parisians and all who watched the cathedral burning soon saw to their horror that it would not. The stained glass windows—the great thirteenth-century rose windows, vulnerable, defining, beautiful—would they melt or shatter? How could they not? And what then? Would the great bells fall? The bells that had rung out for coronations, at the funerals of kings, the bells that had chimed every fifteen minutes from 1856 until this mid-April night. Bells that had rung out to celebrate the armistice of the Great War and the liberation of Paris. If they did fall, would they bring down the bell towers too? Would the Crown of Thorns, relic of the crucifixion—a circlet of rushes braided together with threads of gold wire—survive through the night? It was believed by the devout that the plaited rushes withered each day, then grew again into life the next. The crown carried divine power, believers said, a symbol of life arising from death. The archbishop of Paris sent out a call to the churches: Notre-Dame is burning. Ring the bells.

The bells rang as one, across Paris, across all of France.

The next morning gave the measure of things. The better part of the cathedral stood, but it was badly damaged. The bells and stained glass windows prevailed, the towers held, and the relics—the Crown of Thorns; nails said to have fixed the body of Christ to the cross; a piece of the cross itself—were spared. The 180,000 bees living in hives on the roof of the sacristy seemed little the worse for flame and mayhem. Their survival breathed small hopes into the cathedral (see photo section).

It would be left to architects and time to reckon the losses and determine how to rebuild. Throughout the history of France, President Macron told his fellow citizens, cities and ports and churches had burned to the ground. "Every time, every time, we have rebuilt them." The things we believe to be indestructible, he continued, are not. They are fragile, they must be remembered. "Everything that makes France what it is, materially and spiritually, is alive and, for this very reason, we must not forget it."

We will rebuild the cathedral, he said, and it will be more beautiful than it was. Our loss will be a common thread to the work ahead. The project will be a human one and "passionately French." First, however, the country needed to reflect upon what had happened. Haste was a danger; it would waste the opportunity to learn from grief and from the unity it had brought to the nation. "After this time of testing will come a time of reflection, and then a time of action," the president said. "But let us not mix them up." *Remember, mourn, rebuild.*

In the months after the fire, architects, stone carvers, carpenters, and stained glass conservationists considered the task ahead. Assessing the damage was difficult, delayed by fierce heat, lead contamination, and the lockdown of Paris during the coronavirus epidemic. Engineers and architects tested the cathedral structure. Glass specialists examined stained glass for cracks and removed toxic lead dust. Hundreds of old oaks were cut down in private and public forests across France.

Restoring the spire raised an artistic and historical question: Should it be re-created to the structure that existed before the fire, or should the spire be freshly imagined? Cathedrals are moored in the past; the past may be their essence. Or not. Some architects argued that France should create anew, lean toward the future, and President Macron at first agreed. Proposals for new designs came from more than fifty countries. Brazilian architects suggested a roof and spire to be made entirely of stained glass; Italian architects imagined a spire of Baccarat crystal that would light up the sky. A Paris-based group proposed a giant greenhouse filled with beehives and orchids, and planters for flowers made from reclaimed oak beams from the roof; yet another group proposed a virtual spire made of beams of light. But the consensus of experts, and the French people, argued that the spire and roof should be restored to how they had been in their "last known condition." The spire of Notre-Dame should retain its old design; it should keep to its structural history, hold to its place in the sky. The original design held.

In mid-April 2020, a year exactly after the cathedral had been ravaged by fire, the great bourdon bell of Notre-Dame Cathedral rang out again. The citizens of Paris went to their balconies to acknowledge their gratitude to the doctors and nurses who were treating patients sick or dying from the coronavirus. And they applauded the great bell of their cathedral, the sound of survival. Something ancient, deeply human was to survive.

⟨ornament⟩

Great edifices, like great mountains, are the work of ages. . . . The altered art takes up the fabric, incrusts itself upon it, assimilates it to itself, develops it after its own fashion, and finishes it if it can. . . . It is a graft that shoots out, a sap that circulates, a vegetation that goes forward. . . . Time is the architect, the nation is the builder.

—VICTOR HUGO,
The Hunchback of Notre-Dame

Restoration, whether of stone or soul, offers choices. Is it better to restore only what existed before, to stay within the chalk lines, or to venture into new territory? In the wake of pain comes the opportunity to innovate, and with possibility come questions: what to keep of the past, what to discard; how to scaffold the character and spirit within; whether to go beyond the historical boundaries. There may be but limited time to reflect on how to put the shattered pieces together; how to seek out new ways and places, new ideas and people; how to gather courage for the nights to come.

Healing of this kind is commensurate with the effort put into the endeavor, as well as to other attributes of persistence, imagination, and will. Be it stone or soul, recovery is impossible without hard work. It takes time. Psychotherapy helps, sometimes immeasurably so, but long stretches of the path to healing have to be taken alone. The journey demands work and imagination.

William Osler's observation that work was the "true balm of hurt minds" was not a new thought; putting patients to work had been an important part of healing for thousands of years. The temples of Asclepius were designed as healing environments, as places for therapeutic engagement of body, mind, and spirit. Active engagement in treatment was necessary for healing. Galen, the Greek physician whose ideas, said Osler, were so unassailable that medical thinking stopped for fifteen centuries, agreed with the emphasis on the primacy of work. A disciple of Asclepius, indebted to Hippocrates (Hippocrates sowed, it was said, and Galen reaped), Galen was surgeon to the gladiators and physician to the emperor Marcus Aurelius. Work is "Nature's physician," Galen wrote. It was integral to health, and indispensable to human happiness. In *On the Diagnosis and Cure of the Soul's Passion*, one of the earliest texts to address the practice of psychotherapy, Galen argued that to learn about oneself, to discover what is buried in the mind, one must work. Work affirmed and gave purpose; without it, life stagnated and recovery stalled. Freud, two thousand years later, concurred. Work and love, he said, are the "cornerstones of our humanness." Work and love "are all there is."

Robert Burton, whose *The Anatomy of Melancholy* so influenced Osler, had said much the same thing in the seventeenth century. He wrote at some length about the benefits of flower and fish—"fish that live in gravelly waters, as pike, perch, trout, and herbs such as nepenthe and violets in broth"—but the cure he knew most useful for himself was work. Melancholic patients should be kept active, and diverted from morbid thoughts by "business, exercise, or recreation." The mind put to work, and the body forced into action, heal: "I write of melancholy, by being busy to avoid melancholy," Burton said. Writing drew him away from dark obsession and forced his mind to be active when weighed down by sloth. Writing gave solace, he wrote. It "unladened the abscess in his head." Above all, said Burton, if stricken by melancholy, "be not idle."

Two hundred years later, in nineteenth-century insane asylums, doctors and nurses concurred with the notion; they, too, placed work at the center of treating patients. They imagined a variety of ways for patients to occupy their minds and bodies, to heal through direction and activity. Benjamin Rush, surgeon general for the Continental army and considered to be the "father of American psychiatry," observed in 1812 that mentally ill patients who "assist in cutting wood, making fires, and digging in a garden" were more likely to recover their sanity than those exempted from such activities, who "languish away their lives within the walls of the hospital." To be busy in the external world was to give less opportunity for the growing of a darker, internal one.

In 1855, the Government Hospital for the Insane in Washington, D.C. (known after 1916 as St. Elizabeths Hospital), opened on four hundred acres of land overlooking the City of Washington and the Anacostia and Potomac Rivers. The lands offered "a ramble and pleasure ground for the recreation of the inmates" and initial hopes were high for a humane, therapeutic community to treat the mentally ill. The new hospital was created not just to house the insane, but to heal them. In his State of the Union address in 1853, President Franklin Pierce told Congress that the hospital was to be "an asylum indeed to this most helpless and afflicted class of sufferers." It was to be a "noble monument of wisdom and mercy." Patients were to be active, not packed collectively into a common room. They worked on the hospital farms, in the gardens, and in the apple and peach orchards near the river.

William Whitney Godding, an early superintendent of the asylum, believed that to farm and garden was to keep the mind alive. The time that patients spent looking after the gardens, he said, would "add more to the beauty of the grounds and the pleasure of the inmates than the same amount would yield in almost any other way." It is "not unmeet," he added, "to plant flowers by the pathways of sorrow." Plants brought in from the greenhouses and outside flower beds and taken into the wards "enter into moral treatment of the insane, and so become a medicine to the mind." Vineyards and fig and cherry trees "bring to darkened minds and troubled lives glimpses of sunshine and peace."

Yet another part of the St. Elizabeths therapeutic community was a small zoological garden for rescued bear cubs and other animals collected during expeditions of the Smithsonian Institution. The hospital, which, like most asylums in the nineteenth and twentieth centuries, grew to an unsustainable number of inmates—at one point there were eight thousand patients—continued to add to its occupational and recreational activities: baseball, tennis, dances, concerts, movies, field meets, weaving, art, carpentry, and a circulating library. (In 1928, an article in *The Washington Post* described differences between the patients' library at St. Elizabeths and an average neighborhood library. In the asylum, *The Washington Post* noted, "there is a comparatively greater demand for books of a more serious sort: books on mathematics, philosophy, astronomy, and biography." Books on the topic of the fourth dimension, the article continued, were "in constant demand.")

About the time that the staff at St. Elizabeths was creating its work and recreational programs for patients, the superintendent of a state asylum in Massachusetts spoke to his fellow asylum physicians about how best to heal the mentally ill. "The mind must be managed, hope inspired, and confidence secured," he told them. Insanity was a disease and required medical remedy, but the mind was wounded and must be "diverted, soothed and assuaged." It must be put to good use. He reminded them that the Greeks had advised those who were sick in mind to go to the temple to participate in religious rituals and to avail themselves of the healing power of god, place, and purposeful pursuit. New England alienist and Greek priest alike believed that manual labor and creative work were critical to healing the mind, to turning hard winter into spring. It took effort and time but the dark season would pass.

"The spring would come again," Willa Cather wrote in *O Pioneers!* "The branches had become so hard that they wounded your hand if you but tried to break a twig. And yet, down under the frozen crusts, at the roots of the trees, the secret of life was still safe, warm as the blood in one's heart."

Writing is a form of therapy; sometimes I wonder how all those who do not write, compose or paint can manage to escape the madness, the melancholia, the panic fear which is inherent in the human situation.

—GRAHAM GREENE,
Ways of Escape

Some turn to writing to heal their minds. "How often writing takes the ache away, takes time away," Robert Lowell wrote to a friend. Writing restored a part of him that could not be reached by doctors or medication. Only work could heal the toll exacted by mania and depression, revive purpose. "Up till now I've felt I was all blue spots and blotches inside, more than I could bear really," he said. "So day after day, I wrote." Day after day, he said, he was "under the spell" of lines and rhythm. "I have lived through the unintelligible, have written against collapse and come out more or less healed." Creating gave a ladder up, and out. "By creating I became well," Heinrich Heine said, a belief held by many writers and artists. Writing controls recollection and the flow of horror and despair, keeps depression at bay. Work helps.

Not long after the Great War, playwright J. M. Barrie told students at the University of St. Andrews that the greatest glory he had known was "working till the stars went out." Grief lost some of its sting when he was pursuing new ideas or engrossed in consequential endeavor. Those suffering in the aftermath of war could find a measure of peace in work. It forced engagement with the future, gave some respite from pain, and offered hope that something better lay beyond.

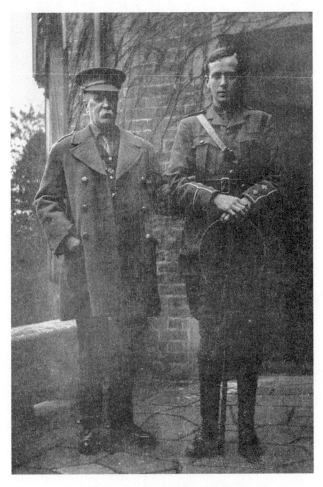

Sir William Osler and his son Revere
Oxford, 1916

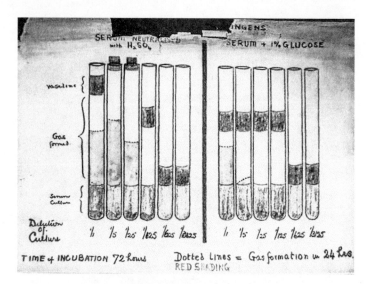

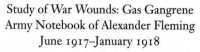

Study of War Wounds: Gas Gangrene
Army Notebook of Alexander Fleming
June 1917–January 1918

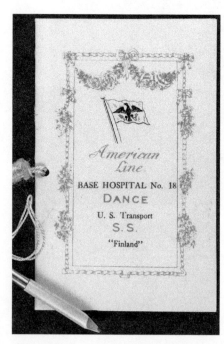

Dance Card, 1917
Transatlantic Voyage to France
Johns Hopkins Base Hospital No. 18

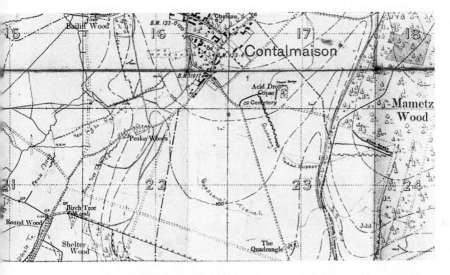

Siegfried Sassoon's Trench Map, 1916

By night each man was back in his doomed sector of horror-stricken Front Line, where the panic and the stampede of some ghastly experience was re-enacted among the livid faces of the dead. No doctor could save him then.

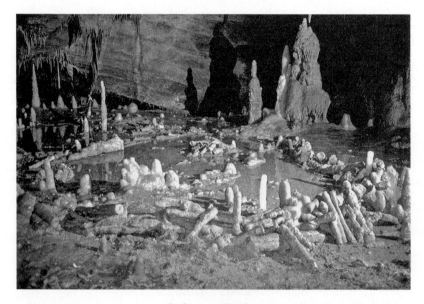

Stalagmite Circles
c. 175,000 BC
Bruniquel Cave, France

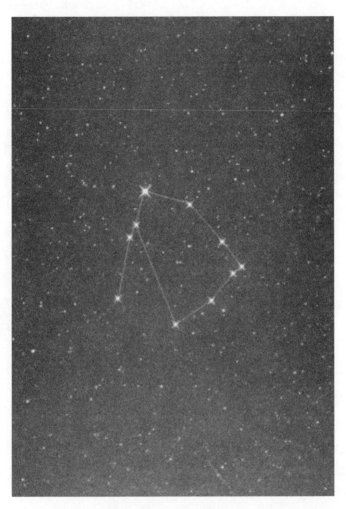

Constellation of Ophiuchus

This is the constellation which is in Scorpion, having in both hands a serpent. It is said, indeed, to be Asclepius whom Zeus, as a favor to Apollo, raised up among the stars.

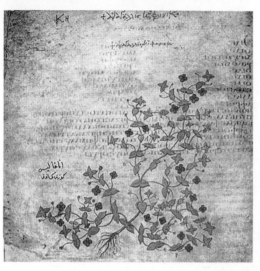

Scarlet Pimpernel
Vienna Dioscurides, c. AD 515

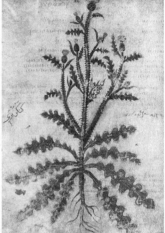

Borage
The Nepenthe of Homer
Vienna Dioscurides, c. AD 515

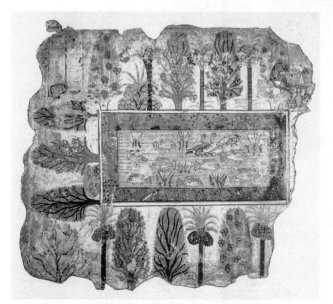

The Garden
Fresco in the Tomb
of Nebamun
c. 1350 BC
Thebes, Egypt

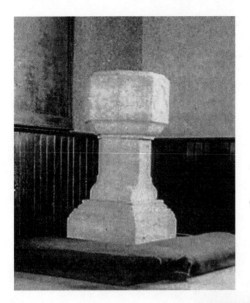

Baptismal font in
Trinity Anglican Church,
Ontario, where William
Osler's father was a priest.

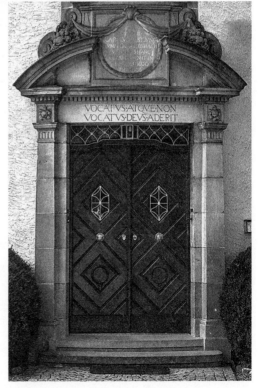

Carl Jung's house in Kusnacht
Carved in the lintel above the door:

> *Vocatus atque non vocatus deus*
> *aderit*
> *'Invoked or not invoked, the god*
> *will be present'*

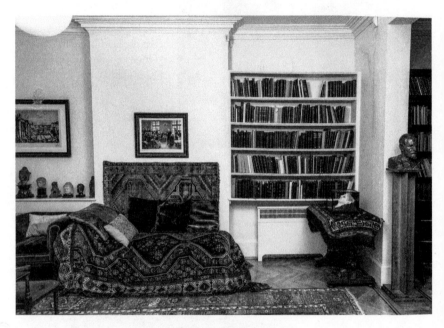

Freud's Study in Hampstead

There was always a feeling of sacred peace and quiet here. The rooms themselves must have been a surprise to any patient, for they in no way reminded one of a doctor's office but rather of an archaeologist's study. . . . Everything here contributed to one's feeling of leaving the haste of modern life behind, of being sheltered from one's daily cares.

SERGEI PANKEJEFF
"The Wolf Man"

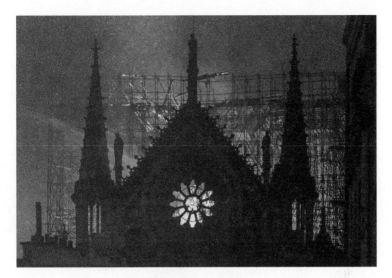

Notre-Dame in Flames
Paris, 2019

Notre-Dame de Paris is our history, our literature, our imagination. . . .
We will rebuild because that is what our history deserves.

EMMANUEL MACRON, PRESIDENT OF FRANCE

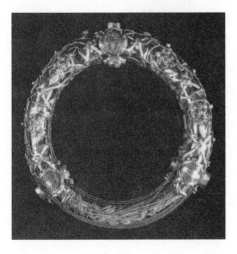

Crown of Thorns
Cathedral of Notre-Dame

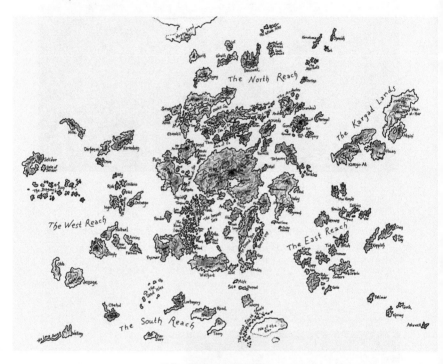

Island Map of Earthsea
Ursula K. Le Guin

*These stories speak of the Islands, of the Outer
Reach of the great rich islands of the Archipelago,
the Inner Lanes, the roadsteads white with ships.*

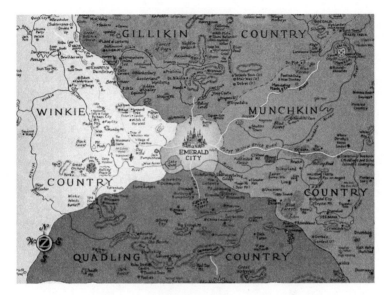

Map of Oz

It is a long way to the Emerald City, and it will take you many days. The Country here is rich and pleasant, but you must pass through rough and dangerous places before you reach the end of your journey.

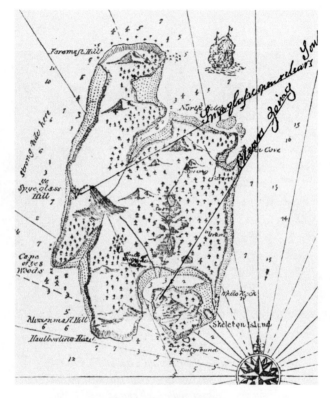

Map of Treasure Island
Robert Louis Stevenson

It contained harbours that pleased me like sonnets.

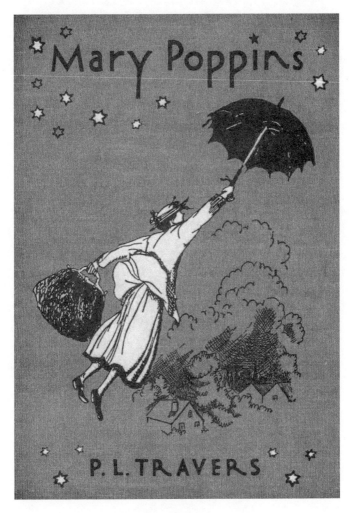

Mary Poppins
P. L. Travers

I'll stay till the wind changes.

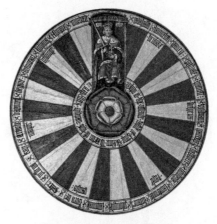

Le Morte d'Arthur
Winchester Manuscript
Sir Thomas Malory, 1485

King Arthur's Round Table
Winchester Castle

And through the puissance of his Table Round,
Drew all their petty princedoms under him,
Their king and head, and made a realm, and reigned.

ALFRED, LORD TENNYSON,
Idylls of the King

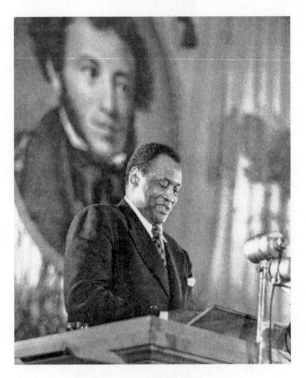

Paul Robeson in Moscow, 1949
Speaking on the 150th Anniversary
of the Birth of Alexander Pushkin

Memorial Stone for Poets of the First World War
Westminster Abbey

Barrie, whose imagination and hard work had brought *Peter Pan* into the world, spoke of how work sustained his life; how it had brought grounding as well as enchantment. And a measure of calm. The playwright was subject to intense mood swings; when melancholic, a friend said, he had "an impenetrable shell of sadness and preoccupation," and was "unreachable," "all grey ashes and devastatingly depressing," like a "full ash-tray and an empty ink bottle." On his good days, however, he was full of charm and life, filled with "a kind of benign wizardry"; he was a "fellow of infinite jest." He worked furiously, till the stars went out, and created new worlds as he did.

Both writing and psychotherapy create stories from the material of life. Whether told to a therapist, or created by a writer, stories give form to the inchoate and construct a path out of confusion and pain. Philip Pullman, author of *His Dark Materials*, describes storytelling as made of "wood and path." The wood is a "wild space . . . an unstructured space." It is a space "where anything can happen." Monsters and strange life-forms live in the wood; it is the place, as Pullman has it, that "contains the history of the character." The path is a structure superimposed on strewn elements; it "leads from here to there." To construct a path through mind and woods is to find a way through pain, to create a life story that is open and honest and well-imagined; it is to begin to heal. The story gives fresh understanding to material long in the mind. It asks, Where do I go next? How shall I get there? What shall I do with what I have learned?

Grief is one kind of story maker. It lays down its own, unsettled path to healing. It is a well-traveled road, some-times brutal, sometimes generous. Several years after my for-mer husband died, I tried to put some of this into words. It was hard but helpful. I wrote about the grace and awfulness of grief, about how it lays waste to denial and gives meaning to loss; how grief carries within its tangle a path to healing. It took a long time to grasp this, and understanding remains imperfect. The lessons were good ones, and they have given much, but they were not sought. In that lies an important part of their value.

Writing about grief forced a distance on death, and some armor against the sadness that comes with it. Writing entangled me once again in life and, in writing about grief, a certain healing came:

> I remember an afternoon at the Natural History Museum in Washington, standing in front of a glass case filled with mummified owls. It seemed a violation of wild things to see such creatures stuffed and fakely perched. Yet had they not been dead and fixed, I could not have seen their wings and claws so clearly; I could not have appreciated the intricate beauty of their feathers and beaks. Had it not been for their deaths, I could not have seen what made them live. I would have preferred to have seen them fly or hunt or take a mouse to beak. But with them dead, I took in— with awe—their parts and proportions, saw in their stillness what made a snowy owl a snowy owl and not an Eastern screech. Death had something to give.

> Grief, lashed as it is to death, instructs. It teaches that one must invent a way back to life. Grief forces intimacy with death; it preserves the salient past and puts into relief our mortal state. All die, says Ecclesiastes. All must die, it is written in the first statute of the Magna Carta. All die, teaches Grief. Grief is at the heart of the human condition. Much is lost

with death, but not everything. Life is not let loose of lightly, nor is love. There is a grace in death. There is life.

A cathedral in flames, asylum patients trapped in madness, hearts paralytic with grief—each calls out for healing. And healing calls for understanding and reflection, followed by the long, hard work of building back.

III

The Healing Arts

Hero, Artist, and Storyteller

CHAPTER 8

Island and Quest

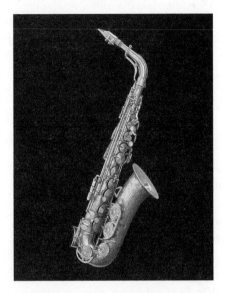

Charlie Parker's alto saxophone

*"If you don't live it, it won't come out
of your horn."*

A little way before him the trees stopped; there was a break in the line of the land like the mouth of a harbour; and the tide, which was then flowing, took him up and carried him through. One minute he was without, and the next within: had floated there in a wide shallow water, bright with ten thousand stars, and all about him was the ring of the land, with its string of palm trees. And he was amazed, because this was a kind of island he had never heard of.

—ROBERT LOUIS STEVENSON,
"THE ISLE OF VOICES"

To be born is to be wrecked on an island," J. M. Barrie wrote. The desire for an island world persists in everyone, he continued, especially writers. On an island "you are constantly making the most delicious discoveries"; and one sets the most marvelous questions: At what age would you want to be wrecked? Raft or not? What kinds of danger? Where would one choose to live: cave, tent, or tree? How would one behave when cast up by the sea? What adventures would one stumble upon? How would one handle fear?

Before I moved to Johns Hopkins, I was director of the UCLA Affective Disorders Clinic, immersed in practicing psychotherapy with patients who had severe mood disorders. Less was known then than now about these illnesses, and the road back for those who had suffered from mania or depression was even harder than it is today. I often said to my patients, most of whom were recovering from psychosis or severe depression: There are many ways to heal your mind, many types of medication and psychotherapy. These will help, time will help, but the yield is less than the hope. There are things that you have to do on your own: Come to terms with your illness, engage the future, take meaning from what you have been through.

Imagine an island of your own making and bring to it what you need to live long and well: Bring love, passion, and friends; bring books and music and work to sustain you. Look at Maui. Everything was brought to the island, whether by man, insect, bird, fire, or wind. Seeds came in on the mud that caked the feet of birds; seeds were borne on the wind and ocean currents. The sea brought life to the islands; tides shaped the sands and bays. We, too, have complicated beginnings. Design your island, populate it with beauty and things that matter to you, that intrigue you. It is your life; it is short. Treat your island with regard. Tides have power; harvest them. Storms have power; take from them. Lava kills, but it brings new land. Do not let your island go to weed; do not give it over to anyone else. No one can cultivate this world but you. Understand the possibilities of your island. Know its dangers. Keep away the ungenerous and the unkind, the duplicitous. "'Tis in ourselves that we are thus or thus," said Shakespeare. "Our bodies are our gardens, to which our wills are gardeners."

At one point, curious about the link between imagination and healing, I asked a few of my patients if they would be interested in creating and describing such imaginary islands, worlds of their own, stocked with sustaining, healing things. We would discuss what they came up with. Most were enthusiastic about the idea and, within short order, had created worlds from scratch, places in which time and geography were theirs alone. Some drew islands that were simple, easy to approach. Others were complex, tangled, and very beautiful. They named the rivers, harbors, and coves on their islands and marked areas of dangerous tides or rocks. All the islands had forests and several had lagoons, harking back to books from childhood.

My patients split their islands into smaller territories: places to explore, or to hide; areas that were quiet places, private, kept for oneself. Books were a critical part of all of the islands—for many, the most important and elaborated part—music was as well. For a long time after, patients showed me additions they had made to their islands, most often new areas for adventure and scrambling about. They talked about lost childhood dreams, forsaken plans, and hopes obliterated by mania, depression, and the passing of time. They talked about filling in lost spaces. There was a sense that they had cobbled together something living, something new.

Did the island exercise have much effect on healing from depression or mania? Seen by itself, probably not. But it did encourage patients to look to their imaginations, and to draw upon them for adventure, escape, or possibility. Conjuring islands was never a consequential part of psychotherapy but it was a different path into my patients' minds: a path into lost fields and yonder ones, forgotten dreams, and abandoned hopes. Creating their own islands, the patients said, allowed them to think in a more protected way about what they had been through when they were ill. Making up stories had been a pleasure that had been left behind with childhood. The exercise encouraged them to mull and to do something new, to create something rather than to obsess. Imagination sets the mind free on alternative paths, paths that can help in grieving lost innocence and lost minds. Imagination didn't cure, but it lent its hand to healing.

There were two patients who distinctly did not feel this way: Their islands were dark and oppressive, empty, and for them the exercise bordered on the absurd; little had come from it. Although all of my patients had experienced severe depression, these were the only ones who had not also experienced mania. Indeed, the patients with the most devastating histories of mania took to the island exercise with the greatest enthusiasm. They, more than the others, saw island-making in the light of a quest or an adventure; they also were more likely to describe their time in psychotherapy as a quest or a journey, rather than as a treatment only.

In "The Man Who Loved Islands," D. H. Lawrence describes island summers of primrose and blackthorn that slid into "dark skies and dampness and rain." And then into autumn and winter. "You felt that your island was a universe, infinite and old as the darkness; not an island at all, but an infinite dark world where all the souls from all the other bygone nights lived on, and the infinite distance was near." Darkness came to the island, and changing skies and seas came too, brought from within the islander as well as the island itself. Mysterious feelings came too, and intimations of the ancient. Islands have their own ways and histories; they are, as James Michener said of the Hawaiian archipelago, "crucibles of exploration and development." There is no certainty in these crucibles, only possibility.

Imagination feeds on itself. Robert Louis Stevenson's *Treasure Island* arose from a map he had drawn of an island, "beautifully coloured" and crossed with roads, and rivers, and "harbours that pleased me like sonnets." It was an island of interest for "anyone who had twopence worth of imagination." As he lost himself in the map he had drawn, the island and the story sprang to life. The imaginary woods, faces, and weapons began to appear from "unexpected quarters, as they passed to and fro, fighting, and hunting treasure, on these few square inches of a flat projection. The next thing I knew, I had some paper before me and was writing out a list of

chapters." From the map in Stevenson's mind came a story of
high adventure shared by millions of us (see photo section).

More than a hundred years later, Scottish poet Douglas
Dunn captured the lasting magic of *Treasure Island* in "Parrot
Islands":

> *Let there be room still for utmost Utopias,*
> *For the back of beyond and the cobbled quays,*
> *The boy and the one-legged pirate, wind-stoked canvas,*
> *Adventure, delight, and doing whatever you please.*
> *In a world of endpaper maps and clear-cut surprise,*
> *There should be such chances, in a world without lies.*

. . . .

> *Pink above turquoise, and purple clouds darkening,*
> *Here is "another sky," beautiful, local, and true.*
> *Someone is dreaming it, a mind on its wing*
> *In search of the life that comes out of the blue.*

"A mind on its wing . . . the life that comes out of the blue":
Imagination. The back of beyond, doing whatever you please.
Life.

Enlisting imagination in the cause of healing is not new.
Nearly five thousand years ago Imhotep, the Egyptian god of
medicine, observed that suggestion heightens the effects of
herbs, spells, and incantations. In the Greek temples of healing, Asclepius and his disciples were adept at using suggestion
to call the imagination into service. Millennia later, physicians

and priests have remained strong in their belief that harvesting the imagination helps to heal the mind. In 1640, Edward Reynolds, bishop of Norwich and author of the influential *A Treatise of the Passions and Faculties of the Soule of Man*, wrote that to alleviate disorders that "darken the serenitie of mans Mind," one must play on imagination to invoke opposing passions, by "scattering and distracting" them, or by mixing them "so they mutually *weaken* one another." Imagination, by awakening opposite mental states, could reconstrue grief and madness: Joy could oust sorrow, desire deflect fear, curiosity eclipse apathy. Robert Burton, a contemporary of Reynolds, argued similarly in *The Anatomy of Melancholy*. Driving out one passion with another, he said, could be likened to forcing out one nail by hammering in another.

Imagination aids healing by offering diverse ways to contend with setback and pain. Usually, imagination serves the imaginer well; it draws toward possibility. "Passion, imagination, self-will, the sense of power, the very consciousness of our existence," wrote essayist William Hazlitt in 1815, "bind us to life, and hold us fast in its chains." We daydream and spin new worlds; expand the territory of our dreams; set out on quests; get lost in books, or write them; emulate the heroic, or fall under their archetypal spell. We find our way through the unexpected and irrational. Through our imagination, or with help from the experience, facility, and imaginings of others, we gather new ideas and ways of doing things; we find solace. Thoreau, observed Emerson, had a deep understanding of this: Imagination not only uplifts, it consoles. Imagining rebuilds self-reliance, shores up the mind in abundant ways. Imagination, Robert Lowell wrote, "catches us and carries us off on the winds of invention." It carries from and to.

We can do some of this alone; we have done so over the centuries. To imagine is to create lands of one's own. It is to immerse oneself in exemplary lives—lives of courage, discovery, and leadership—and to draw upon them for ideas and inspiration. "Literature is full of examples of remarkable cures through the influence of imagination," wrote William Osler. Imagination "is only an active phase of faith." To imagine is to journey.

"I drew the map," wrote Ursula K. Le Guin about creating her fantasy world of Earthsea, a scattering of islands populated by early Iron Age civilizations. "All the islands were on it, but I knew nothing of them except their names, their shapes, the bays and mountains and rivers I had marked, the names of cities on some of them. They all remained to be discovered, one by one." Each island proved to have its own language and dragons, its own ancient texts that carried the history of its race, and wizards that could change the tides or rile the sea. The physician-sorcerers of Le Guin's Earthsea islands used magic spells and chants and brewed cures from the river meadows to heal the sick and troubled in mind. We read about places like Earthsea in order to escape or experience new things. We use them to add scaffolding, ideas and bits of steel, to help us heal (see photo section).

Many of those who write best from the imagination write for children. They understand impressionable minds; they have such minds themselves. They re-create the magic of play and quest, risk and discovery. Children's minds, vulnerable to small wounds, learn in time to be wiser and tougher. Children fall down, get up, look about, and take on the world again. What they see becomes a part of them, to use, to draw upon. Lost innocence cannot be found again, writes Philip Pullman. Nor should one wish otherwise. "The only way is forward, through life, deep into life, deep into the difficulties and the compromises and the betrayals and the disappointments we inevitably encounter." Childhood includes disappointment and betrayal; it also includes love, wonder, and passion. Childhood is its own world and prefigures life to come.

The Wonderful Wizard of Oz is "America's greatest and best-loved fairy tale." Not strictly an island, cut off by desert rather than sea, the land of Oz is a particularly American imagination: exuberant, energetic, optimistic, and lit up in bold colors. Virtue and valor triumph over greed and baseness; moral ambiguity is scarce. It has a midwestern presence, not only in the cyclone that carries Dorothy from the prairies to Oz, and in its landlocked geography, but in the book's underlying values of modesty, loyalty, and love of home. Dorothy, engaging for her independence and grit, is intensely loyal to her new, rather strange friends. She opens herself to winged monkeys, the Emerald City, and witches wicked and good; she travels, in faith and necessity, on a road that goes nowhere, everywhere, and finally home: "If we walk far enough," said Dorothy, "we shall sometime come to some place, I am sure." She is naïve, she learns, she grows (see photo section).

"There was a child went forth every day," Walt Whitman wrote. "And the first object he look'd upon, that object he became. . . . / The early lilacs became part of this child, / And grass and white and red morning-glories, and white and red clover. . . . / The horizon's edge, the flying sea-crow, the fragrance of salt marsh and shore mud." These things, wrote Whitman, become part of the child, who goes forth as impressionable as sealing wax. Impressionable to true things, but also to misperception.

"This is reality, whether you like it or not," wrote Willa Cather in *My Ántonia*. Nature offers truth but it also misrepresents. "All those frivolities of summer, the light and shadow, the living mask of green that trembled over everything, they were lies, and this is what was underneath. This is the truth." The child takes in light and shadow, sees summer for what it is, and recognizes transience. Nothing in life stands still. Seasons pass, knowledge comes, and we grow up.

"One by one," James Barrie said to the boys who inspired *Peter Pan*, "as you swung monkey-wise from branch to branch in the wood of make-believe, you reached the tree of knowledge." Children learn from play, from fantasy, and from improbable leaps of imagination; they learn from "galumphing," as Lewis Carroll had it. Barrie—himself the rare adult who remained a child, wrote Max Beerbohm, "a child who, by some divine grace, can express through an artistic medium the childishness that is in him"—mapped out the imaginary islands, the Neverland, that dwell in the minds of children: the jumbled hours and glorious daydreams, the manicured worlds that revert to wildness; adventures and quests; ambiguities and fleeting moods and wrenching letdowns. The prosaic strands of life that are woven with make-believe. Barrie mapped these shifting islands of childhood:

> I don't know whether you have ever seen a map of a person's mind. Doctors sometimes draw maps of other parts of you, and your own map can become intensely interesting, but catch them trying to draw a map of a child's mind, which is not only confused, but keeps going round all the time. There are zigzag lines on it, just like your temperature on a card, and these are probably roads in the island, for the Neverland is always more or less an island, with astonishing splashes of colour here and there, and coral reefs and rakish-looking craft in the offing . . . and caves through which a river runs.

Life is a journey of chance and waylay; a throw of the stars. Many take their journey with counsel by their side, be it doctor, priest, or teacher. For the young, a guide—a Merlyn, a writer—can make the passage from childhood to maturity less isolated and uncertain, more joyful. Children's books help to make sense of an overwhelming and contradictory world. Their authors go with their readers into dark corners; they encourage exuberance, rather than squelching it. The good storyteller eases the shift from forming to formed. Youth must yield to the expectations of maturity. The adult world demands that we forsake the stuff of daydreams; it expects planning and restraint. Moods narrow, daring tapers. The memory of daring tapers.

Merlyn, tutor to King Arthur, asks Arthur when he is older about his memories of childhood, a time of fabulous magic. Their exchange is recounted by T. H. White in *The Once and Future King*:

> "Do you remember anything about the magic you had when you were small?"
>
> "No. Did I have some magic? I can remember that I was interested in birds and beasts. Indeed, that is why I still keep my menagerie at the Tower. But I don't remember about magic."
>
> "People don't remember," said Merlyn.

Through their characters, writers show us ways to field anxiety, face adversity, and take delight in living. Dorothy, bold and mostly unflappable; the intrepid Jo March in Louisa May Alcott's *Little Women*; and Charlotte, the edgy, inventive spider, size of a gumdrop, in *Charlotte's Web*, all learn over time to deal with hurt and misfortune, to be more fearless and innovative, to swing for the fences. Their influence carries through the generations. My mother, who was president of her fifth-grade Oz Club, passed on her love for Dorothy—the Kansas girl, direct and dauntless and good, who had been left to fare in strange lands with yet stranger creatures—not only to my brother, sister, and me but to the hundreds of elementary school students she taught over the years. Teachers, librarians, and parents who love books, and who know their power for good, pass them on. Books for the young—filled with danger, courage, hope, and adventure—allow children to examine new ideas and worlds under the protective wing of a writer's imagination.

Courage to face that which seems unfaceable is a scarlet thread of inspiration running through many books for children. "Understanding courage is a timeless quest in young people—it always has been so," wrote General Sir Peter de la Billière, a former commander of the British Special Forces. Like de la Billière, my father, a United States Air Force pilot, was interested always in why some have courage and others do not. He told me once while he was reading to me that the Wizard of Oz was correct to counsel the Cowardly Lion that all of us have fear. Everyone, he said emphatically, is afraid in the face of danger. Courage, whether you are a pilot under fire or a fictional character finding your way down a yellow brick road, "is in facing danger when you are afraid." There is no need for courage without fear.

Years later, struggling with my own fears and demons, I read *The Anatomy of Courage* by Lord Moran, Churchill's physician during the Second World War. "Courage is a moral quality," Moran wrote. "It is not a chance gift of nature like an aptitude for games. It is a cold choice between two alternatives, the fixed resolve not to quit." One could aspire to courage; it was not beyond reach. We need courage. We all must grapple with suffering and the fear of death. We need courage to make hard decisions, to contend with what we ordinarily would not, to go to places we would not choose to go.

There are many kinds of courage and quests; some are imaginary, others real. Children most often learn about quests through the lives of heroes. They learn about purpose and risks taken, about dreams lost or met. They come to know the human drive for adventure and knowledge; that failure and death may accompany great accomplishments and that suffering and setback can be used to advantage.

Robert Falcon Scott's 1910–1913 expedition to the South Pole is known as much for its tragedy—the deaths of Scott and four of his men and the disappointment of losing British first-claim to the Norwegian explorer Roald Amundsen—as for its major scientific accomplishments. Yet science remembers the British explorers for what was learned on the ill–fated expedition. Scott and his team of zoologists, oceanographers, meteorologists, and geologists were well-aware of the risks involved in their exploration of the Antarctic. They cast their quest as being a pursuit for scientific knowledge, as well as one for glory, king, and country. The motivations and priorities were mixed, of course. They were bound to be, in that ambitious an undertaking.

"We were primarily a great scientific expedition," wrote Apsley Cherry-Garrard in his extraordinary account of the Scott expedition, *The Worst Journey in the World*. "We had the largest and most efficient scientific staff that ever left England. We were discursive. We were full of intellectual interests and curiosities of all kinds." The expedition was driven to know more, to explore where no one had been before, and to explain to the public the incomprehensible: "Much of that

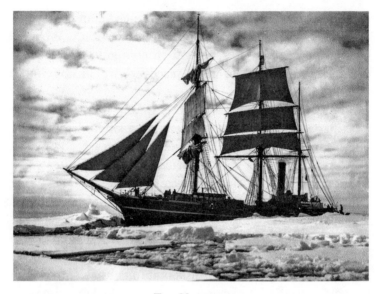

Terra Nova, 1910

I do not regret this journey. . . .
We took risks, we knew we took them; things have come out against us.

—ROBERT FALCON SCOTT, 1912

risk and racking toil had been undertaken that men might learn what the world is like at the spot where the sun does not decline in the heavens, where a man loses his orbit and turns like a joint on a spit, and where his face, however he turns, is always to the North." Scott's team collected tens of thousands of specimens that would be the basis for hundreds of scientific papers. They tracked marine currents and high-altitude winds, and collected rocks that would prove critical to understanding the history of Antarctica. They measured the movement of glaciers and scrambled along ice cliffs in pursuit of penguin rookeries. They sang hymns against the cold.

Their physical and mental suffering could not be told, Cherry-Garrard believed. It was too hard, too brutal. He himself was to be invalided out of the First World War for "nerves" and, later in his life, suffered a prolonged, psychotic depression that left him bedridden for years. His physical and mental courage were beyond question, but his mind was testament to the limits of courage. Mental suffering had been a particularly hard thing. Scott experienced "immense fits of depression," which predated the *Terra Nova* expedition. Scott's triumphs were many, Cherry-Garrard would write, but "the Pole was not by any means the greatest of them. Surely the greatest was that by which he conquered his weaker self, and became the strong leader whom we went to follow and came to love." The struggle and the journey were defining things. So too was what had been learned from them.

Quests are complicated, and how they are seen by others can be more complicated still. No quest is fulfilled until there is a reckoning of it, for good or ill. Cherry-Garrard wrote of the differences between the British and Norwegian expeditions to the South Pole, the differences in their ways of exploration, their successes and failures in what they set out to do, and the extent of their suffering, courage, and knowledge gained:

> I now see very plainly that though we achieved a first-rate tragedy, which will never be forgotten just because it was a tragedy, tragedy was not our business. In the broad perspective opened up by ten years' distance, I see not one journey to the Pole, but two, in startling contrast one to another. On the one hand, Amundsen going straight there, getting there first, and returning without the loss of a single man, and

without having put any greater strain on himself and his men than was all in the day's work of polar exploration. Nothing more business-like could be imagined. On the other hand, our expedition, running appalling risks, performing prodigies of superhuman endurance, achieving immortal renown, commemorated in august cathedral sermons and by public statues, yet reaching the Pole only to find our terrible journey superfluous, and leaving our best men dead on the ice.

~

Writers proffer exemplars who add the heroic, romantic, and courageous to stories. Someone larger than life, with an epic vision. Someone who paints on a great canvas. Someone who will inspire ambition, show ways to overcome setback and pain. "I want to do something splendid," Jo March says in *Little Women*, "something heroic or wonderful,—that won't be forgotten after I'm dead." She refuses the passive lot. "I don't like to doze by the fire. I like adventures, and I'm going to find some." Someone must tell the difficult truths about growing up, and the wonderful ones; help steer through the contradictions that fill a child's world; sort through contrary moods, and provide a primer for the baffling variety of people and situations a child will come across. Someone must encourage children to risk anxiety and failure; to shoot for the stars: to gain familiarity with the vast, know the fever of ambition and excitement of exploration. Stories of imagination and adventure are what make the ageless children's books, the ones that stay. Mine have been the traditional ones of my time and upbringing: the books of Robert Louis Stevenson, J. M. Barrie, Kenneth Grahame, E. B. White,

L. Frank Baum, Louisa May Alcott, Pamela Lyndon Travers, C. S. Forester, and T. H. White. But there is a need for children's writers of all backgrounds, a need that has been filled more recently by many excellent writers who have had different experiences in life, and adventures of a different, more diverse kind.

～

For this was no longer their daytime Park, their intimate ordinary playground. They had never been up so late nor understood that night changes the world and makes the known unknown.

P. L. TRAVERS,
Mary Poppins in Cherry Tree Lane

Pamela Lyndon Travers, author of the Mary Poppins books, wrote her way into children's minds and captured their high dreams, fears, and fantasies. She brought her own life into her books: its odd imaginings and curiosities, her childhood and her parents, and the books she loved. "If you are looking for autobiographical facts," she once said, "Mary Poppins is the story of my life." Imagination was an indispensable part of her childhood, as it is for most of us. It was taken "as a matter of course—another fact, like whooping cough, another fact, like daylight. Every child has it as a natural inheritance":

I remembered how, for a long period in childhood, I was absorbed in the experience of being a bird. Absorbed, not lost, knowing, had I been faced with it, that I was also a child. Brooding, busy, purposeful, I wove the nests and prepared for eggs as though the life of all nature depended on the effort. "She can't come, she's laying," the others would say, arriving for a meal without me. And my mother, deep in her role of distracted housewife, would come and unwind my plaited limbs and drag me from the nest: "If I've told you once, I've told you a hundred times, no laying at lunchtime!"

Not, "You are mad. I fear for your future. We must find a psychiatrist." Simply, not at lunchtime! Could she, too, once have been a bird, I sometimes wonder now?

Often she was left, Travers said, "on her own desert (but by no means unfruitful) island, to work things out" for herself. Her father, an alcoholic, was subject to depression: "I remember his melancholy, which was the other side of his Irish gaiety," Travers wrote. And she knew that "it was catching and inheritable." The pain she saw in him, and the pain she herself experienced, found their way into her books: Her stories make clear that life is more complicated and difficult than some would have you believe. You, she said to parent and child, bear a responsibility to understand this. Indirect lessons are best; when adults explain, they fill in what might otherwise and more profitably be thought up by a child. "Where nobody explains," observed Travers, and "I say this with joy, not sorrow!—children must build life for themselves."

Travers, who was a deeply read scholar of myth and fairy tale, said she found them inseparable from the themes of childhood. Myths, she stated, are fundamental, the "one reality that underlies everything." Myths do many things; they are the stories of a people's history, and ways of explaining how the world began, how its realms fit into the larger cosmos. They are stories that seek to explain the natural world, stories that make sense of the inexplicable. A myth, said W.H.R. Rivers, "is the pure product of the human imagination, an attempt to express the wonderful and the mysterious." The subject of myth is not the habitual, it is the "strangely shaped rocks or dangerous reefs," seen rarely, that light the imagination. Myths and fairy tales are contained by societies in the ancient parts of themselves. They bewitch, pull us in, and tell hard truths: "What *isn't* frightening, after all?" asked Travers. "What *doesn't* carry a stern lesson?" Not surprisingly, Sylvia Plath regarded Mary Poppins as the "fairy godmother" of her youth.

Even the simplest tale has power. Take Humpty Dumpty, Travers said. "All the King's horses and all the king's men couldn't put him together again. That some things are broken irrevocably, never to be whole again, is a hard truth." Stories and fairy tales teach this and other truths. They, and rites and myths, are everywhere. "You only have to open a newspaper to find them crowding into it." They "run around in our blood." They warn. They promise.

Throughout her life, Travers wrote about the human need for myths and fairy tales. As she got older they took on even greater importance. In a talk to the Library of Congress in 1966 she said, "Life, in a sense, is myth, one might say; the one is a part of the other. In both of them, the good and the bad, the dangerous and the safe, live very close together." She told her audience that she had recently read an article in *The New York Times* about eels making their way to the Sargasso Sea to mate and lay their eggs. "Afterwards, they make their long way back to their respective homes [in America and Europe] and apparently feel it was worth it. Well, for me the tales are a sort of Sargasso Sea and I am a kind of eel." A pre-ternatural eel, one who gathered life from the ocean gyre and the great fields of *Sargassum*. Travers took into her stories what she had taken from the Sargasso, a sea of mythic clarity.

P. L. Travers sent Mary Poppins into the world in 1934. The acerbic nanny blows in on the East Wind to Cherry Tree Lane in London; as she does, the trees blow wildly, "looking as though they had gone mad and were dancing their roots out of the ground." She arrives without notice, as she will leave without notice. Her comings and goings are mysterious, as is everything about her. "You'll never leave us, will you?" a child asks her. Her answer is unsettling, Delphic: "I'll stay till the wind changes." I'll stay, until I go. Until the winds gust or a distant door opens (see photo section).

Mary Poppins is unpredictable, acid-tongued, vain, and the hero of her own tales and adventures. She is fearless and implacable. She demands that Michael and Jane, the children in her charge, be well-mannered and mindful of her authority but she leads them into adventures with no rules and where anything can happen. They leap, star to star to star, and press up against the sky; they dance with the moon in their arms. They fly on peppermint-stick horses, step into chalk pictures, and go Christmas shopping with a glittering girl-star from the Pleiades. They dive to the floor of the sea, sown wildly and beautifully with seaweed, ocean daisies, and coral, lit by luminous fish, and they talk with a terrapin who dwells deep in the roots of the world, under cities, hills, and the sea. They watch as fish reel in humans, on hooks baited with strawberry tarts.

Mary Poppins dazzles; she creates a string of magical experiences that loop through the children's minds, lighted up like Chinese lanterns. She teaches, always, and spins magic.

"There was something strange and extraordinary about her," thought Michael. "Something that was frightening and at the same time most exciting."

In each of their adventures, Mary Poppins is the exceptional one, singled out for unique tribute; her specialness is conferred on the children as well. When she and the children fly to join the sun and the constellations, the sun says to her, "For you, Mary Poppins, the Stars have gathered in the dark blue tent, for you they have been withdrawn tonight from shining on the world." The stars blink strangely, brilliantly; the heavens take their breath away. The sun cedes his place to her. It is right and wonderful that a crater on Mercury has been named for Pamela Lyndon Travers.

Mary Poppins is the honored guest at the dancing of the constellations, on the floor of the sea, and at full moon celebrations at the zoo. Creatures and constellations hold her in awe. Each adventure ends with the children back in the nursery brimming with excitement and Mary Poppins denying that anything at all unusual happened. She sniffs indignantly at the children's recollections, but each morning they find a token from the night's happenings that makes clear the adventure was no figment of their imagination—a snakeskin belt shed for Mary Poppins, from their magical evening at the zoo, a small pink starfish that glitters like diamonds from a rapturous trip to the ocean floor, an umbrella filled with stars. The children are left to wonder, to absorb the magic: What really happened? What is real? Does it matter? "Nothing lasts forever," Mary Poppins tells them. "All good things come to an end."

But they don't. The children held onto the memories of their times with her, times that had brought joy, awe, and healing to the hurts and discontents of their childhood. Mary

Poppins left them living in a larger world, a world enhanced by their strange and magical odysseys. She made them think and question. She left them with new ways to create and to contend and to heal, and with places to return to when the mind might need it:

> And the thing they wished was that all their lives they might remember Mary Poppins. Where and How and When and Why—had nothing to do with them. They knew that as far as she was concerned those questions had no answers. The bright shape speeding through the air above them would for ever keep its secret. But in the summer days to come and the long nights of winter, they would remember Mary Poppins and think of all she had told them. . . . Mary Poppins herself had flown away, but the gifts she had brought would remain for always.

The gifts from Mary Poppins went directly from her imagination into that of the children: the trips to the bottom of the sea and into the constellations; the exuberance and adventure; the diversion from sadness. She showed them fresh ways to do things and she taught, in an abiding way, how to dare and why to give in to fantasy. From Mary Poppins they came to understand that being the hero of your own story bestows a certain courage and vision, but it demands answerability as well. Hers was a master class in becoming more than you could have imagined, of learning to rely upon yourself when facing difficulty and of living with uncertainty. To be heroic and to deal with suffering that comes one's way, said Travers, "is to accept everything that comes and make jewels of it . . . You can only be the hero of your own story if you accept it totally."

Mary Poppins left Jane and Michael with the wonder that favors childhood, and skeptical about limits imposed by the rational world. They had flown through cascading trails of stardust, soared over the lampposts and parks of London. They had done impossible things. To sift the real from the fantastic was not always the wisest way to spend one's time. Reality was not everything. P. L. Travers often quoted Theodore Roethke: "I learn by going where I have to go." The journey was the important thing.

P. L. Travers stressed that Mary Poppins was a teacher, the highest of compliments. The best teachers, like the best writers, show us how to spin new worlds and how to go to new places, how to sort through what is important from what is not. Teachers stamp our forming minds and lead us, as books do, to places and philosophies neither familiar nor always comfortable. They acquaint us with images and stories that excite, provoke, and console. One owes an unpayable debt to the best teachers.

Certainly this is true for me. At a critical time in my life, my high school English teacher introduced me to writers and thinkers who were exemplars of courage and determination—Robert Lowell, Siegfried Sassoon, and, through his war memoirs, W.H.R. Rivers. I think my teacher knew I had been very depressed but I had told no one and he said nothing. No one talked about mania or depression in those days. He reached out in the way he knew best, with books that he loved. He lent me his own copies of Lowell's *Life Studies* and *Lord Weary's Castle*, and Sir Thomas Malory's *Le Morte d'Arthur*. He gave me outright his well-read and underlined copy of T. H. White's *The Once and Future King*. These books changed me. They accompany me still, in good mood and dark, and are among the first books I have unpacked whenever I have moved. Passionate teachers, intuitive ones, ensure that great books—with their goadings and pleasures, the worlds they open, and the comfort they give so privately—will continue to inspire, heal, and teach.

~

And therein stuck a fair sword, naked by the point, and letters there were written in gold about the sword that saiden thus:—WHOSO PULLETH OUT THIS SWORD OF THIS STONE AND ANVIL, IS RIGHTWISE KING BORN OF ALL ENGLAND. . . . As Arthur did at Christmas, he did at Candlemas, and pulled out the sword easily.

—SIR THOMAS MALORY,
Le Morte d'Arthur, 1485

To teach is to show, to guide, and to accompany. In early times, the young learned from their elders how to track the stars, to hunt, and to heal wounds as best they could; they were taught to keep watch on slight changes in season and prey. The skill of the first teachers—the shamans and priests, the parents, the tribal elders—would determine whether the young lived and bred, or died. Those early tutors instructed their pupils in the ways of observing and thinking that had been used by their ancestors. The great teacher became the stuff of legend and myth, the guide on quests, often a hero. The renowned magician Merlyn was one of these. Some say he was a Celtic druid and others that he was a poet driven mad by the atrocities of war. For most, he was known simply as tutor to King Arthur.

. . .

The Arthurian legend, "The Matter of Britain," is considered by some to be, with Milton, Shakespeare, and the King James Bible, a foundation stone of English culture and literature. Sir Thomas Malory's *Le Morte d'Arthur*, written in the fifteenth century, Tennyson's *Idylls of the King* published four hundred years later, and T. H. White's *The Once and Future King*, published in four books between 1938 and 1958, are the better-known English accounts of the legend of King Arthur, his life and death, and the lost dream of Camelot. T. E. Lawrence carried Malory's *Le Morte d'Arthur* with him into battle during the Arab Revolt; Siegfried Sassoon, when dying, asked for his worn copy of Malory.

Nothing establishes with certainty that Arthur existed—"no bones, no crowns, no credible documents," as the poet Simon Armitage puts it—but legend prevails over fact. As written by T. H. White, with tribute to Malory, whom White regarded as the "greatest English writer next to Shakespeare," *The Once and Future King* is heartbreaking, noble, and tragic. It is an epic of bitterness and betrayal, of bravery, greatness, and forgiveness (see photo section).

The lyricist Alan Jay Lerner, who, with composer Frederick Loewe, adapted their 1960 musical *Camelot* from *The Once and Future King*, said of the Arthurian legend, "There lies buried in its heart the aspirations of mankind." Therein lies the lasting appeal of King Arthur: his duty to uphold the code of honor and justice by which he himself lived, and by which he expected his knights to live—the calling of Arthur to lead well, to inspire, and to do the right thing, to influence for the good. It is "that subtle force by which the men of the past influence us today," wrote William Osler, that "intangible, mysterious force hard to define but best expressed in the words *noblesse oblige*—that obligation to act in a certain way, to foster certain habits, to conform to certain unwritten laws." It is a code of behavior learned from those before us, those who inspire, those who pass on "certain unwritten laws." Tennyson wrote:

> *And so there grew great tracts of wilderness,*
> *Wherein the beast was ever more and more,*
> *But man was less and less, till Arthur came.*

The Once and Future King portrays Arthur as a king who leads with courage and honor but who fails in much of what he sets out to do. It is also a portrayal of Merlyn, who teaches the young Arthur the meaning of duty and how to contend with suffering. "Merlyn is myself," T. H. White once said. Teaching was essential to who he was. White's own school days had been brutal, marked by sadistic beatings by his schoolmasters, and he was intent on showing his students, and later his readers, why learning is the most serious endeavor, how it salves, protects, and heals. Learning should be a "thirst to throw yourself into life in all its forms," he said. One should be passionate in dealing with life: grapple with it, know it, and master it. Passion and knowledge protect. "When you know a thing, it is subdued, it is in your power, it is yours," White believed. Suffering erodes confidence and self-reliance. Learning builds them up again; it provides diversion, soothes and activates, and draws toward life. Learning prepares the mind. Suffering is inevitable: Prepare for it. Adventure and quest heal in their own right.

"You have to arm yourself against future disasters in which everything can be cut away from under your feet," White said toward the end of his life. "I have had to spend my life foreseeing and preventing catastrophes, and the best way to arm yourself against life is by learning to cope with it, by mastering all the skills you can." Anticipate the future; it will disappoint. There will be grief and suffering. Build sea-walls against them. Learn. In learning is mastery; in mastery is healing.

T. H. White did this. He learned how to fly, plow, hunt with bow and arrow, hunt with falcons, gear himself in medieval armor, and go into the sea in old-fashioned diving suits. He forced himself to be more courageous than he believed himself to be, and to venture where he had not gone before. He read and studied voraciously. He worked on his writing; he sketched. He put into practice his belief that suffering could come to good, and that writing from suffering could help others. (White's gravestone reads, "T. H. White / 1906–1964 / Author / Who from a Troubled Heart / Delighted Others / Loving and Praising / This Life.")

White's life was marked by depression, heavy drinking, and wild enthusiasms; he was, a friend remarked, "chased by a mad black wind. "I think he was 75 per cent of his time unhappy and often *very unhappy;* probably about nothing in particular. Terror and awe mysteriously affected him." The actress Julie Andrews, a close friend of White's from her days portraying Queen Guinevere in *Camelot*, felt, as others did, that White suffered from bipolar illness. He sought medical care and was treated by a psychiatrist from the time he was a young schoolmaster until his death. No doctor, however, could replace myth, religion, and majestic language as the ruling influences in White's imagination. He was "a great man," White said of his psychoanalyst, but "the best psychiatrist in the world can't beat The Book of Common Prayer." Certainly, no psychiatrist could match the power of Cranmer's 1549 prayer book or Sir Thomas Malory's *Le Morte d'Arthur*, the headwaters of White's passion for the Arthurian legend.

To keep depression at bay, White kept his mind and body

ferociously employed. Like Robert Burton, he pitted learning and imagination against melancholy. He lived the counsel his Merlyn gave to King Arthur, that sadness is best fought by learning. The poet and novelist Sylvia Townsend Warner, T. H. White's biographer, described White's restless, electric mind:

> He was studying Erse; he was reading Irish history; he was thinking about becoming a Catholic, and conversing with Father Dempsey; he still had hopes of getting a salmon out of the Boyne; he was keeping a brimming diary, full of conclusions about Irish farming, Irish character, Anglo-Irish relations, which he might make into a book; if he had been committed to Wandsworth Jail, by the end of three months he would have been writing a history of Wandsworth, with sections on its geology, botany, bird-life, etc., together with a dictionary of prisoners' slang and an analysis of what was wrong with the penal system and suggestions how to improve it.

Merlyn, as White wrote him, tutored the young Arthur in the importance of learning, both as preparation for leadership and to steel himself against pain. Merlyn instructed Arthur that he was destined to suffer greatly, and that to be a great king he must work hard, heartbreakingly hard. He would need to find ways to address his own suffering and to console his subjects. He must continue to learn about the world, to hold learning sacred. Learning would heal some of his pain, but not all:

> "The best thing for being sad," [Merlyn said] "is to learn something. That is the only thing that never

fails. You may grow old and trembling in your anatomies, you may lie awake at night listening to the disorder of your veins, you may miss your only love, you may see the world about you devastated by evil lunatics, or know your honour trampled in the sewers of baser minds. There is only one thing for it then—to learn. . . . That is the only thing which the mind can never exhaust, never alienate, never be tortured by, never fear or distrust, and never dream of regretting."

Arthur, not yet king, first met Merlyn while searching for his goshawk, who had flown from his gauntlet to the sky, maddeningly evasive. It was a "quest," he said, that led him to Merlyn. Lost deep in the forest, in pursuit of the hawk, he came upon an old man drawing water from a well; it was the magician who would become his tutor. He was dressed in an odd flowing gown and a pointed hat covered with bits of bones and leaves and stars. His cottage was stuffed with strange, wonderful things: a phoenix "which smelt of incense and cinnamon"; cauldrons and bunsen burners; skulls; live grass snakes; young hedgehogs wrapped in cotton wool; and a chest of drawers "full of salmon flies which had been tied by Merlyn himself." There were badgers; paint-boxes; fossils; an astrolabe; ink bottles "of every possible colour from red to violet"; and, throughout the cottage, thousands of leather-bound books, "propped against each other as if they had had too much to drink and did not really trust themselves."

This "most marvelous room" baptized Arthur into the world of his new tutor. Archimedes, Merlyn's owl—who would initiate him into the ways of hawks and chivalry—taught him now his first lesson, how to approach and touch a wild animal, how to proffer respect. The owl took Arthur's offering of a

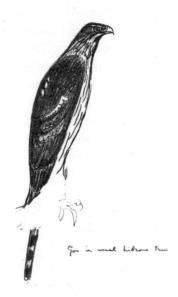

Gos in usual hideous run

From the journals of T. H. White

Each hawk or falcon was a motionless statue
of a knight in armour.

mouse and ate it "with closed eyes and an expression of rapture on his face, as if he were saying Grace, and then, with the absurdest sideways nibble, took the morsel so gently that he would not have broken a soap bubble." As with the other animals to be mustered by Merlyn for Arthur's education—perch, goshawk, ant, badger, and goose—Archimedes would educate Arthur in the small and great ways of nature. Merlyn, Archimedes, and the other animals would instruct him in their distinctive codes of honor, the limits of justice and drawbacks of innocence, how to reign well and fairly, the obligations of leadership, and the danger of power used badly. They would show him the contours of the earth and the pull of tides, and how arbitrary a boundary can be.

Merlyn instructed Arthur in human nature as well, pointed out the dark sides of human character and the cost of ambition. He taught Arthur to encase himself in the wide experiences of the world: To observe it and learn from it. To be thoughtful. To think for himself. Merlyn used his magic to change his young pupil into a multiplicity of species; different animals took him into unfamiliar places: under the water, underneath the ground, into the sky. He learned to move, sense, and hunt differently. These journeys were archetypal quests, deep-rooted and weighted in myth. Arthur entered into extraordinary realms, was tested, and returned with wisdom to rule a kingdom.

For Arthur's first quest Merlyn changed him into a perch. The boy learned to swim weightless and experienced how it was to be water-bound, finned, and tailed. He darted through murky waters where heaven and sky were a small circle overhead, and he swam through great forests of seaweed and water lilies. Merlyn joined Arthur on this first quest and introduced him to the Great Fish, the King of the Moat, a despot "ravaged by all the passions of an absolute monarch—by cruelty, sorrow, age, pride, selfishness, loneliness, and thoughts too strong for individual brains." The only important thing is power, the Great Fish told the boy. "Power is of the individual mind, but the mind's power is not enough. Power of the body decides everything in the end, and only Might is Right." Power was a pitiless thing, to be exercised without reflection or mercy, a contention against which Arthur never ceased to fight. Lessons taken from quests taught not only of ill in the world, but of its promise.

A quest, Merlyn told Arthur, required that he be serious; it required him to face danger and fear and to overcome them. A quest was to be immersed in, and committed to, what was at hand. "You swim along," Merlyn said, "as if there was nothing to be afraid of in the world. Don't you see that this place is exactly like the forest which you had to come through to find me?" Danger must be acknowledged and met. Innocence may come easily, but it comes with risk. Merlyn created quests not just for a boy but for a future king, and he insisted that Arthur travel them in his own way. Merlyn had accompanied Arthur on his first quest into the castle moat as a perch, but "In future, you will have to go by yourself," the magician told Arthur. "Education is experience, and the essence of experience is self-reliance." Time and again Merlyn demanded of Arthur: Rely upon yourself rather than being beholden to the ideas of others. Learn from experience. Reason things through. Inform your decisions with careful and ethical thought. Understand that suffering will come and that you must have the means to deal with it. Understand yourself, understand suffering.

These were the beliefs of many of the classical philosophers and echoed since by other thinkers, including Ralph Waldo Emerson and William James. W.H.R. Rivers agreed. "It is necessary," he said, for the individual who is suffering "to face the facts, get to understand the situation, do his best to meet it in his own strength." The remedies were self-knowledge and self-reliance.

Arthur's transformations into perch, falcon, ant, and goose taught him, each in its own way, that to live wisely was to understand differences in temperament, habit, and capacity. It was to widen one's emotional and physical world and to toughen oneself against trial and pain. He learned from them and from Merlyn that honor defines a person, and that monotony kills. Geese opened him to the glory of the natural world: its great waters and forests, its salt marshes, and the elemental beauty of wind that "came from nowhere and was going through the flatness of nowhere, to no place." He took in the beauty of the world, fresh-found in the "stars of spring and the scent of the currants, the wild cherries, the plums and the hawthorne," newfound in the dark and long flatness of the tides. Geese taught him how to navigate the sky and shared legends of First Goose and the wonder of wing, flight, and sea. They pulled him into the beauty and turbulence of the sky and taught him the features of their synchronized world: "the sea sound . . . darkness, flatness, vastness, wetness: and, in the gulf of night, the gulf stream of the wind." He found hope, if not truth, in their world without boundaries.

In due time, Arthur moved from the freedom of childhood to the doings, anguish, and grandeur of being king. He learned to fence, to joust, and to suit himself in chain mail and greaves. He drew Excalibur from a stone, as he alone could do, and found in it power and unhappiness. He reigned as best he could, ever conscious that he fell short of what he had set for himself. He married Guinevere, and she betrayed him with Lancelot, his closest friend. He and Merlyn conceived the Round Table, "which had no corners, just as the world had none," and chose knights—Galahad, Gawain, Lancelot, Tristan, and others lesser known—who did God's work under Arthur's will and rule of justice. Until, bored and restless, they did not. He made Camelot a court of valor and righteous action. This was a king, as Laurie Lee wrote about a more recent British hero, who drew out what was possible in his subjects, and who could "touch their nerves with fingers of sulphur, stinging them briefly alive into postures of glory, of sacrifice, suffering and triumph" (see photo section).

King Arthur's world, conceived with the highest ideals and endeavor, came to an end, doomed by the nature of man.

Merlyn had taught Arthur to think; he did. He had taught him to be fair and just; he was. But human nature being as it is—flawed, selfish, inflexible—he could not rule the world the way it was; he was constrained by what he thought it ought to be. His education, remarkable though it had been, had left him vulnerable: He had been surrounded by love; he had grown up "without malice, vanity, suspicion, cruelty, and the commoner forms of selfishness." He had grown up naked of the armor that he needed. Guinevere and Lancelot broke faith with him. The queen, sentenced to death for treason, was rescued by Lancelot, but their future was heartbreak. King Arthur slew, and was slain by his own son, a child born of Arthur's unwitting incest with his half sister. It had been done in Arthur's innocence. It was an "Aristotelian and comprehensive tragedy," White writes. "The king had slept with his own sister. He did not know he was doing so, and perhaps it may have been due to her, but it seems, in tragedy, that innocence is not enough."

⟶

The night before King Arthur died in battle he sat alone, broken, in his war tent at Salisbury. The great and tragic king of T. H. White's imagining was old, weary, and in despair. He was surrounded by unread papers of state and unanswered petitions from his subjects; his kingdom, like his papers, was in disarray. A chessboard stood by his bed, the king in checkmate. His country was at war, his Round Table destroyed; his reign seemed without meaning or purpose. Merlyn had taught Arthur to pursue good. To what avail? What good had come from the failure of his reign, what of use had been salvaged from the suffering? The king could not change the fact of war and that he would die. He was spent; he had nothing left to give, only to wait to be taken by barge to Avalon—island of enchantresses and apple trees—to heal his "grievous wound." (Wilfred Owen would draw upon this deeply British imagery during the Great War when he wrote about a hospital barge moving down the Somme, carrying wounded soldiers: "And that long lamentation made him wise / How unto Avalon, in agony, / Kings passed in the dark barge which Merlin dreamed.")

T. H. White does not spare Arthur from suffering or death; instead he confers upon him the possibility of eventual return, and with it the certainty of legend. "There was something invincible in his heart," White wrote about Arthur, as the king sat in his tent before battle. There was "a tincture of grandness in simplicity." The king reaches for the bell to summon his page. The boy enters Arthur's tent, eager to fight for his king; the king commands him otherwise. The boy is to keep alive the legend of Arthur and the knights of Camelot. He is to pass on to all he sees the story that Arthur tells him. The king recounts the history of Camelot and his dreams for it; how he chose his knights for the Round Table, and the chivalrous quests they had undertaken. It had been a noble idea, a magnificent one; it worked for a while. It had aspired to "set the world to right." It failed. But it had aspired.

King Arthur commands the page—whose surcoat bears the Malory name—to be the vessel for his ideas and bearer of his hopes; to be the storyteller who will give meaning to his death and dreams and suffering. "My idea of those knights was a sort of candle," he tells the page. "I have carried it for many years with a hand to shield it from the wind. It has flickered often. I am giving you the candle now—you won't let it out?"

"It will burn," the page tells the king. "It will burn."

Malory ends *Le Morte d'Arthur* as T. H. White ends *The Once and Future King* as unremitting tragedy. The passionate insistence upon learning that Merlyn had passed on to Arthur, the expectation that hard work and valor would provide some protection against suffering, did not save the king. Instead, they gave rise to a legend, one that would inspire the longings and ambitions of others. The king suffered that others might not. Or that they might carry their suffering differently and use it to help others, not only themselves. Malory leavened his bleak thoughts about King Arthur with hope for those who followed:

> Yet some men say in many parts of England that King Arthur is not dead, but had by the will of Our Lord Jesu into another place; and men say that he shall come again, and he shall win the holy cross. I will not say that it shall be so, but rather I will say, here in this world he changed his life. But many men say that there is written upon his tomb this verse: HIC IACET ARTHURUS, REX QUONDAM REXQUE FUTURUS. *Here lies Arthur, the once and future King.*

T. H. White gave King Arthur over to legend and gave him a peace of sorts. "The cannons of his adversary were thundering in the tattered morning when the Majesty of England drew himself up to meet the future with a peaceful heart," wrote White. He ended with the words of Malory: *Here lies Arthur, the once and future King.*

Quests, real or imagined, sow seeds of possibility. And then reap a few of them. They do this imperfectly, and for many, not at all. Yet those who enter into the worlds of exemplars and heroes—whether it is of the flawed, very human Captain Scott, or that of the mythic King Arthur—will be tutored in bravery, in suffering, and in suffering put to purpose.

⌒

High above Port Chalmers in New Zealand, the last port of call for Scott and his men before they left for the South Pole, there is a monument of stones, a cairn, to those who died on the expedition. The inscription ends with words from the book of Joshua:

> *Your children shall ask their fathers in time to come, saying, What mean these stones?*

CHAPTER 9

They Looked to Their Songs

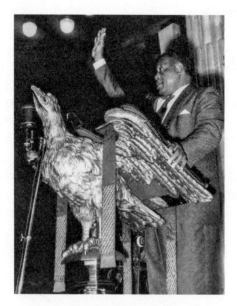

Paul Robeson in 1958
St. Paul's Cathedral, London

*They suffered. They fled to God through their
songs. They sang to forget their chains and misery.
Even in darkness they looked to their songs to work
out their destiny.*

You, Mr. Robeson, embody in your person the sufferings of mankind. Your singing is a declaration of faith. You sing as if God Almighty sent you into the world to advocate the cause of the common man. . . . You have the genius of touching the hearts of men.

—HONORARY DEGREE CITATION,
MOREHOUSE COLLEGE, 1943

Trafalgar Square has been witness to much. Bones of cave lions, hippopotamuses, and a woolly mammoth lie under its stones, as do Bronze Age, Roman, and Anglo-Saxon artifacts. The granite column that dominates the square—Lord Nelson's statue at its top and four bronze lions at its base—is a nation's tribute to Nelson's great victory at sea. Trafalgar Square is in the thick of a rushing city and draws people into it to celebrate and to remember: to see the new year in, watch the Christmas tree lit, mark war's end. Thousands filled the square in 1918 when armistice was declared; a great bonfire was lit.

Trafalgar Square is known as much for protest as for remembrance and celebration. Trade unionists, miners, Irish activists, suffragettes, social reformers, anti-colonialists, anti-apartheid demonstrators, pacifists, and anarchists have all come with placard and bullhorn to speak out against social injustice, petition for reform, or protest government policies. In the summer of 1959 more than ten thousand demonstrators gathered to demonstrate against British policy on nuclear weapons. Many of the founders and supporters of the Campaign for Nuclear Disarmament—Bertrand Russell, Sir Julian Huxley, Kingsley Martin, Benjamin Britten, Doris Lessing, E. M. Forster—were well-known to the public and press; others were not.

During the protest, something caught the attention of an observer. "As London traffic rumbled around the square," he wrote, "a succession of notables addressed the crowd." A tall Black man went to the steps of Nelson's Column and stood in front of the microphone. He spoke for a while, and then he sang.

"Paul Robeson sang," the observer wrote. *"And the buses stopped."*

Paul Robeson was a singer, actor, scholar, lawyer, athlete, and activist. In each field, except the law, which because of

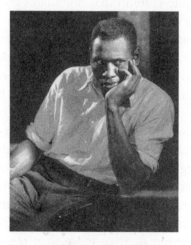

Paul Robeson in 1940

He is one of the few of whom I would say that they have greatness. . . . Paul Robeson strikes me as having been made out of the original stuff of the world . . . a fresh effort of creation.

—Alexander Woollcott

pervasive racism he never practiced, he led with conspicuous talent and bearing. "Before King dreamed, before Thurgood Marshall petitioned," wrote historian Lerone Bennett, Jr., "before the Jim Crow signs came down and before the Civil Rights banners went up . . . there was Paul Robeson." His singing and commitment moved souls. Robeson, wrote James Baldwin, "lives, overwhelmingly, in the hearts and minds of the people whom he touched, the people for whom he was an example, the people who gained from him the power to perceive and the courage to exist." Baldwin had taken his younger sister to hear Robeson sing, he said, because it was important that she "*know* that such a man was in the world."

Paul Robeson's art and music expressed the suffering he saw in others and that he knew for himself; he lent it meaning. He gave a voice to the oppressed, and he made oppression manifest to those who were blind to it:

> *Light*
> *parted from shadow,*
> *day*
> *from night,*
> *land*
> *from the primal waters.*
>
> *And Paul Robeson's voice*
> *separated from silence.*
>
> —PABLO NERUDA

When people heard Paul Robeson sing spirituals, the African American songs of slavery, they didn't forget it. The spirituals, heard first in his home and in his father's church, had been part of Robeson's life for as long as he could remember. His father, born enslaved, had learned them on the plantation in North Carolina. A *New York Times* music critic wrote once that Robeson sang with an "overwhelming inward conviction." It was a "cry from the depths," a cry that "voiced the sorrows and hopes of a people."

Robeson's rare gift touched hearts. He once said that his singing was the "truest expression of himself as a man as well as an artist." Song, he said, had always been a "form of speech" for him. His voice is one of beauty and sorrow, power and persuasion. To the extent that a human voice calls up a sense of deep time, it does. Michael Hersch, a classical composer who often writes for singers, describes Paul Robeson's voice as extraordinary, not only because it is "simply beautiful, with a rare timbre and notable core," but because his "easy, omni-present confidence at once disarms and creates urgency."

Whether Robeson sang in concert halls or churches, to trade unionists or miners, to theater audiences in London or New York, he moved people in a way that was at once deeply emotional and electrifying. He "exuded magnetism and charm and charisma," an observer said. Another remarked that he "strode onto the crowded stage with a combination of dignity, grace and responsive enthusiasm." He was majestic and commanded the room, yet it was "as though each person there had been struck by the lightning of that smile, the gran-deur of that presence . . . He spoke straight to the hearts of all present." Paul Robeson had a common touch and uncom-mon command.

❧

Robeson was five years old when his mother died after a hot coal fell from a stove and set her dress on fire. Those who had known Maria Louisa Bustill Robeson told her young son about his mother's strength of character, how she had fed the poor and tended the sick, and taught many to read. She was strong and gentle, her son wrote, and stunningly intelligent. Because she died when he was so young, his memories of her were few. He was very much his father's son.

"The glory of my boyhood years was my father," Paul Robeson wrote. "I loved him like no one in all the world." Born into slavery, William Drew Robeson escaped to the North when he was fifteen. Twice he went back to take money to his mother, and twice again he made his way north. He worked to pay his way through Lincoln University—later alumni were to include Langston Hughes and Thurgood Marshall—where he studied Greek, Latin, mathematics, botany, chemistry, astronomy, and English literature. He was an honor graduate and a speaker at commencement. After he graduated he enrolled in the divinity school and earned a degree in theology. For the first years of his life, as an enslaved child, William Drew Robeson had had no name, only his age and sex listed in the census; now he had a name and three degrees after it. He became minister at the Witherspoon Street Presbyterian Church in Princeton and later took up the pastorage of an African Methodist Episcopal (AME) church nearby.

The text of his father's life, Paul Robeson wrote later, was loyalty to one's convictions. He had a "rock-like strength and dignity of character." In overtly racist and humiliating situations he showed "no hint of servility." Nor did he complain about the cards he had been dealt. He had a transcendent dignity: "I adored him, would have given my life for him in a flash."

Robeson's father left him with the values by which he would live. You have an obligation to your race. Neither suffering nor compassion is confined to a single people. Be open-minded while taking the measure of another person. React to the actions and ways of individuals, not to whether they are Black or white. Money is not what is important. Your example matters. Pursue truth, live up to your potential. Learn new things. Make the world a place of greater justice. These were what mattered. "I learned that Emancipation—Freedom—meant freedom for all my people, not just for a few wealthy and fortunate Negroes, but for all of us," Robeson once said. "And I've spent my life finding out how to use my own hands—my own talents—for this is a necessary part of the dignity of any people."

Besides intellect, values grounded in respect for others, and discipline, Robeson inherited his father's independence and confidence. "I honestly feel that my future depends mostly upon myself," he wrote when he was in his twenties, "my courage in fighting over the rough places that are bound to come—my eagerness to work and learn. . . . I approach the future in a happy and rather adventurous spirit. For it is within my power to make this unknown trail a somewhat beaten path."

His father's influence continued strong. When Robeson was in his mid-fifties, he still asked himself: "What would Pop think?" His father was true north and reflecting glass. "I often stop and ask the stars, the winds. I often stretch out my arm as I used to, to put it around Pop's shoulder and ask, 'How am I doin', Pop?' " Long after his father's death, and only a few years before his own, a friend brought him a copy of *Ebony;* historians, the magazine reported, had rated Paul Robeson, along with Frederick Douglass, Martin Luther King, Jr., Thurgood Marshall, Malcolm X, and W.E.B. Du Bois, as one of the greatest Black men in American history. On hearing this, "Paul simply said, 'Pop would have been pleased.' "

Paul Robeson's accomplishments were remarkable, in his own or in any time. They were even more so given the racism to which he was subjected. His statewide examination score for entrance to Rutgers was the highest on record. He was twice named All-American in football. Walter Camp, the sportswriter and "father of American Football," wrote that Robeson was "the greatest defensive end ever." He won more than a dozen varsity letters in football, baseball, basketball, and track. He led the Rutgers debating team, won the class oratorial prize, was valedictorian, and gave the commencement address. He played professional football to pay his way through Columbia Law School. He spoke or sang in more than twenty languages, including French, Russian, German, Yiddish, Swahili, Arabic, Gaelic, Chinese, and Norwegian. Robeson, whose father had tutored him in Virgil, Homer, and rhetoric, would sit in a room for hours, said a friend, practicing French verbs or Chinese characters or immersing himself in books about Bach and music theory. He prepared for *Othello* by reading deeply in the English of Chaucer and the medieval poets. His longtime accompanist, Lawrence Brown, remarked, "If he strode in any direction, it was towards knowledge for its own sake. After the greatest ovations, Paul would go home and read or study languages."

Paul Robeson performed in Jerome Kern and Oscar Hammerstein II's *Show Boat* on Broadway, the London stage, and in the 1936 film. Adapted from Edna Ferber's book of the same name, *Show Boat* follows the lives of performers and workers on a Mississippi riverboat as it travels from town to town along the river. The musical, first produced in 1927, broke ground in its depiction of race, poverty, alcoholism, and the plight of Black workers, who find "no rest till the judgment day." Hal Prince, who directed the 1994 revival, said *Show Boat* had influenced everyone who ever wanted to work in musicals "because it was serious and because it was integrated and it was courageous."

Robeson's singing of "Ol' Man River" is the quick, and the throughline of *Show Boat*. Jerome Kern said he had conceived the melody after hearing Robeson speak, and "Ol' Man River" would be associated with Robeson from his first performance of it to his death. And since. The song shares qualities with spirituals; it is a song of burden, struggle, race, of workers "aching and racked with pain." "Ol' Man River" reprises at different points, as the musical threads its way through the years and lives of its characters. The river is all-seeing, indifferent, an ever-changing constant, and Robeson, said a critic, expressed "a sorrow which seemed to know no end."

Edna Ferber described the response of the audience when she saw Robeson perform in *Show Boat*. "I went in, leaned against the door and looked at the audience at the very moment when Paul Robeson came on to sing 'Ol' Man River.'" In all her years of going to the theater, she said, "I have never seen an ovation like that given any figure of the stage, the concert hall, or the opera." The audience "stood up and howled. They applauded and shouted and stamped." Then, she said, the show stopped. Robeson sang "Ol' Man River" once more. The show stopped again and, once again, the audience went wild. *Show Boat* changed musical theater and it changed the life of Paul Robeson. *Show Boat*, he said at the time, "is the most interesting thing I have done."

Robeson's acclaim on the dramatic stage was yet greater. His *Othello* continues to hold the Broadway record for the longest run of any production of Shakespeare. On opening night in 1943, observers wrote that the applause and "bravos" were deafening, and the number of curtain calls unprecedented. The audience, they said, "cheered the roof off." One prominent New York theater critic said that it was "one of the most memorable events in the history of the theater." Never in his life, he said, had he seen an audience "sit so still, so tense, so under the spell of what was taking place on the stage." Another reported that Robeson's *Othello* premiere was the moment when "the American theatre opened for the Negro people."

The Broadway production of *Othello* toured North America for two years. The audiences, Robeson wrote in *The American Scholar*, felt the play's contemporary power and "clash of cultures," its personal and universal tragedy:

> It was deeply fascinating to watch how strikingly contemporary American audiences from coast to coast found Shakespeare's *Othello*—painfully immediate in its unfolding of evil, innocence, passion, dignity and nobility, and contemporary in its overtones of a clash of cultures, of the partial acceptance of and consequent effect upon one of a minority group. Against this background the jealousy of the protagonist becomes more credible, the blows to his pride more understandable, the final collapse of his personal, individual world more inevitable. But beyond the personal tragedy, the terrible agony of Othello, the irretrievability of his world, the complete destruction of all his trusted and sacred values—all these suggest the shattering of a universe.

Robeson's art was personal and universal, no more so than in his singing of African American spirituals:

There is a balm in Gilead
to make the wounded whole;
There is a balm in Gilead
to heal the sin-sick soul.

Some times I feel discouraged,
and think my work's in vain.
But then the Holy Spirit
revives my soul again.

"My cradle song" is from Africa, Paul Robeson wrote; the music is "in my soul and in my hearing." In the Black churches and in his childhood home "there was a warmth of song. Songs of love and longing, songs of trials and triumphs, deep-flowing rivers and rollicking brooks, hymn-song and ragtime ballad, gospels and blues, and the healing comfort to be found in the illimitable sorrow of the spirituals . . . I heard these songs in the very sermons of my father. . . . The great, soaring gospels we love are merely sermons that are sung." Spirituals portrayed "the hopes of our people who faced the hardships of slavery," he said. "They suffered. They fled to God through their songs. They sang to forget their chains and misery. Even in darkness they looked to their songs to work out their destiny and carve their way to the promised land." The songs of the people—their spirituals, work songs, folk songs, gospel—are "sometimes of quiet meditation—sometimes of momentary thunder—sometimes of terrifying beauty for the faint of heart. Songs bursting through the bar-lines, calling for love . . . for freedom."

Robeson's friend, the historian, activist, and sociologist W.E.B. Du Bois, wrote in "The Sorrow Songs" that spirituals come from sorrow but they have within them also the power of comfort. Sorrow can give way to hope and faith:

They that walked in darkness sang songs in the olden days—Sorrow Songs—for they were weary at heart. . . . [They] tell in word and music of trouble and exile, of strife and hiding; they grope toward some unseen power and sigh for rest in the End. . . .

Through all the sorrow of the Sorrow Songs there breathes a hope—a faith in the ultimate justice of things. The minor cadences of despair change often to triumph and calm confidence. Sometimes it is faith in life, sometimes, a faith in death, sometimes assurance of boundless justice in some fair world beyond.

The spirituals came from a deep place; in times of suffering they could be summoned for solace. To the questions of Jeremiah—"Is there no balm in Gilead? / Is there no physician there?"—Robeson answered through his art. Spirituals were born in pain; they could alleviate pain. Music, Robert Burton had written, is the "sovereign remedy against despair and melancholy." It is a "tonick to the saddened soul," a balm to the wounded.

When Paul Robeson was in his thirties he visited Canterbury Cathedral in England, a place of towering stone and glass, the site of Thomas Becket's martyrdom, and of the miracles claimed from Becket's blood. The miracles, rendered into the stained glass windows, were of healing the mind, as well as the body. Robeson, his son recounts, went to the foot of the altar and stood in silence, "lost in his own reverie." Then he looked upward and, with his head thrown back, began to sing. The desolate beauty of "Were You There (When They Crucified My Lord)" filled the cathedral.

"He seemed transfixed by the fusion of his own spirituality and the majesty of the surroundings," said his son. So too were the other visitors to the cathedral, caught by surprise, and privy to an extraordinary gift of private beauty made open. "Were You There"—the first spiritual to be published in a major American hymnal, that of the Episcopal Church— was one of the earliest spirituals recorded by Robeson. When Robeson sang this "old plantation song," a critic wrote, it was with "emotional burning." It was "elemental, agonizingly poignant . . . as startling and vivid a disclosure of reverent feeling of penetrating pathos as one could imagine."

Spirituals were in the blood for Robeson. Instinct and intuition, the power of music and the irrational, had been eclipsed by rationality, he said. Somewhere we lost the substance:

> Somewhere, sometime—perhaps at the Renaissance, but I think much earlier—a great part of Religion went astray. A blind groping after Rationality resulted in an incalculable loss in pure Spirituality. Mankind placed a sudden dependence on that part of his mind that was brain, intellect, to the discountenance of that part that was sheer evolved instinct and intuition; we grasped at the shadow and lost the substance . . . and now we are not even altogether clear what the substance was.

Paul Robeson, in 1925, was the first soloist to perform an entire concert program of spirituals and Black secular songs. By the 1930s and 1940s he was the leading concert singer in the world. "He is without doubt," W.E.B. Du Bois said, "the best known American on earth, to the largest number of human beings. His voice is known in Europe, Asia and Africa, in the West Indies and South America and in the islands of the seas."

As his fame spread Robeson put his success at risk in order to pursue justice for those who had been left behind. Spirituals and folk songs fueled his political and social activism. "My art is a weapon in the struggle for my people's freedom and the freedom of all people," he told a meeting of workers. "I mean to continue as long as the breath stirs within me." "Why should we not sing during war?" Lloyd George had asked his fellow Welshmen at the Eisteddfod during the First World War. "War means sorrow. Darkness has fallen . . . but it has been ordained that the best singer amongst the birds of Britain should give its song in the night, and according to legend that sweet song is one of triumph over pain." Song could heal; it could unite and defy: "Why should we not sing?"

⟋

I am a citizen of the world as well as a singer, and I have the right to say what I think.

—PAUL ROBESON, 1939

Paul Robeson's political activism came early to him and grew as he grew. It was inevitable. His father's life bore witness to the human cost of slavery and, once he had escaped, to the human cost of racism in the North. Robeson knew racism well himself. As a child in Princeton, he said, he had lived "for all intents and purposes on a Southern plantation. And with no more dignity than that suggests—all the bowing and scraping to the drunken rich, all the vile names, all the Uncle Tomming to earn enough to lead miserable lives." In sports at Rutgers, he had been taunted, attacked, cleated, and slurred.

He was admired and well-liked, but still he was excluded from close relationships with white students. He was not allowed to attend social functions or travel with the glee club. "There was a clear line beyond which one did not pass," he wrote forty years after his college years at Rutgers. He was denied accommodation by hotels and restaurants, seated at tables away from public view, or made to eat in the kitchen, and told to take the freight elevator rather than the public one. He gave up the practice of law after a stenographer refused to take dictation from a Black man and his law firm told him that his race would keep him from succeeding as an attorney. He received death threats. Most film roles that he was offered were stereotypic and demeaning. During a social conversation with a psychiatrist in the late 1940s, Robeson remarked that he found it difficult to "control his rage over a lifetime of feeling and being treated as an inferior." Robeson was a "very proud person and unable to tolerate humiliation," the doctor observed. What he had experienced was "a pain so intense he felt it could kill him."

Other people, Robeson made clear on many occasions, had it far worse than he did. They faced poverty as well as prejudice, and they'd had neither the joy he had in his work, nor the acknowledgment. The dehumanizing Jim Crow laws, unchecked racism in the United States, and flagrant injustice against workers and minority groups grew intolerable. He used his concert performances to express his political beliefs and to raise money for social causes. He was unwilling to wait for change that was too long and too little in the coming:

> We must wait, we are told, until the hearts of those who persecute us have softened—until Jim Crow dies of old age. This idea is called "Gradualism." It is said to be a practical and constructive way to achieve the

blessings of democracy for colored Americans. But the idea itself is but another form of race discrimination: in no other area of our society are lawbreakers granted an indefinite time to comply with the provisions of law. There is nothing in the 14th and 15th Amendments, the legal guarantees of our full citizenship rights, which says that the Constitution is to be enforced "gradually" where Negroes are concerned.

Patience wears thin, he said. "It is easy for the folks on the top to take a calm, philosophical view and to tell those who bear the burden to restrain themselves and wait for justice to come." Robeson would not wait. "How long?" he asked. "*As long as we permit it.*"

In June 1937, Paul Robeson spoke and sang at a fundraiser to benefit refugee children from the Spanish Civil War. The event, held at the Royal Albert Hall in London, was sponsored by artists and intellectuals who supported the Republican cause in Spain, including Virginia Woolf, Henry Moore, E. M. Forster, H. G. Wells, and W. H. Auden; Picasso donated a drawing for the front cover of the program. Robeson's fiery speech was wildly cheered by the audience and described by the British and international newspapers as the most powerful and moving part of the evening. His remarks, his credo, that the artist must be an active voice in society and serve as its conscience, that the artist must be passionately engaged in the fight against fascism, set down a marker:

> Every artist, every scientist, must decide *now* where he stands. He has no alternative. There is no standing above the conflict on Olympian heights. There are no impartial observers. Through the destruction—in certain countries—of the greatest of man's literary

heritages, through the propagation of false ideas of racial and national superiority, the artist, the scientist, the writer is challenged. The battlefront is everywhere. There is no sheltered rear.

The challenge must be taken up. Time does not wait. The course of history can be changed, but not halted. Fascism fights to destroy the culture which society has created; created through pain and suffering. . . .

The artist must take sides. He must elect to fight for freedom or slavery. I have made my choice. I had no alternative.

At the end of his speech, Robeson sang "Ol' Man River" and ended it with words he had substituted for the original lyrics from *Show Boat*. Instead of "I gets weary and sick of tryin' / I'm tired of livin' and scared of dyin'," he sang, "I must keep fightin' / Until I'm dyin'." Robeson, and the power of the song that for so many defined him, had a message that carried. Harry Belafonte, the singer and activist, was to say later that Paul Robeson taught him that "the purpose of art is not just to show life as it is, but to show life as it should be. And that if art were put into the service of the human family, it could only enhance their betterment."

In 1938, Robeson traveled to Spain to support the Republican forces and to sing for soldiers in the field. At one point the fighting stopped while troops on both sides drew quiet and listened to him sing. He campaigned and sang for many groups, including trade unionists, longshoremen, cooks and stewards, miners, civil rights activists, anti-colonialists, anti-apartheid activists, and the Aboriginal Australians. He was active in establishing an alliance between Blacks and American Jews, as well as contributing to the anti-fascist movement in other ways. He supported Jewish publications that fought fascism. He created and led the American Crusade Against Lynching to protest the murder of thousands of Blacks, to protest the escalation in mob rule, and to prevent Ku Klux Klan members from election to Congress.

In September 1946, on the anniversary of Lincoln's preliminary Emancipation Proclamation, Robeson and other activists met in the White House with President Truman. The president objected to Robeson's unbending language on the federal government's inaction about lynching, and to Robeson's statement that it "seemed inept for the United States to take the lead in the Nuremberg trials and fall so far behind in respect to justice to Negroes in this country." When Truman told the petitioners that the United States and England were the "last refuge of freedom in the world," Robeson pointed out that England had been "one of the greatest enslavers of human beings in history." He warned that Blacks could not promise the patience counseled by the government. Truman ended the meeting. (The Emmett Till Antilynching Act, which makes lynching a federal hate crime, was signed into law in 2022, more than seventy-five years after Robeson met with President Truman.) In 1951, Robeson and other activists presented a petition, "We Charge Genocide," to the United Nations. It accused the United States government of being in violation of the U.N. Genocide Convention by turning a blind eye to lynching

Robeson's temperament and thinking were more in line with Frederick Douglass than with those who cautioned a slower pace. "If there is no struggle there is no progress," Douglass said before the Civil War. "Those who profess to favor freedom and yet deprecate agitation are men who want crops without plowing up the ground; they want rain without thunder and lightning." Robeson had no problem plowing up the ground.

It was not long, however, before Robeson's left-wing political causes and his increasingly open support for the Soviet Union made him a target of Senator Joseph McCarthy, the FBI, and the House Un-American Activities Committee. In his autobiography, *Here I Stand*, Robeson explained his refusal either to acknowledge or to deny membership in the Communist Party, a statement demanded by the government. The question was un-American, he said, and to answer it would be a betrayal of American values. "In 1946, at a legislative hearing in California, I testified under oath that I was not a member of the Communist Party, but since then I have refused to give testimony or to sign affidavits as to that fact. . . . An important issue of Constitutional rights was involved in the making of such inquiries." In fact, there is not evidence that he was ever a member of the Communist Party.

The government was unrelenting. They revoked his passport in 1950 and the FBI kept him under surveillance for decades. They tapped his telephone, monitored his daily activities, and took down the license plate numbers of those who attended his concerts. They obtained access to his medical and legal records. He was blacklisted for years; he could not perform in concert halls or record his music. From 1949 to 1950 alone, eighty-five of his concerts were canceled. He went from being the best-paid concert singer in the world to earning little. Without a passport he could not travel to Europe, where his audiences had been overflowing and enthusiastic. The surveillance, blacklisting, and revocation of Robeson's passport were undertaken by the American government despite the fact that he was never charged, arrested, or put on trial. "What they have done to Paul," said W.E.B. Du Bois, "has been the most cruel thing I have ever seen."

In 1956, Robeson was summoned to Washington to testify before the House Un-American Activities Committee. It was an unequal confrontation, the greater weight of intellect, integrity, and wit lying with Robeson's side of the table. A few of the exchanges:

Mr. Arens. Are you now a member of the Communist Party?
Mr. Robeson. Oh please, please, please.
[. . .]
Mr. Arens. Are you now a member of the Communist Party?
Mr. Robeson. Would you like to come to the ballot box when I vote and take out the ballot and see?
[. . .]
Mr. Robeson. You are the author of all of the bills that are going to keep all kinds of decent people out of the country.
The Chairman. No, only your kind.
Mr. Robeson. Colored people like myself . . . and just the Teutonic Anglo-Saxon stock would you let come in.
The Chairman. We are trying to make it easier to get rid of your kind.
[. . .]
Mr. Robeson. In Russia I felt for the first time like a full human being. . . . I did not feel the pressure of colored as I feel in this committee today.
Mr. Scherer. Why did you not stay in Russia?
Mr. Robeson. Because my father was a slave, and my people died to build this country, and I am going to stay here and have a part of it just like you. And no Fascist-minded people will drive me from it. Is that clear?

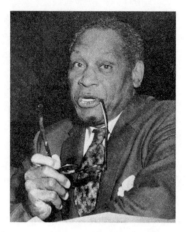

Paul Robeson in 1956
Testimony before the House Un-American
Activities Committee

*My father was a slave, and my people died to build
this country, and I am going to stay here and have
a part of it just like you. And no Fascist-minded
people will drive me from it. Is that clear?*

Inexplicably, while making clear his love for the Russian people, their music, and their open, very public love for him, Robeson never acknowledged Stalin's killing of more than one million of his own people. He would not talk about the purges at the congressional hearings nor to journalists. It is hard to understand why Robeson, who fought against fascism, which he abhorred, and against racism and other forms of oppression for most his life, would remain so silent. It is unlikely that he was not aware of Stalin's purges, even though Soviet officials tried to conceal the truth from him. He and many artists and intellectuals of the time took far too long to lose faith in a political state that was betraying their ideals.

The only thing wrong with Paul Robeson, W.E.B. Du Bois

had said, was "having too great faith in human beings." Like his father, Robeson was proud, private, and reluctant to discuss things close to his heart. He was disinclined to turn his back on his beliefs and dreams, however unrealized; all the more so because he knew that his criticism would be used by those who had tried to silence him. He made this clear in his congressional testimony. "Whatever has happened to Stalin, gentlemen," he said to the committee members interrogating him, "is a question for the Soviet Union. . . . You are responsible and your forebears for 60 million to 100 million Black people dying in the slave ships and on the plantations, and don't you ask me about anybody, please."

Robeson, not always a man at peace, had found a measure of peace and acceptance in his trips to the Soviet Union and he felt strong affinity for Russian culture, folk songs, and music. The Russian people opened their hearts to him with warmth of a kind he had not known. Mountain climbers discovered a new peak in a land of apricot trees, glaciers, and snow leopards; the mountain was named for him, Mount Robeson. The Russian people loved and appreciated him and his art. This acceptance had not been his experience for most of his life. On his way by train in 1934 to visit the Soviet Union for the first time, Robeson spent a day in transit in Berlin. Stormtroopers glared at him with open revulsion and hatred. Marie Seton, a film critic who was traveling with Robeson, described his "terrible fury struggling with a desperate fear." He was trembling with fear and anger, she said. "This is like Mississippi," he told her. "It's how a lynching begins" (see photo section).

In Moscow, he was in a different world. He went to Pushkin Square, one of the busiest city squares in the world, and looked up for a long time at the statue of Russia's national poet, Alexander Pushkin. Pushkin was the great-grandson of a slave and it was said that his "Negro blood had given a vast empire its tongue of today." "Could I find a monument to Pushkin in a public square in Birmingham or Atlanta or Memphis, as one stands in the center of Moscow?" Robeson asked. "No. One perhaps to Goethe, but not to the dark-skinned Pushkin." (Once, when Robeson was asked in a radio interview why his spoken Russian was flawless, he said that he "had family in the Soviet Union." The interviewer looked startled until Robeson laughed and said, "Alexander Pushkin of course.") Later, he played in the snow with young children, who "fell in love with him on sight." They grabbed his hands, tried to climb up his towering body, and were dismayed that he had to leave, that he no longer could play with him. "They have never been told to fear black men," Robeson told Marie Seton. "I would like [my son] to come here; it would protect him from being hurt." Regardless of the Soviet leaders, there was a bond between Robeson and the Russian people that was in all ways contrary to his experience in Berlin. And America.

He explained some of this to Russian filmmaker Sergei Eisenstein. "Maybe you'll understand—I feel like a human being for the first time since I grew up. Here I am not a Negro but a human being. Before I came I could hardly believe that such a thing could be. In a few days I've straightened myself out. Here, for the first time in my life I walk in full human dignity. You cannot imagine what that means to me as a Negro."

Helen Rosen, a progressive activist and wife of a prominent New York surgeon, one of Robeson's closest friends, spoke to his deeply affectionate and meaningful relationship with the Russian people. "I think he felt that he had walked there in dignity and respect, and there was something about the warmth of the Russian people and the language that he liked. . . . I think he'd had sort of this idea of what the world could be, and he thought that maybe it was going to happen there and probably was vastly disappointed. But if he had spoken out against [them] in his time, it might have seemed as if he were praising some of the things in America which he abhorred. But he wouldn't join the crowd in that anti-Soviet way."

In 1958, the Supreme Court ruled that the government could not deny a passport to any American citizen because of belief or association and Robeson's world reopened, at least for a while. He published *Here I Stand* and performed before wildly enthusiastic audiences in California, Chicago, and New York's Carnegie Hall. He went on an extended concert tour of London, Wales, Europe, the Soviet Union, Australia, and New Zealand. He received awards, honorary degrees, and tributes for his work as an artist and activist. Those who had been silent when they could have spoken up, spoke now.

In 1963, fifteen years before he died, he retired from public performances on account of poor health. He rarely sang in front of an audience again.

$\sim$

. . . the irretrievability of his world, the complete destruction of all his trusted and sacred values—all these suggest the shattering of a universe.

—PAUL ROBESON, 1945

When Paul Robeson retired from public singing, his health had been deteriorating for several years, eroded by unrelenting government persecution, the State Department's refusal to issue him a passport, FBI surveillance, and blacklisting. The shame and restrictions imposed by the government were all the more powerful for being inflicted on someone who was particularly proud, who delighted in people and performing, and who was vulnerable to depression. Helen Rosen said that the "conspiracy of the government to make him and keep him a nonperson was very successful. A man who loved to sing, who loved people, loved to travel, loved to learn, to give, was very much kept down, enslaved in a way. . . . I think he had a streak of sadness in him which was engaged and increased with the years. . . . And that [sadness] had a tendency to reappear, that kind of streak of sadness as he grew older." ("I'm a very melancholy person by nature," Robeson had told a journalist many years before.)

Robeson's struggle with depression began most recognizably in 1931 when he was a young man acting in a Eugene O'Neill play in London. One evening after a performance, he unexplainably began to yell; suffering from "strain and nerves" and exhaustion, he was admitted to a nursing home for a week. The next year, following a romantic breakup with the woman he described as the one he most loved in his life, he refused to see anyone for six weeks, would not go out or talk to anyone, and stayed alone in his room with the curtains drawn. Yolande Jackson, a British actress, his besetting passion, told him that she would not marry him because he was Black. (He had made plans to divorce his wife, Eslanda Robeson, a highly accomplished anthropologist, chemist, and civil rights activist; she managed Robeson's concert and acting career, but not his heart.) Rejection by Jackson was devastating. He came very close to killing himself, a friend said.

In 1956, Robeson had a "complete emotional collapse," later to be diagnosed as manic-depressive illness, now known as bipolar disorder. He was manic, agitated, delusional, and disheveled. He became obsessed with developing a universal music theory and was convinced that he could solve the riddles of Bach, and thereby the problems of the world. This period of frenzied expansiveness, impulsiveness, and agitation was followed by a deep depression. Thereafter, his moods continued to swing erratically, with periods of incessant talking, struck through with uncharacteristic boasting and self-absorption; these periods were interspersed with exhaustion, despair, and paranoia.

In 1961, Paul Robeson cut his wrists in a hotel room and was found on the bathroom floor "semiconscious and incoherent." "One could see the scars," Helen Rosen recalled later. "I used to feel them and they were so obvious, the scars, but we never talked about it." He was admitted to a hospital for several months and treated with antipsychotic medications, but it was not long before he relapsed, to be found "huddled in a fetal position, tangled up in the bedsheets, positively cowering in fear." Robeson's illness grew worse. He was admitted to hospitals in England, the Soviet Union, Germany, and the United States.

One admission, which was involuntary, was to the Priory Hospital in London, where he was diagnosed with "endogenous depression in a manic-depressive personality," a descriptive if not recognized diagnosis. (His physician wrote in his clinical notes that Robeson was a "cyclothymic personality," who had been throughout his marriage "morose, depressed and elated at times." His admitting diagnosis was "chronic depressive state with severe delusional background with marked apprehension." Robeson, according to his doctor, was suicidal as well.) He was agitated, profoundly depressed, and had delusional thoughts about being unworthy. He received an extended series of electroconvulsive (electroshock) treatments, or ECT, which was then, and is still, the treatment of choice for delusional bipolar depression. He was given more than fifty ECT treatments, which relieved his symptoms, but only in the short term. At different times and in different hospitals, Robeson received insulin coma therapy; chlorpromazine and other antipsychotic medications; barbiturates in high doses; multiple drugs for sleep and agitation; and several kinds of antidepressants. The antipsychotic medications prescribed to him were often in heavy doses, presumably to control or to prevent mania. It is not clear from the record. There is no indication that he was prescribed lithium, although it would have been available during the latter years of his life.

Robeson said that he could not imagine getting well, that he expected just to "wither away." He continued to lose weight, sleep poorly, and to experience periods of deep depression—lethargy, withdrawal, apathy, suicidal thinking and behavior, and agitation—followed by times when he engaged with friends and seemed himself. On his sixty-fifth birthday—agitated and insistent that he would never be able to sing or speak in public again—he said, "I'll never be well. . . . Maybe some sympathetic understanding doctor will give me something." Two years later his son found him in his bedroom, "his face blank with terror, holding a double-edge razor."

Robeson passed the final ten years of his life living with his sister in Philadelphia. He went out seldom, and was visited by only close friends and members of his family. Not long before he died, Robeson told his son, "I'm just putting in time, waiting to go. I would have checked myself out long ago, but for you, the grandchildren, the family and the public. Anyway, if this is the way I'm to pay for my sins, so be it." The FBI, still tracking him, wrote in their field notes that he was "very ill."

Toward the end of Robeson's life, Harry Belafonte visited him in Philadelphia. "I looked at him, and I said, 'Paul, I must know. Was all that you have gone through really worth it? Considering the platform you had gained, and how easy life could have been for you, was it worth it?' And he said, 'Harry, make no mistake: there is no aspect of what I have done that wasn't worth it. Although we may not have achieved all the victories we set for ourselves—beyond the victory itself, infinitely more important, was the journey.'" Robeson's journey continued through the lives of others. John Lewis, who had been beaten nearly to death at Selma, one of the great moral leaders of the civil rights movement, approached Helen Rosen and asked to meet Robeson: "Would you introduce me to Paul Robeson?" he asked her. "That would be the greatest thing that could ever happen to me." When Lewis finally met Robeson, he said, "Paul, this all started from you."

Robeson's life was one of great gift, marked by a generous but broken realization of that gift, an infectious joy, love and deep friendships, courage, and purpose. It was also a life of not infrequent pain and, as he had written about *Othello*, the shattering of a universe. Most lastingly it was the life of a serious man, as W.H.R. Rivers would have it, a life given to the common good. Robeson inspired and gave balm to those who suffered more than he. He healed through his example and music. He accompanied the vulnerable. "He knew the price he would have to pay and he paid it," his son, Paul Robeson, Jr., said. "He never regretted the stands he took "because almost forty years ago, in 1937, he made his basic choice. He said then, 'The artist must elect to fight for freedom or slavery. I have made my choice. I had no alternative.'"

Going home, going home, I'm a going home;
Quiet-like, some still day, I'm just going home.
It's not far, just close by,
Through an open door.

Paul Robeson died in January 1976, when he was seventy-seven years old. Five thousand people came to his funeral on a rainy winter night in Harlem. It was held at the Mother AME Zion Church, founded in 1796, Robeson had said, by "free Negroes who refused to be part of the church of the Christian slaveholders." Sojourner Truth had been an early member, and Frederick Douglass and Harriet Tubman had "played their part in the freedom-striving tradition of this church." Robeson's brother had been pastor at the church for nearly thirty years, and Robeson, a member, had given concerts there to pay down the mortgage. Harlem and Mother AME Zion Church had been sanctuary to him; for a year he had lived in his brother's parsonage. Elsewhere, he said, he had heard the "baying of the lynch-mob, the cries for my life shrilled from hate-twisted mouths," but in Harlem he felt the "caress of love." He was known and held there with value and affection: " 'Hello, Paul—it's good to see you!' the people say as I walk in their midst and as they take my hand in theirs."

In his eulogy for Paul Robeson, the presiding bishop said, "He bore on his body marks of vengeance." He likened him to Saint Paul, who carried the marks of whip and shipwreck and had proclaimed, "Henceforth, let no man trouble me, for I bear on my body the marks of Jesus." Years earlier, Robeson's brother had cast his brother as martyr and healer: "Paul is medicine to me—the music of his soul has cured me of many maladies." Their father's death and "the war with its shattering of dreams [have] plunged him into the depths of something he is just now beginning to fathom. . . . He is bearing the cross of a despised, oppressed and neglected people; he is voicing the heartaches of the years that he has seen." It is written in Isaiah: "He hath borne our griefs, and carried our sorrow," and by his wounds are we redeemed. By his suffering, the pastor seemed to say, we are healed. And by his art.

A soloist sang a hymn that had been sung achingly, beautifully, by Robeson. Its refrain speaks to the end of the journey, and to weariness known. At its heart are the words from Saint Matthew: "Well done, thou good and faithful servant." Well done.

> *Oh, when I come to the end of my journey,*
> *Weary of life and the battle is won;*
> *Carrying the staff and the cross of redemption,*
> *He'll understand, and say, "Well done."*

Pallbearers carried Paul Robeson's coffin out of the church; as they did, his voice singing "Deep River" came over the loudspeakers, a spiritual, as he had said, of "illimitable sorrow."

Paul Robeson was the first Black person to stand behind the lectern of St. Paul's Cathedral in London. It was in October 1958; four thousand people packed the cathedral, five thousand more listened outside. Robeson sat in the front row for the evening service. He was led three times by the verger to the lectern, first to read from the Old Testament, twice to sing. His voice, a journalist wrote, "soared 100 feet high to the very roof of the great Dome, to the farthest shadowed corners."

Robeson's long fingers rested on the lectern and now and

again his foot tapped in rhythm as he sang a selection of spirituals: "We Are Climbing Jacob's Ladder" and "Go Down,
Moses," "Sometimes I Feel Like a Motherless Child," "Balm
in Gilead." No one coughed, it was said. No child fidgeted,
no pages rustled. The choir boys were unearthly still, caught
in the moment. So too was Robeson. In the vestry after the
service he said to the group assembled there, "This has been
one of the great honors of my life." It was "a wonderful thing
for me . . . something I shall never forget. I am close to tears."

Beneath Robeson as he sang was the crypt of St. Paul's,
holding the tombs of Nelson, Wellington, and Christopher
Wren, the architect of the cathedral. The epitaph for Wren
ends: *Here in its foundations lies the architect of this church and
city, Christopher Wren, who lived beyond ninety years, not for his
own profit but for the public good. Reader, if you seek his monument, look around you.*

Paul Robeson's monument lies in many places. It lies in
the thousands who listened to him in St. Paul's that evening
in the heart of White Establishment Protestantism, and it
lies with those to whom he lent his voice and time and power.
It lies in those who had been forgotten, but whose memory
he kept, and in those he helped to heal of America's original
sin. It lies with the beaten and the lynched. Paul Robeson was
a wounded healer, and the more powerful because of that.
His monument lies with the artists and activists he inspired,
and the tens of thousands of others to whom he gave strength
and hope. "Get them to sing your song," he told Harry Belafonte. "They will want to know who you are. And if they
want to know who you are, you've gained the first step in
bringing truth and bringing insight that might help people
get through this rather difficult world."

"You never gave up your song," Pablo Neruda wrote in
his ode to Paul Robeson. "Man stumbled and you lifted him."

Gwendolyn Brooks, too, wrote of Robeson's bonds to humanity: "The major Voice. / The adult Voice . . . / Warning, in music-words / devout and large, / that we are each other's / harvest: / we are each other's / business: / we are each other's magnitude and bond." When Robeson died, Andrew Young, the first Black to represent the United States as ambassador to the United Nations, said, "I can never forget . . . the magnificent voice that helped to soothe our collective sorrow. I can never forget the melodious words that helped to sweep away our bitter tears. I can never forget the strength of conviction that helped to stiffen our backs."

"We know enough of history," Paul Robeson said, "to be aware that great cultures do not completely die, but are soil for future growths." Inspiring where hope and purpose are lost enriches that soil of future growth; it stiffens the back and gives strength to face pain in the moment and in times to come. Lives tangle and touch one another. We stay long enough, Robert Lowell wrote, "to pass something on that someone else catches by his fingertips."

Robeson's father had passed on his convictions to his son. Throughout his life Robeson continued to ask, "What would Pop think?" Margaret Burroughs, an artist, teacher, and the founder of Chicago's DuSable Museum of African American History, said much the same about Robeson's influence upon her when she was a young woman. "Whenever faced by grave and serious decisions, I would ask myself: What would Paul Robeson do or decide in this case? What would Paul Robeson think of this? What side of the question would Paul Robeson take?"

Robeson's monument also lay in a young Los Angeles girl who became a poet, Leah Zazulyer. Confused and conflicted about being a Jew in the years following World War II, she attended a Paul Robeson concert with her parents. Robeson, she remembers, spoke for a while, and then sang spirituals and folk songs. "To my utter amazement," Zazulyer recalled, "he began to sing all the Jewish songs I had ever heard my Mother sing to me at bedtime, or softly to herself at the kitchen sink! He who spoke perfect English was singing in Yiddish":

> As he sang, I forgot. About Hitler, about McCarthy. As the Yiddish proverb says, "He crawled into my heart with both feet," and in so doing displaced much, somehow making room for me to forgive my enemies, love my parents, their friends, their stories, their language, and myself.

"It was a sort of power of getting into another man's life and treating it as if it were his own," a colleague had said about W.H.R. Rivers. "And yet all the time he made you feel that your life was your own to guide, and above everything that you could if you cared make something important of it." A trade unionist who met Paul Robeson described the "warmth and love" he felt from him, even in a brief encounter. Robeson, he said, "stands like a giant, yet makes you feel, without stooping to you, that you too are a giant and hold the power of making history in your hands as well." When Robeson died, Bill Brown, a Black prisoner in Illinois, wrote about Paul Robeson's constancy and courage and how they lived on in him. He enclosed a poem in a letter he gave to a judge:

> *They knocked the leaves*
> *From his limbs,*
> *The bark*
> *From his*
> *Tree*

But his roots
were
so deep
That they are
a part of me.

"They looked to their songs to work out their destiny," Robeson said of those who sang the spirituals born in "anguish and longing." They looked to their songs "to carve their way to the promised land."

We all look in our different ways to find the way back from pain, to find the way to peace and redemption. We look for purpose, for the rock that is higher than us. We look to healers for courage and the way forward. We look to them for convoy and toughness, for knowledge and humanity. We seek the balm in Gilead that makes the wounded whole.

CHAPTER 10

Ashen Roots

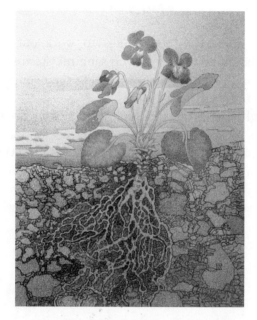

By ashen roots the violets blow.

—Alfred, Lord Tennyson,
In Memoriam

We obtained in the island of Eddystone a long account
of the destination of man after death. We were told
that he stays in the neighbourhood of the place where
he died for a certain time until spirits arrive in their
canoes from a distant island inhabited by the dead to
fetch the ghost to his new home.

—W.H.R. RIVERS, 1912,
"THE PRIMITIVE CONCEPTION OF DEATH"

Siegfried Sassoon and W.H.R. Rivers outlived the war.
When armistice was declared in November 1918, Sassoon was walking through the Oxford water-meadow. It was
"impossible to realise," he wrote in his diary. "A jolly peal
of bells was ringing from the village church . . . the war is
ended." He stood still for a while, "with a blank mind, listening to the bells which announced our deliverance," and
then made his way to London to observe the celebration. He
was appalled by the "outburst of mob patriotism," and the
"masses of people in streets and congested Tubes, all waving
flags and making fools of themselves." Like many who had
fought in the war, he felt the uncrossable distance between
himself and those who had not. He believed his jaded reaction to armistice carried a certain "moral authority" because
he had served at the Front, but it put him at odds with the
exuberant celebration of his countrymen. "It was a wretched
wet night, and very mild," he wrote. "It is a loathsome ending
to the loathsome tragedy of the last four years."

W.H.R. Rivers was in his mid-fifties when armistice
was declared. Sassoon dined with him in London the next
evening and they talked about the celebrations of the night
before. Rivers, he said, was "an ideal moderator of victorious

agitations. He had watched the wild scenes in the streets with ethnological eyes. It was more or less what he'd expected, he remarked, while admitting that mass-emotion was definitely overdoing it." Years of treating the shell-shocked and the insane had left him, like Sassoon, disinclined to celebrate.

Rivers returned to Cambridge after the war to teach and write. He and Sassoon kept in touch, occasionally dining together in London or Cambridge. In early June 1922, Rivers was suddenly taken ill in his rooms at St. John's College and died in the hospital the next day. Sassoon was shattered. "I feel / His influence undiminished," he wrote in a poem dedicated to Rivers: "And his life's work, in me and many, unfinished / . . . Selfless and ardent, resolute and gay, / So in this hour, in strange survival stands / Your ghost, whom I am powerless to repay." The night before Rivers's funeral, he wrote down in his diary the final lines of Hardy's novel *The Woodlanders:* "For he was a good man, and did good things."

~

The funeral of Rivers was held on an early June afternoon in 1922 in St. John's College Chapel in Cambridge. An anthropologist and the son of a priest, Rivers had maintained a keen interest in the rites of death, including those he chose for himself. The procession through the college grounds had been rehearsed by several of his closest friends. "It was a day of brilliant sunshine and cool breezes," wrote Sassoon on the evening of Rivers's funeral. "The single bell tolled at long intervals. . . . There was a hush. And then, while we all stood up, from the college courts there came a sound of distant singing. As the procession entered the chapel, the singing swelled to a joyous triumph. It was all up with me as soon as I heard that music." The coffin, covered in crimson pall, was followed by young men carrying wreaths. The ceremony, Sassoon said, was sublime. The "whole college seemed to be absolutely one with the ceremony. It had lost something which was an intense factor in its communal existence. But, in the presence of death, it was alive."

Rivers is buried in a Cambridge graveyard close to other great names of Cambridge—explorers, classicists and mathematicians, astronomers and philosophers—in the midst of beech and lime trees, and yews, symbol of death and resurrection. The inscription on his gravestone, at the foot of a Celtic cross, is simple:

WILLIAM

HALSE RIVERS RIVERS

FELLOW OF ST. JOHN'S COLLEGE

BORN MARCH 12TH 1864

DIED JUNE 4TH 1922

The epitaph gives no notion of what Rivers did in his life, what fields he pioneered, what he taught, or what minds he saved. His contributions to anthropology, psychology, and medicine, regarded as groundbreaking while he was alive, are less remembered now. Indeed, advances in science and medicine are inevitably overtaken. Methods improve and new ideas supplant standing theories. What do survive are the names of those healers who, by personality, intrepid intellect, clinical acuity, character, and integrity, made their world a notably better place.

Healers like W.H.R. Rivers and William Osler take on a legendary quality less for their contributions in the sciences than for their influence on the minds and lives of those they cared for and taught. Great doctors are remembered for extraordinary clinical skills and for teaching that leaves an abiding mark. Their work is kept alive through the practice and writing of others. Rivers had his Boswell in Sassoon, who captured for generations how an extraordinary doctor in extraordinary times changed him and gave him purpose. The poet repaid his debt.

Rivers, Sassoon wrote, "exists only in vigilant and undiminished memories, continuously surviving in what he taught me." Rivers had made him aware of the desultory nature of his life before the war, Sassoon wrote, brought him to recognize the shallowness of an existence centered on country houses, cricket, and fox-hunting. "He had shown that he believed me to be capable of achieving something useful. He had set me on the right road and made me feel that if the War were to end to-morrow I should be starting on a new life's journey." Rivers had taught him that "a strenuous effort must be made to take some small share in the real work of the world."

"Every Toda has two funerals," Rivers observed in his study of the Nilgiri Hills people of southern India. "Soon after death the body is burned with many ceremonies, and this is known as the 'green funeral.' Weeks or months later certain relics from the first occasion—some hair and a piece of skull—are burned and the ashes buried, and this is called the 'dry funeral.'" The rituals of death, extended over time— the sacrifice of a sacred buffalo; music and dancing; feasting— sustain the spiritual presence of the dead. To be burned once and then a second time would seem final. But it is not the end, and what remains lasts.

Rivers had died, but for Siegfried Sassoon, he was, in his pervasive influence, still alive. In a poem dedicated to Rivers, he wrote: "What voice revisits me this night? What face / To my heart's room returns? . . . Hastes he once more to harmonize and heal? / I know not. Only I feel / His influence undiminished." Undiminished. Again. Lasting. Healing. "*And still*

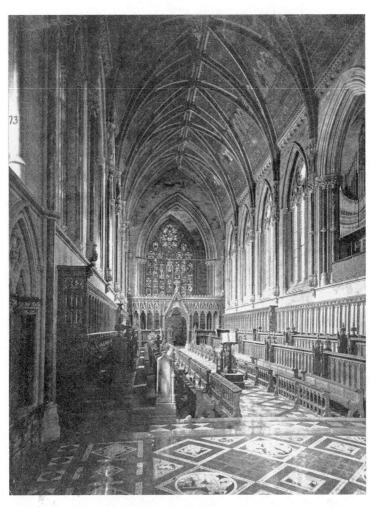

St. John's College Chapel, Cambridge

*He aroused in those who came into contact with him a passionate consciousness
of the significance of life and the beauty of organized knowledge.*

he comes uncalled to be my guide / In devastated regions / when the brain has lost its bearings in the dark."

It was likewise with Robert Graves, friend and fellow soldier of Sassoon, who had intervened with military authorities to send Sassoon to Craiglockhart War Hospital rather than held in prison or hanged for his statement protesting the war. Graves was a poet, novelist, and classicist and, like Sassoon, the author of a powerful war memoir, *Goodbye to All That*. In his book, a bitter, unsentimental account of war, atrocity, and death, Graves described a letter he had received from Sassoon quoting the French writer and war surgeon Georges Duhamel. "It was ordained that you should not suffer without purpose and without hope, but I will not let all your sufferings be lost in the abyss." For both Sassoon and Graves the trauma from the war lasted long after it had ended. For many others, it lasted a lifetime. Years after the armistice, T. E. Lawrence wrote to Graves asking why he, Graves, and Sassoon "can't get away from the War? Here you are riddled with thought like an old table-leg with worms." Sassoon was "yawing about like a ship aback . . . what's the matter with us all? It's like the malarial bugs in the blood, coming out months and years after in recurrent attacks."

Although Graves was never treated by Rivers, he consulted him after the war about his "black depressions" and recurrent fears of going mad. Rivers, whom Graves believed was "by far the greatest living psychiatrist," encouraged him to use the traumatic memories of his war experience, which he thought a likely wellspring for poetry, in his work. He told Graves that writing would help him heal. He was correct. Writing did help, and Graves felt a debt to Rivers for inspiring him—"still in a neurasthenic state from my own war experiences"—to write his "therapeutic poems."

Rivers taught Graves to see that shell shock gave him

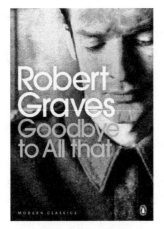

I will not let all your sufferings
be left in the abyss.

"special powers to draw upon as a poet," writes Miranda Seymour, a biographer of Robert Graves. "In Rivers' view, the neurasthenic state which [Graves] had tried to suppress was his most potent creative source. Pain was the key. The cure was to write out of his unconscious and then use the poems to examine his state of mind." Graves incorporated many of Rivers's ideas about psychology and psychotherapy into his writing about language and poetry, admiring the wide-ranging medical and anthropological scholarship that Rivers joined to scientific discipline. Graves dedicated his book *On English Poetry* to two of his time's most restless thinkers, both of whom had redrawn the borders of mind and country. "To T. E. Lawrence of Arabia and All Souls College, Oxford," Graves wrote, "and to W.H.R. Rivers of the Solomon Islands and St. John's College, Cambridge." (Rivers wrote to Graves that he was "delighted" with the dedication and to have it associated with that of Lawrence, "one of my heroes of the war.")

Graves, like Sassoon, was hit hard when Rivers died. Not long afterward he wrote a poem that drew back to the warmth, acceptance, and ease he had felt with Rivers:

I stood quite dumb, sunk fast in the mire,
  Lonely as the first man, or the last man,
  Chilled to despair since evening began,
Dazed for the memory of a lost desire.

But a voice said "Easily," and a voice said "Come!"
  Easily I followed with no thought of doubt,
  Turned to the right hand, and the way stretched out;
The ground held firmly; I was no more dumb.

For that was the place where I longed to be
  And past all hope there the kind lamp shone.

For Robert Graves and Siegfried Sassoon the death of Rivers, their "kind lamp" and doctor, was a break in the journey, but not the end. For Sassoon, it was the death of a doctor who had seen him through a conflicted war and a differently conflicted peace. He kept Rivers alive: in his memory and poetry, and, perhaps, most powerfully, through his war memoirs. Sassoon and Graves were able to engage with Rivers's mind and values through a shared world of literature, class, and tough expectation. But others, perhaps not so deft with symbol or metaphor, also benefited from Rivers's capacity to heal. The librarian at St. John's College, Cambridge, remembered Arnold Middlebrook, who served as a junior officer in the 4th Battalion of the East Yorkshire Regiment. "He was treated for shellshock by W.H.R.R. at Craiglockhart Hospital in September 1917," the librarian said, and had visited the library in 1963 and on at least two previous occasions. "Each time he asked to see the portrait of Rivers. He would stand, at the salute, and thank Rivers for all he did for him. On his last visit he was obviously in poor health and finished with the words 'goodbye my friend I don't suppose we shall ever meet again.'"

What does Keats have to teach me of rifle and machine-gun drill . . . how will Shelley show me how to hate or any poet teach me the trajectory of the bullet?

—WILFRED OWEN, 1916

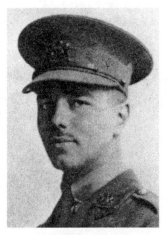

Lieutenant Wilfred Owen, 1916

These are men whose minds the Dead have ravished.

Very dear Siegfried . . . The boy by my side, shot through the head, lay on top of me, soaking my shoulder, for half an hour. . . . Can you photograph the crimson-hot iron as it cools from the smelting? That is what Jones's blood looked like, and felt like. My senses are charred. I shall feel again as soon as I dare, but now I must not. I don't take the cigarette out of my mouth when I write Deceased over their letters.

—WILFRED OWEN, 1918,
LETTER TO SIEGFRIED SASSOON

In June 1917 Wilfred Owen, widely regarded as the finest of the war poets, was admitted to Craiglockhart War Hospital suffering from shell shock. In France, asleep on a riverbank, Owen had been blown into the air by a shell that exploded not far from his head. He spent the next several days buried next to the dismembered remains of a fellow officer. Owen described the time leading up to the explosion and after: "For twelve days I did not wash my face, nor take off my boots, nor sleep a deep sleep. For twelve days we lay in holes, where at any moment a shell might put us out. . . . A big shell lit on the top of the bank just 2 yards from my head. Before I awoke, I was blown in the air right away from the bank! I passed most of the following days in a railway Cutting, in a hole just big enough to lie in." A brother officer lay opposite him covered in earth. "No relief will ever relieve him," Owen wrote. "Nor will his Rest be a 9 days-Rest." His body "lay in various places round about." The doctor who treated Owen at the time forbade him to go back into battle—"he is nervous about my nerves," Owen told his mother—and diagnosed him with neurasthenia. "My nerves," Owen noted, "have not come out without a scratch." He was not having a breakdown, he tried to reassure her, "simply *avoiding* one."

Not long afterward, Owen's commanding officer reported that Owen was shaking, confused, and behaving oddly. He was sent to the 13th Casualty Clearing Station and treated by Dr. William Brown, one of the leading specialists in trauma. (During his time as a doctor in France, Brown evaluated or treated between two and three thousand soldiers suffering from shell shock.) Brown's therapeutic philosophy, which he held in common with W.H.R. Rivers, included a deeply sympathetic attitude toward soldiers who had suffered severe trauma, which Brown described as the "petrification of terror," and the belief that long talks between doctor and patient would lead to greater self-knowledge and self-reliance. Like Rivers, Brown believed that expecting the patient to recover and imparting hope to him were essential to healing. And, like Captain A. J. Brock, who was to be Wilfred Owen's psychiatrist at Craiglockhart, Brown supported the "gospel of work."

Owen first met Siegfried Sassoon in August 1917 when both were patients in Craiglockhart. They differed in class, background, and temperament but were bound by books and writing, by having fought in the trenches, and by having known the responsibility of command. Their psychiatrists had different personalities, as well. Evaluations of the medical staff at Craiglockhart made these differences clear. Sassoon's doctor, W.H.R. Rivers, was described as warm, lively, highly respected, and affectionately regarded by staff and patients. He had a quick wit, and was notably gracious to those below him in rank. Owen's doctor, Arthur J. Brock, was different. Notes in the Craiglockhart Hospital records describe him as "Very tall, thin, hunched up shoulders, big blue hands, very chilly looking, with a long peaked nose that should have a drip at the point. High pitched voice suggestive of Arctic regions. Full of energy." Warmth and humor were not words that colleagues or patients used to describe A. J. Brock. Yet both doctors helped their patients. Rivers, as we have seen, shepherded Sassoon through his painful war experiences and his decision to return to the war. Psychotherapy was key to this, the "gospel of work" less so. Sassoon spent much of his time at Craiglockhart golfing, reading, and writing.

Captain Arthur Brock, son of a farmer and a poet, a Scot, translator of Galen, a humanist, and proponent of the "work cure," believed that it was vital for psychiatric patients to "go back to the land" and to engage in activities that would connect them more intimately to the world. Rigorous physical activity, long walks in the hills near Edinburgh, and direct contact with nature and the arts were central to his treatment of Owen. "The minds of these patients were fragmented," Brock wrote of his shell-shocked patients. "Their memories held such a painful content that they tended to let the past slip altogether." They lost their bearings and their contact with their world.

The basic clinical goal, as Brock saw it, was to rebuild the body and mind, grapple with the horror of war, and teach his patients once again to rely upon themselves. Brock believed that patients could cure themselves with hard work, purposeful activity, and a closer bond with nature. Work kept people alive, gave them a sustaining purpose. He was not alone among the war doctors in his enthusiasm for work therapy; many felt as he did, including Rivers to an extent. The chief psychiatric consultant in the American Expeditionary Force, Colonel Thomas Salmon, who stated that occupational therapy would "one day rank with anesthesia in taking the suffering out of sickness."

Not long after Wilfred Owen arrived at Craiglockhart, his letters home began to reflect his jammed days at the hospital. He belonged to the Natural History Club and was lecturing on topics such as "Do plants think?" and "Soil" and "Mosses in the District." "I held my own in the matter of Water Plants," he wrote to his mother. He had had tea with the Astronomer Royal, visited schools and slums and factories in Edinburgh, been swimming in the public bath, taught English literature to schoolboys, gardened, gone on group expeditions to the zoo, trekked in the hills and walked along the sea, gone to concerts and acted in plays, and taken on the editorship of *The Hydra*, the magazine of the Craiglockhart War Hospital.

Brock encouraged Owen in his poetry and pushed him to examine the causes of his breakdown and psychological trauma. Nightmares, he said, could be used by taking them into poetry; mastery of them could make art, and could help him heal. Like Rivers, Brock felt strongly that life was a serious enterprise and that it should be strenuously engaged. Like Rivers in his relationships with Sassoon and Graves, Brock encouraged Owen to put his suffering to use. Art should be more than a refuge, Brock believed; it should be a way back into life. At Brock's and Sassoon's urging, Owen increasingly wrote his terror and disillusion into his poetry. "In the powerful war-poems of Wilfred Owen," Brock wrote later, "we read the heroic testimony of one who[,] having in the most literal sense 'faced the phantoms of the mind' . . . had all but laid them ere the last call came; they still appear in his poetry but he fears them no longer."

When Wilfred Owen met Siegfried Sassoon at Craiglockhart, he was already in awe of, and in debt, to Sassoon's work. "Nothing like his trench life sketches has ever been written or ever will be written," Owen said in one of many bursts of admiration. Later, he wrote to Sassoon, "I held you as Keats + Christ + Elijah + my Colonel + my father-confessor" (a telling phrase, the one Sassoon applied to his own relationship with Rivers). Brock liked his patients to work in pairs, acting as one another's doctors. Sassoon did this with Owen in an informal way. In him, Owen found not only a friend and fellow poet, but someone as well who helped heal his mind. Sassoon urged him to face his war experiences head-on. He read Owen's poems with a critical but encouraging eye, and kept at him to strip his poems of language that softened the brutality of war. Owen, Sassoon reiterated, should write from the horror of his experience. This he did. In "Mental Cases," a poem about the mad and the madness of war, the atrocity of war, and those accountable for its hell, he wrote in part about the things he had seen in war and known at Craiglockhart:

> —*These are men whose minds the Dead have ravished.*
> *Memory fingers in their hair of murders,*
> *Multitudinous murders they once witnessed.*
> *Wading sloughs of flesh these helpless wander,*
> *Treading blood from lungs that had loved laughter.*
> *Always they must see these things and hear them,*
> *Batter of guns and shatter of flying muscles,*
> *Carnage incomparable, and human squander*
> *Rucked too thick for these men's extrication.*
>
> *Therefore still their eyeballs shrink tormented*
> *Back into their brains, because on their sense*
> *Sunlight seems a blood-smear; night comes blood-black;*
> *Dawn breaks open like a wound that bleeds afresh. . . .*

Sassoon's influence on Owen was deep but not entire. Owen was not new to suffering, nor innocent of how hard it was to heal the mind. He "put the suffering of his fellow soldiers front and centre," according to the poet Andrew Motion. In this he was like Sassoon. The poetry of Keats, Motion believes, persuaded Owen "long before the outbreak of the war that he needed to confront the brutal realities of experience, and to render them in ways that allowed him to become a physician [as Keats had been] to all men." The image of the poet as doctor is storied and powerful. "I came out in order to help these boys," Owen wrote, "directly by leading them as well as an officer can; indirectly, by watching their sufferings that I might speak of them as well as a pleader can." Owen, who demonstrated physical as well as moral courage, was awarded the Military Cross, as Sassoon had been, "for conspicuous gallantry and devotion to duty." But the critical thing for Owen was to put into words what he had experienced: to watch, to take on, to speak for the suffering and dying soldiers. It was to grieve for what might have been, what should have been.

From "Futility," written in 1918:

> *Move him into the sun—*
> *Gently its touch awoke him once,*
> *At home, whispering of fields unsown.*
> *Always it woke him, even in France,*
> *Until this morning and this snow.*

Both Owen and Sassoon wrote in the strange refuge of a shell shock hospital and protected time, wrote in the peculiar peace that Craiglockhart gave them. They wrote some of their best poetry during this period—away from the guns, under the care of good doctors and nurses, near the hills and sea, and in the company of one another. The therapeutic expectations of Captain Brock—that he live and write seriously; remake suffering into art, engage exuberantly with the world—made for a strikingly creative time for Owen. That Sassoon, too, took Owen seriously as a poet was critical. "And you have *fixed* my Life—however short," Owen wrote to him in November 1917, a few days after leaving Craiglockhart. "You did not light me: I was always a mad comet; but you have fixed me. I swung round you a satellite for a month, but I shall swing out soon, a dark star in the orbit where you will blaze." And so he did.

Siegfried Sassoon, W.H.R. Rivers, and A. J. Brock survived the war. Wilfred Owen did not. He returned to the Front and was killed in action in France a week before the war ended. The church bells in his village were ringing to celebrate armistice when the telegram arrived.

Earlier in the year, Owen had written to his mother about having at last become a poet, about his troops, and about the strange, incomprehensible faces of war:

> I go out of this year a Poet, my dear Mother, as which I did not enter it. I am held peer by the Georgians; I am a poet's poet.
>
> I am started. The tugs have left me; I feel the great swelling of the open sea taking my galleon.
>
> Last year . . . I lay awake in a windy tent in the middle of a vast, dreadful encampment. It seemed neither France nor England, but a kind of paddock where the beasts are kept a few days before the shambles. . . .
>
> I thought of the very strange look on all faces in that camp; an incomprehensible look. . . . It was not despair, or terror, it was more terrible than terror, for

it was a blindfold look, and without expression, like a dead rabbit's.

It will never be painted, and no actor will ever seize it. And to describe it, I think I must go back and be with them.

Six weeks before he was killed, Owen sent Sassoon the draft of what was to be his last poem. From "Spring Offensive":

> *So, soon they topped the hill, and raced together*
> *Over an open stretch of herb and heather*
> *Exposed. And instantly the whole sky burned*
> *With fury against them; earth set sudden cups*
> *In thousands for their blood; and the green slope*
> *Chasmed and steepened sheer to infinite space.*
>
> *Of them who running on that last high place*
> *Leapt to swift unseen bullets, or went up*
> *On the hot blast and fury of hell's upsurge,*
> *Or plunged and fell away past this world's verge,*
> *Some say God caught them even before they fell.*

"My subject is War, and the pity of War," Wilfred Owen wrote shortly before he was killed: "The Poetry is in the pity" (see photo section).

After the war, Siegfried Sassoon edited Owen's poems for a posthumous volume. He ended his introduction to the book with lines from "Strange Meeting." The poem was, he said, Owen's "testament, his passport to immortality, and his elegy for the Unknown Warrior of all nations":

> *Courage was mine, and I had mystery,*
> *Wisdom was mine, and I had mastery.*

CHAPTER II

The Eleventh Hour

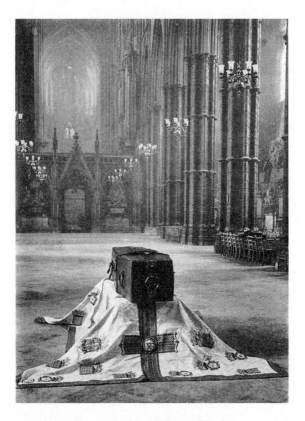

The coffin of the Unknown Warrior
Westminster Abbey, November 1920

But death replied: "I choose him." So he went,
And there was silence in the summer night;
Silence and safety; and the veils of sleep.
Then, far away, the thudding of the guns.

—Siegfried Sassoon

In all the woods where the fighting was most severe not a tree is left alive, and the trunks which still stand are riddled with shrapnel and bullets and torn by fragments of shell, while here and there unexploded shells may still be seen embedded in the stems. Aveluy Wood, however, affords another example of the effort being made by Nature to beautify the general scene of desolation. Here some of the trees are still alive though badly broken, but the ground beneath is covered with a dense growth of the Rose-bay Willow Herb (*Epilobium angustifolium*) extending over several acres. Seen from across the valley this great sheet of rosy-pink was a most striking object, and the shattered and broken trees rising out of it looked less forlorn than elsewhere.

—CAPTAIN ARTHUR HILL, 1917,
"THE FLORA OF THE SOMME BATTLEFIELD"

At eleven o'clock on the eleventh day of November in 1918 the guns fell silent. Six hours earlier the Conditions of an Armistice with Germany had been signed in the Forest of Compiègne, forty miles north of Paris. In this favorite hunting ground of the French kings, battles between kingdoms had come and gone, Julius Caesar had led thirty thousand Roman troops to victory over the Gauls, and emperors had entertained with abandon. In the same place in the forest where the Germans surrendered in 1918, Adolf Hitler took the surrender of France in 1940.

Armistice, when it came, was met variously with relief, joy, weariness, or disillusionment. With the peace came respite, but the suffering did not end. Hundreds of thousands

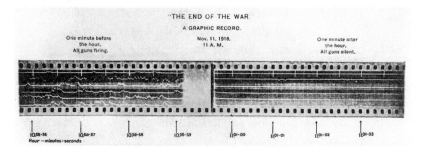

The Armistice:
Seismographic recording of the end of the war

mourned their dead. For some, the end of the war suggested the possibility of new life, an Aveluy Wood, fresh growth in the midst of shattered and broken trees. For many others, armistice was a no-man's-land between past and future, a time of dread and uncertainty.

For most of the doctors and nurses who served in the war, armistice was a relief and a time to think about the future. Nurses differed in their reactions to the armistice, consistent with differences in temperament, background, and what they had seen and done during the war. For all of them, there had been a toll taken. Mary Borden described her psychological exhaustion as a nurse at the Front:

> *Come to me quickly and take me away from my*
> *wounded men—*
> *I cannot bear their pain anymore—*
> *Come quickly and take me away out of this place*
> *Give me rest*
> *Give me strength then, give me cleanness and joy for*
> *one hour—*

I am suffocating—
I cannot get away—
They cling to my skirts, my arms
My hands—
They clutch at my strength
They call my name—They keep calling me—
They cry to me to undo their pain and let them free—
I cannot set them free.
They throw themselves onto my breast, to die—
I cannot even let them die—

Alice Fitzgerald, the Johns Hopkins nurse who had left her Baltimore society life of "tulle and orange blossom" to train as a nurse, was in Paris when the war ended. Her reaction was typical of many, less complicated than some. "At 11 A.M. on the morning of November 11, 1918," she wrote in her diary, "the cannons began to roar, the sirens screeched, the bells chimed in. . . . The War was over! The sorrow and anxiety of four hideous years were suddenly transformed into irrepressible joy." The lights of Paris seemed on fire after so many years of night-masking: "Paris wore her brightest jewels—the sky blazed with the lights so long shrouded in fear from enemy planes"—and for Fitzgerald, along with tens of thousands of others in the streets, "Yesterday was forgotten; tomorrow's problems had not arrived. For that one day and night we lived absolutely and entirely for the joy of the moment."

Helen Boylston, a nurse from Massachusetts General Hospital who had served in France, had a more ambivalent response. She drew a stark line between the war years, now past, and the future that she believed would lack the purpose and excitement she had known during the war. "In ten minutes the war will be over," she wrote in her diary. "I lay awake all last night, thinking. What are we all to do now?" The intensity of the war years would fade, and she would return to the "never ending, never varying routine" of civilian life. The feverish pace of her work as a nurse anesthetist—"We admitted eleven-hundred [patients] in twenty-four hours, and we are averaging ninety operations a night," she wrote at one point—had suited her well. Now the bells, the drums, the cheering. What did it mean? "The war is over," she wrote, "and I never felt so sick in my life. Everything is over." At home in Boston a year later, she reminisced about the odd glory of war. She and the other nurses and doctors had given everything they had to give; the future could not compete with the adrenaline and purpose she had felt during the war. "The scream of shells; and the horror and pity of it, and the wild joyous youth of us all," she wrote. "Even numbed with fatigue as we were, we knew it was glorious."

Harvey Cushing, senior consultant in neurosurgery for the American Expeditionary Forces in Europe, was in France on November 9 when he and his staff heard rumors that the war was to end. Their responses were restrained. "We have received the news of a possible armistice with a peculiar indifference almost amounting to a stupefaction," he wrote in his journal. "No shouts or throwing up of hats . . . This contest has been too appalling for that kind of thing, and there's a lot yet for everyone to do." Two days later he heard the official announcement of the armistice. "Thus the Great War ends. . . . How still it must be with the guns silent." He jotted down words from "Flanders Field," written by his friend and fellow doctor John McCrae: They can sleep now, he wrote, they can sleep "amid the crosses row on row."

Cushing, unlike most of the nurses, did not see a break

between the end of war and his own future. The war had given nurses independence and clinical opportunities impossible before the war. Cushing was older, a man and a surgeon, and he came from social and academic privilege. He would return to privilege and would resume his professorship at Harvard. "There will be much celebrating," Cushing wrote, "and drawing of corks—but perhaps not so much after all." In the afternoon of the armistice he, his head nurse, and a chaplain had tea before a wood fire "wondering what the future held in store for us." This was followed by a long and "serious discussion of religion."

On his way home to Boston two months later, Cushing stayed with William and Grace Osler in Oxford and read Whitman's *Memoranda During the War*, given to him by Osler. Cushing, who had operated on and attended the deaths of thousands of young men, including Osler's son, marked passages from Whitman that underscored the atrocity and futility of war and its "sheer stupidity, extravagance, waste."

Grace Revere Osler, who later would ask Cushing to write a biography of her husband (which received the Pulitzer Prize in 1926), wrote about the end of the war not as a doctor or nurse, but as a mother who had lost her only child. She described a gray world filled with grief and unnerving quiet. "It is very strange here—no training in the Parks—no flying over head. The Calm is very oppressive after four years of noise. I can hardly imagine what it must be at the front. . . . What a sad world it has been and is. . . . Even in all the rejoicing—tears are flowing—Even the soldiers do not seem very gay and the homecoming men are so weary they can hardly stumble along." Her husband, she said, remained desolate.

So they gave their bodies to the commonwealth, and received, each for his own memory, praise that will never die, [and] a home in the minds of men. . . . For the whole earth is the sepulchre of famous men; and their story is not graven only on stone over their native earth, but lives on far away, without visible symbol, woven into the stuff of other men's lives.

—THUCYDIDES,
"FUNERAL ORATION OF PERICLES," 431 B.C.

❧

Remembrance of the First World War continues to this day, long after the signing of the Conditions of Armistice in the Forest of Compiègne. Its carnage and sacrifice remain deeply personal for millions, marked each year by tightly held rituals. On the eleventh of November 2018, my husband and I attended a service in our church in Washington to mark the centenary of the end of the First World War. It was hosted by the British Embassy and included representatives of the countries that had fought in the war, including Germany. The hymns and recitations were Protestant, English, Greek, and German; the words were familiar, like those of carols and prayer book, and consoling in that familiarity.

At the 11th hour of the 11th day of the 11th month, the Invitatory Prayer began, *the guns fell silent on the Western Front, bringing to an end the First World War*. Then, in the Act of Remembrance, familiar from public recitation and school, followed the words of Laurence Binyon: *They shall grow not old, as we that are left grow old: / Age shall not weary them, nor the years condemn. / At the going down of the sun and in the morning / We will remember them.* The Last Post. The piper's lament, "Flowers of the Forest." The Silence. The Official Remembrance of the German War Graves Commission: *Today we remember . . . We mourn . . . We remember.* The repeated call to remember: *We remember them. We mourn. We remember. We will remember them.*

Most in the church had a personal association with the war. My husband was one. His father, Thomas Cathcart Traill, was a fourteen-year-old cadet at the Royal Naval College in Dartmouth when "a bugler on the cricket ground sounded the end of my school days." Within days he was a midshipman on HMS *Lord Nelson.* Like many, he was fresh and enthusiastic to serve king and country. "We had read the brass letters on the Quarterdeck every day, 'Fear God—Honour the King': We had been schooled and trained in the idea that the real and desirable virtues are courage, loyalty to King and Country, devotion to duty, and service in and to the Royal Navy. Now here we were with England in peril and a ship to serve, a ship that stood for home as well as for King and Empire." He was doing what he was meant to do, he wrote in his schoolboy diary.

At fifteen he was on the beach at Gallipoli, slipping, scrambling along the beach, "revolver in hand, looking for our soldiers: calling quietly, 'Anybody about?,' and hoping the reply would not be in Turkish." He transferred from the Royal Navy into the Royal Flying Corps and then, when it came into existence in 1918, the Royal Air Force. By the time he was nineteen he had crash-landed several times, shot down eight German planes, and been awarded the Distinguished Flying Cross. Like most who served in the war, he was incomprehensibly young for what he had been asked to do and, like tens of thousands of other soldiers and pilots who fought in the First World War, he would fight again in the Second.

Traill's reaction to armistice was not a disillusioned one, like that of Sassoon. It was instead the reaction of many who fought in the war: relief, a kind of happiness, and a continuing, if tempered, belief in king and country. He described it in his diary: He was returning to England on leave, grateful "to be almost sure of living for another fortnight, to be free from fear and dawn patrols and Fokkers at 18,000 feet waiting for you," when the blare of the ship's sirens announced the end of the war. "I took a taxi across London, still with a feeling of unreality, had a glimpse of the excited thousands in Trafalgar Square, and caught a train for home. My parents knew I was about due for leave again, but did not know when it would come, so when I walked in on the afternoon of armistice day it seemed to us that nothing much better had ever happened." War had ended for him and for millions of others. Suffering and remembering had not.

⌒

In the funeral procession cypress coffins are borne in carts, one for each tribe; the bones of the deceased being placed in the coffin of their tribe. Among these is carried one empty bier decked for the missing, that is, for those whose bodies could not be recovered.

—THUCYDIDES, C. 471–C. 404 B.C.,
History of the Peloponnesian War

Grief had been thick in Europe's marrow since 1914. At the end of the war memory and ritual were to be critical in healing the immensity of this grief: What was best to remember, what best to lay aside? How did one move forward without forsaking the past? Rivers had taught that repression of atrocity and suffering was ill-advised in treating shell-shocked soldiers. It was better to transform the horror into manageable grief, if necessary and if possible, through psychotherapy. But then grief itself called for healing. How did a parent or a wife or a child contend with the death of a person whose life was everything to them? How did one contend with personal loss when the entire nation was grieving? How did one remember the dead, keep faith, and yet go forward? *Have you forgotten yet?* Sassoon asked. *Look up, and swear by the green of the spring that you'll never forget.*

How too did one grieve for the soldiers whose bodies were never identified or found? Of the British and empire military personnel who were killed in the Great War, historian John Keegan estimates that five hundred thousand bodies were never found or identified. "Their bodies had been blown to pieces by shell fire and the fragments scattered beyond recognition. Many other bodies could not be recovered during the fighting and were then lost to view, entombed in crumbled shell holes or collapsed trenches or decomposing into the broken soil left behind." Without a body or a grave, grief became that much more awful.

In 1916, an Anglican army chaplain on the Western Front struggled to find a way to heal this grief. "Every Padre serving with infantry brigades was bombarded after each publication of casualties with at least this request," he wrote. "Where—exactly where—did you lay to rest the body of my son? Can you give me any further information? I have been officially notified that he is 'missing, believed killed.'" The chaplain, David Railton, after conducting a burial service for a British soldier, came across a white wooden cross in a French garden; penciled into it was, *An Unknown British Soldier*. "So I thought and thought and wrestled in thought. What can I do to ease the pain of father, mother, brother, sister, sweetheart, wife and friend? Quietly and gradually there came out of the mist of thought this answer clear and strong, 'Let this body—this symbol of him—be carried reverently over the sea to his native land.'"

Railton, not long before the second anniversary of the armistice, wrote to the Dean of Westminster and asked whether he would consider burying the remains of an unknown soldier in Westminster Abbey, one soldier to represent the hundreds of thousands who had died in the war. The Dean was encouraging but the king less so, as his private secretary conveyed. "His Majesty is inclined to think that nearly two years after the last shot fired on the battlefields of France and Flanders is so long ago that a funeral might now be regarded as belated, and almost, as it were, re-open the war wound, which time is gradually healing." The prime minister, Lloyd George, the Dean of Westminster, and British senior military staff strongly backed the idea, however, and the king, once persuaded, became the symbolic leader of what was to be one of the most important ceremonies of remembrance and healing in the history of Britain.

The choice of the Unknown Warrior to be buried "amongst the Kings" in Westminster Abbey, and the journey of his remains from the battlefields of France to England, drew deep from history, church, and military tradition. Four bodies, sufficiently decomposed as to be unidentifiable, were disinterred from battlefields at Ypres, the Somme, Aisne, and Arras. At midnight on November 7, 1920, the commanding officer of the British forces in France and Flanders entered a makeshift military chapel in St. Pol, lifted his lantern, reached out, and put his hand on one of the bodies. This body, placed in a temporary coffin, was now the Unknown Warrior; the bodies not chosen were reburied. The permanent coffin, made of oaks from the grounds of Hampton Court Palace, was banded with iron, and a sixteenth-century sword given by the king was laid on top. The coffin was placed aboard a Royal Navy destroyer, which was met in the middle of the Channel by another six destroyers. Together they accompanied the coffin into home waters.

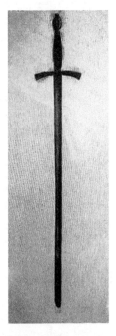

Sword given by King George V
For the coffin of the Unknown Warrior

*They buried him among the Kings because he
Had done good toward God and toward
His house.*

On the morning of the eleventh of November 1920, the coffin of the Unknown Warrior was placed on a gun carriage and drawn through immense, silent crowds to the newly unveiled cenotaph at Whitehall. The king placed a card, and a wreath of laurel and red roses, on top of the coffin. (Laurel, or bay leaves, Sir Thomas Browne had said, are "a singular emblem of the resurrection, for the leaves that seeme dead and drie will revive into a perfect green if theire roote bee not withered, as is observable in bay trees after hard winters.") The king's card read, "In proud memory of those Warriors who died unknown in the Great War. Unknown and yet well-known; as dying, and behold they live." So it was throughout the day's commemoration: words of death and resurrection, symbols of dying into life. A perfect green after a hard winter. Grief was made less terrible when graced with the honor due it and shared by a nation.

Ritual offers balm. The selection of the body of the Unknown Warrior, its somber sea-borne transport across the English Channel, and its burial in Westminster Abbey: All detail was taken from myth and history. Grief was lashed to duty and national purpose; the days of elevated ceremony honored honor itself. The ceremony existed for those who were grieving, and for the nation as well: It healed by its words, music, pathos, and beauty.

In 431 B.C., Pericles addressed the parents of the Athenians who died in the first year of the Peloponnesian War. Honor and love of country seem weak reeds toward which to swim when mourning, but they were what Pericles offered on behalf of Athens. "You must feed your eyes upon Athens," he told the grieving, "till love of her fills your hearts; and then when all her greatness shall break upon you, you must reflect that it was by courage, sense of duty, and a keen sense of honor in action that men were enabled to win all this." Athens had no need for a Homer as eulogist, he said. "We have forced every sea and land to be the highway of our daring." It is only the love of honor that never grows old, he said. "So died these men as became Athenians."

—

So it was with the ancient rituals and music used during the burial service in Westminster Abbey. "We all were made one people, participants in one act of remembrance," wrote a correspondent for *The Times*. "Here was one of ourselves, one of the people, one of the hundreds of thousands of all sorts and of all conditions, who had laid down his life for us." It was many brought to one. "Here all was planned and as in a great piece of music, and all of us were members of the orchestra we had, each, his part in the expression of this grief and pride without discord or difference or failure."

The Silence—two minutes of silence observed by the congregation and the entire nation, and a part of Remembrance Sunday services to this day—was described by a journalist. "For a little while the bereaved of a nation walked in spirit through the cemeteries of France and Flanders, Gallipoli and Mesopotamia, and stood before faraway wooden crosses. The tension was almost too great. . . . At last a woman sobbed."

During the hymn "Lead, Kindly Light"—the great hymn of desolation and faith—the Union Jack, helmet, sidearm, and king's wreath, which had been placed on the top of the coffin, were removed. The king sprinkled a handful of earth from France onto the coffin and the Dean committed the body to the ground of the abbey. Later the grave would be filled with sandbags of earth from the major battlefields of the war.

The Burial of the Unknown Warrior, said *The Times*,

"was the most beautiful, the most touching, and the most impressive that in all its long, eventful story this island has ever seen." There is competition for this and not all felt the sacrifice was warranted. But, in her "long, eventful story," Britain held to the rituals of tragedy and in doing so had a profound effect on healing the minds of those devastated by death. *We remember. We mourn. We remember.*

Chesapeake

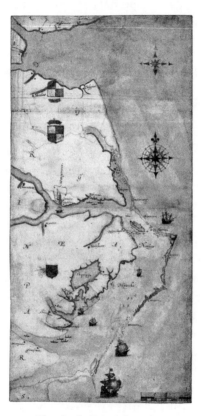

Chesapeake Bay, 1585–1593

*As for your feares that I will lose my selfe
in these unknown large waters, or be swallowed
up in some stormie gust . . . there is as much
danger to returne, as to proceede.*

—Captain John Smith, 1608

The young forest below the embankment was still almost bare, as in winter. Only in the buds, which were spattered all over it like drops of wax, was something superfluous setting in, some disorder, a sort of dirt or swelling, and this superfluous thing, this disorder and dirt, was life, enveloping the first opening trees of the forest in the green flame of foliage.

—BORIS PASTERNAK, *Doctor Zhivago*

The Chesapeake Bay finds its way to the open sea in a manner known only to God. Like the young forest in *Doctor Zhivago*, it is dirt, disorder, and life: water-meadows and star grass; persimmon, honeysuckle, and black walnut. Wild plum. Crabs. Oysters, geese, and blue heron. The bay is abundant. Its mid-Atlantic rivers evoke the life and commerce of a younger America: the York, the James, and the Potomac; the Susquehanna and Rappahannock. The Sassafras, Tred Avon, and Choptank. And so many more.

Life flows in and out of the bay, irregular and unpredictable. "The many Rivers, Creeks, and Rivulets of Water," wrote a clergyman in 1699, are tangled like "veins in humane Bodies." The estuary tides can be treacherous. The salt level, upon which the bay's variety of life depends, fluctuates from low at the freshwater river inlets to highest where the Atlantic seawater enters the mouth of the bay. The Chesapeake water, stirred by action of man and rhythm of nature, is capricious, a place of danger and bounty. It can be navigated only if you know its shoals and narrow channels, its dissolving islands, and gusts that rise up from nowhere.

If the Chesapeake water can be treacherous, it is majestic and generous as well. In 1624, Captain John Smith wrote that

"Heaven and earth never agreed better to frame a place for man's habitation." It was a "faire Bay, compassed but for the mouth . . . [a] delightsome land." Early settlers who fished the bay and farmed its surrounding lands reaped extravagant harvests of crab, fish, tobacco, and oyster. But danger countervailed bounty. Hurricanes breached seawalls and swept away bridges; ships wrecked and their crews drowned. Great trees snapped and tobacco barns were wrested from their foundations. Ice in the bay cracked the hulls of ships; vessels were blown inland, to be discovered later in corn or tobacco fields. Wind and water brought life into the bay; their brute force took life from it. Islands disappeared, as they are doing still. Geese, hundreds of thousands of them, fly to the bay, their waters since earliest times. Inlets and coves of the bay give them shelter, seed, and grasses; the water and its banks provide runway and landing field. These are their home waters.

Most of us have home waters, a bay or river, a sea, to which we return in fact or longing. We call up the beauty and nostalgia that infuse them; we use memory of them as a measure of passing time. The Chesapeake has been my home waters since I was a child. When I was young, and summers seemed forever, I sailed the bay with friends, confused by its ragged geography but smitten by its beauty and in awe of its squalls that turned the sky and water black. In the fall, flocks of geese flew overhead, loud and thick in their formations, bound on paths they have flown for years, long before man came to the bay.

In those summers of innocence, the irregularity of the bay, its incomprehensibility, its dotting of coves and islands, were an easy fit with my mind. Restless and various: My mind was at home. These were days far distant from the convulsive moods that I would later know. A place innocent of pain draws one back, and I have gone to the bay often since to mull and renerve, to think and write, and to spend the most joyous honeymoon and long days of happiness with my husband. The bay has lost none of its magic; it couldn't, not with the geese honking overhead, the taste of salt and sensual draw of the sun, and the storms that seem the *Dies irae*. Things that delighted me when I was young give pleasure still, as well as a peace that is welcome, a peace not so needed when one was young.

The islands I imagined as a child, not of the Chesapeake but my own conjuring, are with me still, somewhere—with their lagoons, books, wild and uninhabitable places—but they are layered over with life. Less quirky, less free, but by no means boring. So many things come back from one's younger days to give pleasure and meaning: books, music, the lives of explorers and writers who provide rare company in blithe times, and distracting, deepening company in darker ones; the kindness of strangers, the love of friends and the understanding of teachers. All have given company, ideas, and heart.

I set out to write a book about healing and instead I have written more about healers. This was perhaps inevitable. Healers leave their mark. When I was young, mania and depression forced me to seek a doctor's help. I was lucky; he was a consummate healer. Part of getting well was learning about healing from someone who was so good at it. He knew clinical medicine and psychopathology well. And he understood, respected, and took delight in the magnificent oddities of human nature. He took life with the gravity it warrants. He was intelligent in his use of medicine and judicious in his use of expectation. He probed my fears with subtlety, kindness, and persistence. He taught me to expect that things would be hard, and that there was no way to face mental illness except with courage that I was not sure I had. He was clear he would be there for a harsh but interesting journey. Along the way, I was to rely upon myself and my better instincts, yet be open to change and to other ways of seeing life. It would require that I take real risks. It was necessary for a serious life.

In a hard time, I had to do things I doubted I could do. I dipped more deeply, took to heart the bold acts of others. I imagined throwing a summer wreath over an unclimbable fence in impassable weather. The way over the fence would be difficult, but curiosity and necessity would lure me on. My doctor expected I could do it, gave me hope that I could do it, and I did it. Drawing upon things I loved from the past allowed me to reach the future. I had been advised that the work of life, and of contending with madness and depression, would be within my reach. I was told, and it was true, that healing would be hard. I was told as well that the journey would bear benefit of a sort I could not imagine. This too was true.

The Chesapeake Bay makes its way inlet to inlet, filled with the river waters of Maryland and Virginia. At Harpers Ferry, the Shenandoah joins the Potomac, and joined they flow into the bay. It is a beautiful place, where two great rivers meet. The Shenandoah, of a beauty all its own, is taken by its sister river from fresh water to salt. Different waters, past and future, mix and tumble together, complicated and extraordinary. When I was a girl I took an uncomplicated pleasure in these home waters. I could wish to experience them now as I experienced them then. But as an adult I needed to know, was forced to know, more of the darker waters, more of their capacity to hurt as well as to teach. Dark waters have mixed with the lighter ones, giving a fuller measure. Knowledge accrues, not always without pain, not always without grace. We have a covenant with life to make of it something serious and wonderful. There is a cost for this, and to redeem it we look to our healers.

Acknowledgments

I am indebted to several people who were kind enough to read early drafts of this book: Donald Graham, Dean Jamison, Stuart Kenworthy, Daniel Auerbach, Andrew Motion, Arthur Kleinman, Andrew Solomon, Leo Kottke, Mark Anderson, James Potash, Helen Vendler, Erica Richards, Leslie Jamison, Joanne Leslie, David and Linda Hellmann, John Mann, Jeffrey and Kathleen Schlom, Tim Page, Jeremy Waletzky and Susan Clampitt, Erwin and Stephanie Greenberg, and Robert and Mary Jane Gallo.

I am also indebted to the following librarians, archivists, and libraries: Lily Szczygiel, Rare Books and Special Collections, Osler Library of the History of Medicine, McGill University; Andrew Harrison, archivist, Alan Mason Chesney Medical Archives, Johns Hopkins Medical Institutions; Micah Connor, library associate, Maryland Center for History and Culture; Harvey Williams Cushing Papers, Yale University Library; Dr. Adam Crothers and Mrs. Fiona Colbert, the Library, St. John's College, Cambridge University; Frank Bowles, Department of Archives and Modern Manuscripts, Cambridge University Library; the Reverend David Green, Rector, and Michael Rowe, historian, Parish of St. Michael and All Angels Church, Offham, Kent; W.H.R. Rivers collection, McMaster University Library; Haddon

Papers, Cambridge University Library; Papers of Siegfried Sassoon, Cambridge University Library; Henry Head archive, Wellcome Library, the Wellcome Trust; the London Library; Private Papers of Siegfried Sassoon, Imperial War Museum; Siegfried Sassoon Papers, Beinecke Rare Book & Manuscript Library, Yale University; Wilfred Owen Collection, Harry Ransom Humanities Research Center, University of Texas at Austin; Robert Graves Papers, Morris Library Special Collections Research Center, Southern Illinois University; First World War Poetry Digital Archive, University of Oxford.

The Rivers family and the National Museum of the Royal Navy generously gave me permission to use photographs of the Rivers gunnery book from HMS *Victory*. Richard Valente, whose father's wonderful photograph of Paul Robeson is in the collection of the National Portrait Gallery, was also generous in allowing me to use his photograph; Chris Rogers, program director of the Paul Robeson House and Museum, provided my husband and me with a very helpful and enjoyable tour of Paul Robeson's house in Philadelphia and answered many of our questions.

The Dalio Foundation and the support of Ray and Barbara Dalio and Paul and Kristina Dalio have made my book possible, and I am grateful to them for their friendship and belief in my work. Michael Hersch, chair of the composition department at the Peabody Institute, was kind enough to give me valuable insight into the unique musical gift of Paul Robeson. Alain Moreau did the artwork for the chapter openings "Big Sur" and "Ashen Roots," which have added greatly to the book. I am indebted to Robert Barnett and Emily Alden of Williams & Connolly, and to my editor at Knopf, Deborah Garrison, for her many helpful suggestions and her support; to Zuleima Ugalde for all her help shepherding my manuscript along; to Muriel Jorgenson, who copyedited my manuscript; to those responsible for the book design and production, Melissa Yoon, Soonyoung Kwon, John Vorhees, and Lorraine Hyland; and to those overseeing publicity and marketing, Josefine Kals, Andreia Wardlaw, and Matthew Sciarappa.

William Collins, Ioline Henter, and Sharon Blackburn have been the most involved in putting the book together. They have been excellent in everything they have done: word processing, tracking down references and permissions, and graphic design. Luke Henter was also very helpful. I cannot thank them enough. "Island and Quest" is dedicated to the memory of my sister, Phyllis Temple Jamison, who died not long before this book was finished. "The Night Nurse" is dedicated to my friends and colleagues at Johns Hopkins, Mary Beth Cogan, RN, Barbara Schweizer, RN, and Karen Swartz, MD. "Ashen Roots" is for Douglas Dunn, a great poet and a wonderful friend.

My deepest thanks go, as always, to my husband, Tom Traill. I could not have written this book without him. He has read, revised, and made my manuscript more eloquent and thoughtful than it otherwise would have been. Like me, he believes that doctors and psychotherapists learn their clinical skills best by working with those who are preeminent in diagnosing, treating, and healing patients. I could not have learned about healing from a better source. Our discussions about medicine have been a rare education. I am grateful to have learned about the art and science of healing from him; I am more grateful still for the love, happiness, and peace he has given me.

Notes

EPIGRAPH

vii "Psycho-therapeutics would seem": W.H.R. Rivers, "Psychotherapeutics," in *Encyclopedia of Religion and Ethics*, ed. James Hastings, vol. 10 (Edinburgh: T. and T. Clark, 1918), 433.

vii "Fires in the dark": Siegfried Sassoon, "To a Very Wise Man," in *Siegfried Sassoon: Collected Poems, 1908–1956* (London: Faber and Faber, 2002), 97.

vii "Accompaniment": Paul Farmer, "Accompaniment as Policy," Commencement Address, Harvard Kennedy School, May 25, 2011.

PROLOGUE: THE OLDEST BRANCH OF MEDICINE

3 "Rivers was intolerant": Sir Frederic Bartlett, "Obituary: W.H.R. Rivers," *The Eagle* (St. Johns College, Cambridge), 43 (1923), 14.

5 "between medicine on the one hand": W.H.R. Rivers, "Psycho-therapeutics," in *Encyclopedia of Religion and Ethics*, ed. James Hastings, vol. 10 (Edinburgh: T. and T. Clark, 1918), 433.

5 "if the remedies of": Rivers, "Psycho-therapeutics."

5 "Your soul is full of cities": Siegfried Sassoon, "To a Very Wise Man," in *Siegfried Sassoon: Collected Poems* (London: Faber and Faber, 2002), 97.

5 "out beyond the boundaries": Sassoon, "To a Very Wise Man," 98.

6 "Do you remember": Siegfried Sassoon, "Aftermath," in *Siegfried Sassoon: Collected Poems*, 110.

8 "I will not leave you": Gospel of St. John 14:18.

8 "Often the best part": Sir William Osler, "The Master-Word in Medicine," talk delivered at the University of Toronto, 1903, in *Aequanimitas: With Other Addresses to Medical Students, Nurses*

and Practitioners of Medicine, 3rd ed. (New York: McGraw Hill, 1951), 368.

8 "comfort and help": Osler, "The Master-Word in Medicine," 369.

8 "true balm of hurt minds": Osler, "The Master-Word in Medicine," 357.

9 "takes the ache away": Letter from Robert Lowell to Frank Bidart, September 4, 1976, in *The Letters of Robert Lowell*, ed. Saskia Hamilton (New York: Farrar, Straus and Giroux, 2005), 656.

10 "devastated regions": Siegfried Sassoon, draft version of "Revisitation," a poem dedicated to W.H.R. Rivers. Final version of the poem omits these lines. "Revisitation (W.H.R.R.)," in *Siegfried Sassoon: Collected Poems* (London: Faber and Faber, 2002), 205.

11 "lowering of the sail": Dante, *Cantica I: Hell (L'Inferno), The Comedy of Dante Alighieri*, Canto XXVII, trans. Dorothy Sayers (London: Penguin, 1949), 242.

> But when I reached the age when it is meet
> For every mariner, with his port in sight,
> To lower sail and gather in the sheet.

12 "Rivers came in": Siegfried Sassoon, *Sherston's Progress* (London: Faber and Faber, 1983; first published 1936), 149.

CHAPTER I: THE SHADOW OF A GREAT ROCK

15 "Live in the ward": William Osler, quoted by William Sydney Thayer, in Thayer, *Osler and Other Papers* (Baltimore: Johns Hopkins Press, 1931), 1.

16 "It is a hard matter": William Osler, "The Treatment of Disease," *Canada Lancet* 42 (1909): 899–912.

16 "Theirs was, I think": Sir John Slessor, *These Remain: Memories of Flying, Fighting and Field Sports* (London: Michael Joseph, 1969), 23. Slessor saw action of the Western Front in the First World War; later, he was Marshal of the Royal Air Force and Chief of the Air Staff.

16 A recent study: S. Rourke and G. Ellis, "The Most Influential Physicians in History, Part 4: The Top Ten," *Medscape*, March 18, 2016.

17 "unduly sentimental": Slessor, *These Remain*, 25.

17 "hell where youth": Siegfried Sassoon, "Suicide in the Trenches," in *Siegfried Sassoon: Collected Poems* (London: Faber and Faber, 1984; first published 1947), 72.

> *You smug-faced crowds with kindling eye*
> *Who cheer when soldier lads march by,*
> *Sneak home and pray you'll never know*
> *The hell where youth and laughter go.*

17 "above all to whose": Slessor, *These Remain*, 21.

17 "a strange Oxford": Slessor, *These Remain*, 30.

17 "Not an inch of earth": Letter from Revere Osler to his father, William Osler, November 14, 1916. Osler Library Archives, P417 Harvey Cushing Fonds.

18 "old helmets": Letter from Revere Osler to his mother, Grace Revere Osler, October 29, 1916. Osler Library Archives, P417 Harvey Cushing Fonds.

18 quiet world of Oxford: Letter from Revere Osler to his father, William Osler, December 27, 1916. "I never knew how much I loved you all and Oxford before now. All this worry and trouble will make things doubly pleasant afterwards—whatever the result of the war." Osler Library Archives, P417 Harvey Cushing Fonds.

18 "His nerves are A.1.": William Osler, quoted in Harvey Cushing, *The Life of Sir William Osler*, vol. 2 (Oxford: Clarendon Press, 1925), 569.

18 "No regrets cloud": Letter from William Osler to his son, Revere Osler, December 28, 1916. Osler Library Archives, P417 Harvey Cushing Fonds.

18 "Every bed, every aisle": George Crile, *George Crile: An Autobiography*, vol. 1 (Philadelphia: J. B. Lippincott, 1947), 301.

18 "did a hundred operations": Crile, *An Autobiography*, vol. 1, 302.

19 "The surgeon is barraged": Crile, *An Autobiography*, vol. 2, 312.

19 "Sir Wm. Osler's son": Harvey Cushing, *From a Surgeon's Journal: 1915–1918* (Boston: Little, Brown, 1936), 197.

19 "Revere seriously wounded": Cushing, *From a Surgeon's Journal*, 197.

19 "Obviously all was lost": Crile, *An Autobiography*, vol. 2, 308.

20 "I thought about": Crile, *An Autobiography*, vol. 2, 308–9.

20 "We saw him buried": Harvey Cushing, *From a Surgeon's Journal: 1915–1918* (Boston: Little, Brown, 1936).

20 "4:15 pm": William Osler, entry in his day book, August 1917. Osler Library (McGill University).

22 "The physician's work": William Osler, *Science and Immortality* (London: Archibald Constable, 1906), 11.

22 "Pathology is the basis of": Quoted in Michael Bliss, *William Osler: A Life in Medicine* (Oxford: Oxford University Press, 1999), 88.

22 "In seeking": William Osler, "Aequanimitas," in *Aequanimitas: With Other Addresses to Medical Students, Nurses and Practitioners of Medicine*, 3rd ed. (New York: McGraw Hill, 1932), 7.

24 "I have careful records": Osler, *Science and Immortality*, 36–37.

24 "In Flanders Fields": John McCrae wrote "In Flanders Fields" in May 1915; it was published in *Punch* on December 8, 1915.

25 "long association": Quoted in Bliss, *William Osler*, 425.

25 "as if last year's blood": Jerdan William, ed., *Letters from James Earl of Perth, Lord Chancellor of Scotland, to His Sister, the Countess of Erroll, and Other Members of His Family* (London: John Bower Nichols and Son, 1865), 28.

25 "fertilised by twenty thousand": Thomas Babington Macaulay, *The History of England, from the Accession of James the Second*, vol. 7 (Leipzig: Bernhard Tauchnitz, 1855), 222. Macaulay also quotes a letter from Lord Perth to his sister, June 17, 1694.

25 "The earth was disclosing": Isaiah 26:21.

25 "scouring the fields": Cushing, *From a Surgeon's Journal*, 280.

25 "diverse straunge": D. Murray Angevine, "John McCrae: Pathologist, Poet, Soldier, a Man Among Men, 1872–1918," *Archives of Pathology* 88 (1969): 456.

26 "God have them": Angevine, "John McCrae."

26 "Medicine is a science": William Osler, quoted in W. B. Bean, *Sir William Osler: Aphorisms from His Bedside Teachings and Writings* (Springfield, Ill.: Charles C. Thomas, 1968), 129.

27 "You are in this profession": William Osler, "The Reserves of Life," in *St. Mary's Hospital Gazette* 13 (1907): 95–98.

27 "His very presence": C. B. Farrar, "I Remember Osler, Psychotherapist," *American Journal of Psychiatry* 121 (2006): 761.

27 "immediate unplanned": Farrar, "I Remember Osler."

27 "an emanation": C. B. Farrar, "Osler at Johns Hopkins," read at the Osler Society Banquet, March 8, 1950, *University of Western Ontario Medical Journal* (1950): 131.

28 "If you want a profession": William Osler, quoted in Thomas McCrae, "The Influence of Pathology on the Clinical Medicine of William Osler," bulletin no. 9 of *International Association of Medical Museums and Journal of Technical Methods*, ed. Maude E. Abbott, Sir William Osler Memorial Number: Appreciation and Reminiscences (Montreal: Privately issued, 1926), 39.

28 "No two individuals": William Osler, "On the Educational Value of the Medical Society," in *Aequanimitas*, 331.

28 "taught us": William Thayer, "Reminiscences of Osler," in *Osler and Other Papers* (Baltimore: Johns Hopkins Press, 1931), 34.

28 "nothing human": Letter from William W. Frances to Palmer Howard Futcher, 1953, cited in P. H. Futcher, "William Osler's Religion," *Archives of Internal Medicine* 107 (1961): 475–79.

29 "I affirm": Correspondence (email) from David Hellmann, MD, and Thomas Traill, FRCP, to the author, August 2, 2021. In 2000, David Hellmann, MD, professor of medicine at Johns Hopkins School of Medicine and program director of the Osler House Staff Program, and Thomas Traill, FRCP, professor of medicine at Johns Hopkins and firm faculty leader for the Osler House Staff, conferred and decided that, in addition to their recitation of the Hippocratic Oath on graduation from medical school, senior residents in medicine should additionally pledge themselves to the principles and practice of medicine as taught by William Osler. Traill wrote the version of the oath that has been used at Johns Hopkins since. The substrate, a pledge adapted by the American College of Physicians, was modified to be, in Traill's words, "less like a declaration for hospital privileges and more like what physicians really aspire to be and do."

29 "pestilence of darkness": "Not for the pestilence that walketh in darkness; nor for the destruction that wasteth at noonday" (Psalm 91:6).

29 "And a man shall be": William Osler, "Man's Redemption of Man," a Lay Sermon delivered at McEwan Hall, University of Edinburgh, July 2, 1910 (London: Constable, 1918), 5. From Isaiah 32:2.

30 "It is astonishing": William Osler, "Books and Men," a talk given at the Boston Medical Library, January 12, 1901, in *Aequanimitas*, 211.

30 "essential melancholy": Charles Singer, cited in James A. Knight, "William Osler's Call to Ministry and Medicine," *Journal of Medical Humanities and Bioethics* 7 (1986): 11.

31 his most precious book: William Osler, "An Address on Sir Thomas Browne," *British Medical Journal* 2 (1909): 993–98.

31 "in the presence of sublime imagination": Virginia Woolf, "The Elizabethan Lumber Room," in *Collected Essays*, vol. 1 (London: The Hogarth Press, 1924), 53.

31 "All was mystery": Woolf, "Elizabethan Lumber Room," 51.

31 "I that have examined": Sir Thomas Browne, *Religio Medici* (Cambridge: Cambridge University Press, 1953), 63.

31 "discourse of humane": Sir Thomas Browne, "Hydriotaphia, or Urne-Buriall," in *Religio Medici and Urne-Buriall*, ed. Stephen Greenblatt and Ramie Targoff (New York: New York Review Books, 2012; first published 1658), 94.

31 "As a long-winged hawk": Robert Burton, "Cure of Melancholy,"

The Anatomy of Melancholy, pt. 2, sec. 2 (New York: New York Review Books, 2001; first published 1621), 34.

31 "a tissue of many languages": Samuel Johnson, *Sir Thomas Browne: The Major Works*, ed. C. A. Patrides (London: Penguin, 1977), 508.

32 "By compassion": Sir Thomas Browne, *Religio Medici: The Religion of a Doctor—A Classic Treatise of Spiritual and Philosophical Self-Reflection, Dating to 1642* (Morrisville, N.C.: Lulu Press, 2018), 52.

32 greatest medical treatise: William Osler, "Robert Burton: The Man, His Book, His Library," based on lectures delivered at Yale, April 20, 1913; reprinted in *Selected Writings of Sir William Osler, 12 July 1849– 29 December 1919* (London: Oxford University Press, 1951), 90.

32 "serious in purpose": Osler, "Robert Burton," 86.

32 "presents such a stage": Osler, "Robert Burton," 86.

32 "I was fatally driven": Burton, *Anatomy of Melancholy*, 35.

32 "To ease my mind": Burton, *Anatomy of Melancholy*, 20–21.

32 "an antidote": Burton, *Anatomy of Melancholy*, 21.

32 "Undertaken partly": Osler, "Robert Burton," 89.

32 "desirous to be unladen": Burton, *Anatomy of Melancholy*, 21.

33 "If unhappy—have hope": In fact, Burton had written "Sperate Miseri, / Cavete Felices" [Hope, Ye unhappy ones; ye happy ones, fear]. Robert Burton, *Anatomy of Melancholy*, pt. 3, sec. 4, 432.

33 "We have been preparing": Letter from William Osler to Mabel Brewster, August 30, 1917. Cushing Papers, Osler Library, McGill University.

33 "Our boy has gone": Letter from Grace Revere Osler to Marjorie Futcher, September 2, 1917. Futcher Papers, Osler Library.

33 "sobbing hour after hour": Letter from Grace Revere Osler to Marjorie Futcher, September 2, 1917.

33 "Cushing was with him": Letter from William Osler to William Halsted, September 6, 1917. Osler Library Archives, P417 Harvey Cushing Fonds.

33 "We are taking": Letter from William Osler to C. D. Parfitt, November 14, 1917. Cushing Papers, Osler Library.

33 "he went through the wards": Nancy Astor, quoted in Harvey Cushing, *The Life of Sir William Osler*, 580.

34 "It is Mr. Revere": Quoted in J. George Adami, "Sir William Osler: The Last Days," bulletin no. 9 of *International Association of Medical Museums and Journal of Technical Methods*, ed. Maude E. Abbott, Sir William Osler Memorial Number: Appreciations and Reminiscences (Montreal: Privately issued, 1926), 422–33.

34 "put every halfpenny": Letter from William Osler to the mayor of Oxford, May 1, 1919. Osler Library.

34 "work is the true balm": William Osler, "The Master-Word in Medicine," *Aequanimitas*, 357.

34 "there was a subdued": William Thayer, "Reminiscences of Osler," 40.

35 "Bearing the bandages": Walt Whitman, "The Dresser," in Walt Whitman, *Drum-Taps, The Complete 1865 Edition*, ed. Lawrence Kramer (New York: New York Review Books, 2015), 37–39.

36 "Such was the War": Walt Whitman, *Memoranda During the War* (New York: Oxford University Press, 2004), 7.

36 "unending, universal mourning-wail": Whitman, *Memoranda During the War*.

36 "The war is surely over": Harvey Cushing described the January 9, 1919, dinner with William Osler in slightly different words in his journal and in his biography of Osler. Cushing, *From a Surgeon's Journal*, 506; and Cushing, *The Life of Sir William Osler*, vol. 2, 630–31.

36 "a hot water bottle": Cushing, *The Life of Sir William Osler*, vol. 2, 630–31.

36 "The marrow of the tragedy": Harvey Cushing, epigraph to *From a Surgeon's Journal*. Wording is changed slightly from Whitman's original in *Memoranda During the War*, 6–7.

37 "thin light of winter": J. George Adami, "Sir William Osler: The Last Days," 425.

37 "The Cathedral was packed": Letter from Grace Revere Osler to Featherston Osler, January 1, 1929. Osler Library Archives, P417 Harvey Cushing Fonds.

37 "under the arched roof": Letter from Grace Revere Osler to Featherston Osler, January 1, 1929. Osler Library Archives, P417 Harvey Cushing Fonds.

CHAPTER 2: THE NIGHT NURSE

38 "What have all these": Mary Borden, *The Forbidden Zone* (London: Hesperus Press, 2008; first published 1929), 83.

39 "He was taken": Alice Fitzgerald, "Memoirs of an American Nurse," April 4, 1916, unpublished manuscript (Maryland Historical Society, n.d.), 38.

39 "The world is drunken": William Osler, *Science and War*, an address delivered at the University of Leeds Medical School on October 1, 1915 (London: Oxford University Press, 1915), 1.

39 "thick layers of the dead": Osler, *Science and War*, 19–20.

39 "spread out for miles": Osler, *Science and War*, 26.

40   "made slaughter possible": Osler, *Science and War*, 15, 20.

40   Yet as Henry Adams: Henry Adams, *The Education of Henry Adams: An Autobiography* (Boston: Houghton Mifflin, 2000; first published 1907), 249.

40   "has its shadows": George Crile, *George Crile: An Autobiography*, vol. 2 (Philadelphia: J. B. Lippincott, 1947), 312.

40   "If he wants": Crile, *An Autobiography*, vol. 2.

40   "incomparable opportunities": Harvey Cushing, "Neurological Surgery and the War," *Boston Medical and Surgical Journal* 181 (1919): 550.

41   "crackling and smell": Ellen N. La Motte, *The Backwash of War: The Human Wreckage of the Battlefield as Witnessed by an American Hospital Nurse* (New York: G. P. Putnam's Sons, 1916), 25.

41   "The wound stank": La Motte, *The Backwash of War*.

41   "took a curette": La Motte, *The Backwash of War*.

42   "Surrounded by all": Alexander Fleming, quoted in André Maurois, *The Life of Sir Alexander Fleming: Discoverer of Penicillin*, trans. Gerard Hopkins (London: Jonathan Cape, 1959).

42   "vast crucible": W.H.R. Rivers, *Instinct and the Unconscious*, 2nd ed. (Cambridge: Cambridge University Press, 1924), 252.

43   "to play a role": Sigmund Freud, cited in R. Cooter, "Malingering in Modernity: Psychological Scripts and Adversarial Encounters During the First World War," in R. Cooter, M. Harrison, and S. Sturdy, eds., *War, Medicine and Modernity* (London: Sutton, 1995), 130.

44   "We all met": *World War One Nurse, a War Nurse's Diary: Sketches from a Belgian Field Hospital* (New York: Macmillan, 1918), 6.

44   "It is one of": Edith Wharton, *Fighting France: From Dunkerque to Belfort* (London: Hesperus Press, 1915), 68.

45   "suppressed excitement": J.M.T. Finney, *A Surgeon's Life: The Autobiography of J. M. T. Finney* (New York: G. P. Putnam's Sons, 1940), 157.

45   "acute sense of high adventure": Thomas B. Turner, *Heritage of Excellence: The Johns Hopkins Medical Institutions, 1914–1947* (Baltimore: Johns Hopkins University Press, 1974), 32.

46   "They must be able": Violetta Thurstan, *A Text Book of War Nursing* (London: G. P. Putnam's Sons, 1917), 13.

46   "to dance well": Fitzgerald, *Memoirs of an American Nurse*, 4–5.

47   "I have lived a week": Fitzgerald, *Memoirs of an American Nurse*, July 4, 1916, 52–53.

47   "We had a frightful": Fitzgerald, *Memoirs of an American Nurse*, November 7, 1916, 89.

47 "The patients are kept": Fitzgerald, *Memoirs of an American Nurse*, 66.

47 "Is a man sane": Fitzgerald, *Memoirs of an American Nurse*, 100.

47 "essential players": William Osler, "Doctor and Nurse," talk given at Johns Hopkins Hospital, 1891, in *Aequanimitas: With Other Addresses to Medical Students, Nurses and Practitioners of Medicine*, 3rd ed. (New York: McGraw Hill, 1951), 19.

48 "This is the Backwash": La Motte, *The Backwash of War*, 7.

48 "When he could stand it": La Motte, *The Backwash of War*, 8.

48 "It was an expensive business": La Motte, *The Backwash of War*, 9.

48 "given to reflection": La Motte, *The Backwash of War*, 10.

49 "Ten kilometres from here": Mary Borden, *The Forbidden Zone* (London: Hesperus Press, 2008; first published 1929), 79–80.

50 "We could revive": Borden, *The Forbidden Zone*, 95–96.

50 "I possessed": Baroness de T'Serclaes (Elsie Knocker), *Flanders and Other Fields* (London: Harrap, 1964).

50 "It was very frightening": Louie Johnson, oral history interview, Imperial War Museum, London, quoted in Christine E. Hallett, *Containing Trauma: Nursing Work in the First World War* (Manchester: Manchester University Press, 2009), 96–97.

51 "When the poor soul": Louisa May Alcott, *Civil War: Hospital Sketches* (Mineola, N.Y.: Dover, 2006; first published 1863), 69.

51 "He was quite conscious": Mary Borden, letter posted May 26, 1917. Papers of Edward Spears, Churchill College, Cambridge, SPRS 11/1/1.

51 "shocking scenes": Penny Starns, *Sisters of the Somme* (Stroud, Gloucestershire: History Press, 2016), 57.

52 "the gift of understanding": Thurstan, *A Text Book of War Nursing*, 3.

52 "It was my business": Borden, *The Forbidden Zone*, 95.

53 "A nurse comes along": Borden, *The Forbidden Zone*, 43.

53 "As soon as routine": Gavin Maxwell, *Ring of Bright Water* (New York: Penguin, 1996; first published 1960), 105.

54 "Mighty dread": Beatrice Hopkinson, *Nursing Through Shot & Shell: A Great War Nurse's Story*, ed. Vivien Newman (Barnsley, South Yorkshire: Pen and Sword Military, 2014), 73–74.

54 "Winter may rise": Edward Thomas, "The Grave of Winter," in *In Pursuit of Spring* (Beaminster: Little Toller, 2016; first published 1914), 115.

55 "The war has done": J. M. Barrie, "Courage," rectorial address delivered at the University of St. Andrews, Scotland, May 3, 1922; reprinted in J. M. Barrie, *The Works of J. M. Barrie*, vol. 9 (New York: Charles Scribner's Sons, 1930).

55   "The crown of the hill": Enid Bagnold, *A Diary Without Dates* (London: William Heinemann, 1918), 96–97.

55   "though they escaped": Erich Maria Remarque, *All Quiet on the Western Front* (New York: Ballantine Books, 1982; first published 1928), epigraph.

55   "Our knowledge of life": Remarque, *All Quiet on the Western Front*, 264.

56   "These are wonderfully care-free": Remarque, *All Quiet on the Western Front*, 9.

56   "What will happen afterwards?": Remarque, *All Quiet on the Western Front*, 264.

56   "He fell in October": Remarque, *All Quiet on the Western Front*, 296.

CHAPTER 3: RIVERS

57   "The problem": W.H.R. Rivers, "The Repression of War Experience," *The Lancet* 191 (February 2, 1918): 174.

58   "If imagination is active": W.H.R. Rivers, *Instinct and the Unconscious* (Cambridge: Cambridge University Press, 1924), 226.

58   Captain W.H.R. Rivers: W.H.R. Rivers deeply influenced many individuals, several of whom left accounts of their relationship with him. (Rivers himself left very little record of his personal life.) Siegfried Sassoon's diaries, letters, and memoirs—especially *Memoirs of an Infantry Officer: Siegfried's Journey, 1916–1920;* and *Sherston's Progress*—remain the most important account of Rivers as a doctor and psychotherapist. Robert Graves, who knew Rivers through Sassoon's relationship with him, also described his literary and psychological debt to Rivers. Rivers's colleagues and friends—anthropologist Alfred Cort Haddon, neurologist Sir Henry Head, Egyptologist Sir Grafton Elliott Smith, physicians Sir Walter Langdon-Brown and Charles Samuel Myers, psychologists Sir Frederic Bartlett and T. H. Pear, and those who wrote obituaries for him after his early death—provide highly descriptive and warm accounts of Rivers as an intellect, doctor, teacher, and friend.

Richard Slobodin's *W.H.R. Rivers* gives a general introduction to Rivers's life; it focuses on Rivers's work as an anthropologist but also gives an overview of his work in psychology and medicine. Novelist Pat Barker's widely read *Regeneration* centers on Rivers, Siegfried Sassoon, and Craiglockhart Hospital during the First World War. Several historians and scholars have written about Rivers, including Arthur Kleinman, *What Really Matters;* Paul Fussell, *The Great War and Modern Memory;* Elaine Showalter, *The Female*

Malady; Ben Shephard, *A War of Nerves* and *Headhunters;* and John
Forrester and Laura Cameron, *Freud in Cambridge.*

58   "root and branch": W.H.R. Rivers, testimony before the War Office
     Committee of Enquiry into "Shell-Shock," report presented to Par-
     liament (London: His Majesty's Stationery Office, 1922), 55.

58   "last straw": Rivers, Testimony, 55.

58   The term "shell shock": "Shell shock," as used by psychiatrists dur-
     ing the First World War, meant many different things. (This confu-
     sion is even more true for the term currently used, "post-traumatic
     stress syndrome," which is defined and applied in an exception-
     ally broad way.) For accounts and definitions of "shell shock" that
     were used during the First World War, see: Charles S. Myers, "A
     Contribution to the Study of Shell Shock," *The Lancet* 185 (1915):
     316–20; G. Elliot Smith and T. H. Pear, *Shell Shock and Its Lessons*
     (Manchester: Manchester University Press, 1917); Elmer Ernest
     Southard, *Shell-Shock and Other Neuropsychiatric Problems* (Boston:
     W. M. Leonard, 1919); Charles S. Myers, *Shell Shock in France,
     1914–18: Based on a War Diary* (Cambridge: Cambridge University
     Press, 1940); Martin Stone, "Shellshock and the Psychologists," in
     The Anatomy of Madness, vol. 2, ed. W. F. Bynum, R. Porter, and
     M. Shepherd (London: Tavistock, 1985).

58   "wound": Rivers, Testimony, 56.

59   "If you think about": Rivers, Testimony, 58.

59   "altogether unsuited": Rivers, Testimony.

59   "Put it out of": Rivers, Testimony.

60   "familiarity which": W.H.R. Rivers, "Freud's Psychology of the
     Unconscious" (originally published in *The Lancet,* 1917), in Rivers,
     Instinct and the Unconscious, 168.

60   "in a position": Søren Kierkegaard, "The Rotation Method: A Ven-
     ture in a Theory of Social Prudence," in Kierkegaard, *Either/Or,*
     vol. 1 (Princeton, N.J.: Princeton University Press, 1944), 291.

60   "brood upon feelings": W.H.R. Rivers, "The Repression of War
     Experience," *The Lancet* 191 (February 2, 1918): 177.

60   "intolerable memories" . . . "controlled reflection": These ideas are
     discussed at length in W.H.R. Rivers, *Instinct and the Unconscious*
     (Cambridge: Cambridge University Press, 1924); and Rivers, "The
     Repression of War Experience."

62   "The past was still": Siegfried Sassoon, *Sherston's Progress* (New
     York: Penguin Classics, 2013; first published 1936), 33.

62   "[Rivers] was intensely": Henry Head, "Obituary for W.H.R. Rivers,
     M.D., D.Sc., F.R.S.: An Appreciation," *British Medical Journal* 1
     (June 17, 1922): 977–78.

63 His detailed account: Tim Clayton and Phil Craig, *Trafalgar: The Men, the Battle, the Storm* (London: Hodder & Stroughton, 2004).

63 complicated kinships: W.H.R. Rivers, *The Todas* (London: Macmillan, 1906); W.H.R. Rivers, "Geneaologies, Kinship, Regulation of Marriage, Social Organization," in *Sociology, Magic, and Religion of the Eastern Islanders: Reports of the Cambridge Anthropological Expedition to Torres Straits*, vol. 6 (Cambridge: Cambridge University Press, 1908); W.H.R. Rivers, *Kinship and Social Organization* (London: Constable, 1914); W.H.R. Rivers, *The History of Melanesian Society* (Cambridge: Cambridge University Press, 1914).

64 "I woke up": Letter from Robert Lowell to Harriet Winslow, July 31, 1961, in Saskia Hamilton, ed., *The Letters of Robert Lowell* (New York: Farrar, Straus and Giroux, 2005), 385.

65 "might be regarded": W.H.R. Rivers, *Conflict and Dream* (London: Kegan Paul, Trench, Trubner, 1923), 131.

65 "preeminently 'hidden source'": Rivers, *Conflict and Dream*.

65 "Also I am ancestral": Siegfried Sassoon, "Microcosmos," in Siegfried Sassoon, *Collected Poems, 1908–1956* (London: Faber and Faber, 1984), epigraph page.

66 "His study was like": Frederic C. Bartlett, "Cambridge, England: 1887–1937," *American Journal of Psychology* 50 (1937): 91–110, 104–5.

66 "At Cambridge": Bartlett, "Cambridge, England."

66 "Rivers came out": Bartlett, "Cambridge, England."

67 "boundless enthusiasm": T. G. Platten, correspondence to Frederic Bartlett, cited in Bartlett, "Obituary: W.H.R. Rivers," *The Eagle* (St. John's College, Cambridge), 43 (1923), 11.

67 "When students no longer": W.H.R. Rivers, quoted in Robert H. Thouless, *How to Think Straight* (New York: Simon and Schuster, 1950), 74.

67 "leads his pupils": W.H.R. Rivers, "Education and Mental Hygiene," in Rivers, *Psychology and Politics* (London: Kegan Paul, Trench, Trubner, 1923), 104.

67 "not by asking": H. Finer, "Dr. W.H.R. Rivers: Labour Candidate for London University," *The Times* (London), June 7, 1922.

67 "It was his belief": Bartlett, "Obituary: W.H.R. Rivers," 14.

68 "One of the strongest elements": Rivers, *Conflict and Dream*, 85.

68 "I got into such a state": W.H.R. Rivers, untitled and undated manuscript. Haddon Collection, University of Cambridge Library, MS Haddon, 12004.

69 "always had to fight": Letter from Sir Grafton Elliot Smith, in War-

ren Dawson, ed., *Sir Elliot Smith: A Biographical Record by His Colleagues* (London: Jonathan Cape, 1938), 79.

69 periods of depression: L. E. Shore, "W.H.R. Rivers," *The Eagle* (St. John's College, Cambridge, 1922), 2–12.

69 "nervous exhaustion": Queen Square records indicate that Rivers resigned his post at the National Hospital in 1892, likely due to a nervous breakdown. Cited in Ben Shephard, *Headhunters: The Pioneers of Neuroscience* (London: Vintage, 2015), 276.

69 "more common": Shephard, *Headhunters*, 276.

69 "horrible weariness": Bartlett, "Obituary: W.H.R. Rivers," 14.

69 "Sometimes when I": Bartlett, "W.H.R. Rivers," *The Eagle* (St. John's College, Cambridge), 62 (1968), 159.

69 "A spontaneous remembrance": Sassoon, *Sherston's Progress*, 19.

70 "Fear and its expression": W.H.R. Rivers, "War-Neurosis and Military Training" (first published in *Mental Hygiene*, 1918), in W.H.R. Rivers, *Instinct and the Unconscious*, 208.

70 "The public school boy": Rivers, "War-Neurosis and Military Training," 209.

70 "to set an example": Rivers, "War-Neurosis and Military Training," 218.

71 "The officer shall": Rivers, "War-Neurosis and Military Training."

71 "The soldier should": Rivers, "War-Neurosis and Military Training," 226.

71 "think horribly": Rivers, "War-Neurosis and Military Training."

71 "*futurorum malorum*": See Seneca's *Moral Epistles* and *Letters from a Stoic*, as well as the *Meditations of Marcus Aurelius*.

71 "pass unscathed": Rivers, "War-Neurosis and Military Training," 226.

71 "If imagination is active": Rivers, "War-Neurosis and Military Training."

71 "perturbed and disturbed": Arthur Kleinman, *What Really Matters: Living a Moral Life Amidst Uncertainty and Danger* (New York: Oxford University Press, 2006), 215.

71 "an exemplar": Kleinman, *What Really Matters*, 207.

72 "unlovely struggle": Siegfried Sassoon, *Memoirs of an Infantry Officer* (London: Penguin Classics, 2013; first published 1930), 156.

72 "the times are so ominous": W.H.R. Rivers, Letter of Acceptance for the Representation of the University of London in the House of Commons. Quoted in Prefatory Note by Elliot Smith, in W.H.R. Rivers, *Psychology and Politics*, v.

73 "gift of co-ordinating": Arnold Bennett, "W.H.R. Rivers: Some Recollections," *The New Statesman*, June 17, 1922, 290.

73   "beauty of organized": Henry Head, "Obituary: W.H.R. Rivers,"
       977–78.

73   "Rivers," said a colleague: Anonymous, "Obituary for Dr. W.H.R.
       Rivers: A Noted Anthropologist," *The Times* (London), June 5,
       1922.

74   "a history of the movement": W.H.R. Rivers, "The Unity of
       Anthropology," Presidential Address to the Royal Anthropologi-
       cal Institute, *Journal of the Royal Anthropological Institute* 52 (1922):
       15–25.

74   "They went as physiologists": Walter Langdon-Brown, "To a Very
       Wise Man," *St. Bartholomew's Hospital Journal* (November 1936):
       29–30.

74   "regarded all human conditions": A. C. Haddon, "Obituary: W.H.R.
       Rivers," *British Medical Journal*, June 10, 1922, 937.

74   "Every form of social activity": W.H.R. Rivers, quoted in
       J. L. Myres, "W.H.R. Rivers," *Journal of the Royal Anthropological
       Institute of Great Britain and Ireland* 53 (1923): 14.

74   "I should go in for insanity": W.H.R. Rivers, diary entry, 1892. This
       diary, the only found in Rivers's papers, has been lost. See Richard
       Slobodin, *W.H.R. Rivers* (New York: Columbia University Press,
       1978), 13.

76   "sits about": Case record of Alice Meek, who was a patient at Beth-
       lem Royal Hospital from April 15, 1893, to March 27, 1894. She
       was readmitted on July 16, 1894, and then discharged, "uncured,"
       on June 26, 1895. Bethlem Royal Hospital Casebook 146 (Female,
       1893). See also Colin Gale and Robert Howard, *Presumed Curable:
       An Illustrated Casebook of Victorian Psychiatric Patients in Bethlem Hos-
       pital* (Petersfield, Hampshire: Wrightson Biomedical, 2003).

77   "excited . . . gushing": Case record of Alice Meek.

77   "excess of spirits": Case record of Alice Meek.

78   "perhaps no man": C. J. Seligman, "Dr. W.H.R. Rivers." Haddon
       Collection, University of Cambridge Library, MS Haddon 12081a,
       162–63.

78   "It was not really until the war": Langdon-Brown, "To a Very Wise
       Man," 29–30.

79   "one of that brilliant band": Head, "Obituary: W.H.R. Rivers,
       M.D., D.Sc., F.R.S.: An Appreciation," 977–78.

79   "what seemed to me": T. H. Pear, "Some Early Relations Between
       English Ethnologists and Psychologists," *Journal of the Royal Anthro-
       pological Institute of Great Britain and Ireland* 90 (1960): 231.

79   "like priests, of mysteries": Pear, "Some Early Relations Between
       English Ethnologists and Psychologists," 232.

79   "five thousand years": Siegfried Sassoon, "Early Chronology," in
     Siegfried Sassoon: Collected Poems, 1908–1956, 149–50.

80   "The war has been a vast crucible": W.H.R. Rivers, "Psychology
     and the War," in Rivers, *Instinct and the Unconscious*, 252.

80   "The war has shown": Rivers, "Psychology and the War," 252–53.

80   "hope and promise": W.H.R. Rivers, "Psychiatry and the War," *Sci-
     ence* 49 (1919): 367.

80   "uncompromising hostility": Rivers, "Psychiatry and the War,"
     368.

81   "sift the grain from the chaff": Rivers, "Psychiatry and the War."

81   "taken its place": Rivers, "Psychiatry and the War."

81   "a thing which has not": Sigmund Freud, "Analysis of a Phobia in a
     Five-Year-Old Boy," in *The Complete Psychological Works of Sigmund
     Freud*, vol. 10 (London: Hogarth Press, 1909), 123.

81   "material of morbid complexes": W.H.R. Rivers, "Freud's Psychol-
     ogy of the Unconscious," *The Lancet*, June 16, 1917, 913.

81   "and to a large extent Freud": Rivers, "Freud's Psychology of the
     Unconscious."

82   "a regular part of my treatment": W.H.R. Rivers, "The Dream-
     Work," in *Conflict and Dream* (London: Kegan Paul, Trench, Trub-
     ner, 1923), 35.

82   "undermined my treatment": Rivers, "The Dream-Work," 36.

82   "There were enthusiastic psychotherapists": Langdon-Brown, "To
     a Very Wise Man," 30.

82   "My own standpoint": W.H.R. Rivers, "Freud's Psychology of the
     Unconscious," 914.

83   "He was wearing the King's uniform": T. H. Pear, "Some Early
     Relations," 235.

83   "brought me into contact": Quoted in Langdon-Brown, "To a Very
     Wise Man," 30.

84   "I think it was because": Langdon-Brown, "To a Very Wise Man."

84   "The War was too big": Sassoon, *Memoirs of an Infantry Officer*, 152.

86   "Lit by departing day": Siegfried Sassoon, *The Weald of Youth* (Lon-
     don: Faber and Faber, 1986; first published 1942), 277–78. Major
     biographies of Siegfried Sassoon include John Stuart Roberts, *Sieg-
     fried Sassoon* (London: Richard Cohen Books, 1999); Max Egre-
     mont, *Siegfried Sassoon: A Life* (New York: Farrar, Straus and Giroux,
     2005); Jean Moorcroft Wilson, *Siegfried Sassoon: Soldier, Poet, Lover,
     Friend* (New York: Overlook Duckworth, 2014). (Wilson's biogra-
     phy of Sassoon is a one-volume publication that includes her exten-
     sive, previous writing on Sassoon.)

86   "Afterwards I went": Sassoon, *Memoirs of an Infantry Officer*, 7–8.

87   "There is a sense": Sassoon, *Memoirs of an Infantry Officer*, 8.

87   "conspicuous gallantry": "Military Cross citation for 2nd Lt. Siegfried Lorraine [*sic*] Sassoon," Supplement 29684, July 25, 1916, *The London Gazette*, 7441.

87   "One cannot be a good soldier": Siegfried Sassoon, June 15, 1918, in *Siegfried Sassoon Diaries, 1915–1918*, ed. Rupert Hart-Davis (London: Faber and Faber, 1983), 271.

88   "I am making this statement": Siegfried Sassoon, June 15, 1917, *Siegfried Sassoon Diaries, 1915–1918*, 173–74.

89   "Three evenings a week": Sassoon, *Sherston's Progress*, 6–7.

90   "mental collapse": Robert Graves wrote that when Sassoon went for a walk he on occasion "saw corpses lying about on the pavements . . . He was beastly weak and in a rotten state of nerves." Robert Graves, *Goodbye to All That* (London: Penguin Classics, 2000; first published 1929), 211–12.

90   "His conversation is disconnected": Medical Board examining Siegfried Sassoon, July 20, 1917. Public Record Office / Wo339 / SI440 / 49289.

91   "There was never any doubt": Sassoon, *Sherston's Progress*, 3.

91   "wash-outs and shattered heroes": Siegfried Sassoon, October 4, 1917, in *Siegfried Sassoon Diaries, 1915–1918*, 189.

91   "a live museum of war neuroses": Sassoon, *Sherston's Progress*, 4.

91   "I went to Rivers' room": Sassoon, *Sherston's Progress*, 3.

91   "From childhood he has written": Imperial War Museum, London: Documents / 9059 / A.

93   "He discusses his recent actions": Imperial War Museum, London: Documents / 9059 / A.

93   "From an early stage": Imperial War Museum, London: Documents / 9059 / A.

93   "mark time": Sassoon, *Sherston's Progress*, 4.

93   "I asked him whether": Sassoon, *Sherston's Progress*.

94   "lost control": Sassoon, *Sherston's Progress*, 40–41.

95   "cloudless weather": Siegfried Sassoon, *Memoirs of a Fox-Hunting Man* (New York: Penguin Classics, 2013; first published 1928), 231.

95   "It was my own countryside": Sassoon, *Memoirs of a Fox-Hunting Man*, 66.

95   "My intellect was not": Sassoon, *Memoirs of a Fox-Hunting Man*, 7.

96   "Some of the modern measures": W.H.R. Rivers, "Psycho-therapeutics," in *Encyclopedia of Religion and Ethics*, ed. James Hastings, vol. 10 (Edinburgh: T. and T. Clark, 1918), 440.

96   "again bringing religion": Rivers, "Psycho-therapeutics," 440.

96   "cities with dead names": Siegfried Sassoon, "To a Very Wise Man,"

in Sassoon, *Collected Poems: 1908–1956* (London: Faber and Faber, 1984), 97.

96   "largely ascribed": Rivers, "Psycho-therapeutics," 436.

97   "Fires in the dark": Sassoon, "To a Very Wise Man," 97–98.

97   "There is all the difference": Rivers, "Psycho-therapeutics," 438.

98   "enveloped by a sense": Rivers, "Psycho-therapeutics," 437.

98   "Autognosis": *Siegfried Sassoon Diaries, 1920–1922*, ed. Rupert Hart-Davis (London: Faber and Faber, 1981), 47.

98   "My brain is screwed up": Siegfried Sassoon, April 24, 1917, in *Siegfried Sassoon Diaries, 1915–1918*, 161.

99   "it follows the grim reality": W.H.R. Rivers, "Affect in the Dream," in Rivers, *Conflict and Dream*, 67.

99   "different from any known": Rivers, "Affect in the Dream," 66.

99   "The dream ends": Rivers, "Affect in the Dream."

99   "dread of its repetition": Rivers, "Affect in the Dream."

99   "The Artilleryman's Vision": Walt Whitman, "The Artilleryman's Vision," in Walt Whitman, *Leaves of Grass*, ed. Sculley Bradley and Harold W. Blodgett (New York: W. W. Norton, 1973; first published 1865), 317–18.

100 "The garden waits for something": Siegfried Sassoon, "Repression of War Experience," in *Collected Poems* (London: Faber and Faber, 1984), 82.

100 "No, no, not that": Sassoon, "Repression of War Experience," 82.

101 "Repression of War Experience": W.H.R. Rivers, "The Repression of War Experience," *The Lancet* 191 (1918): 173–77. Rivers's *Lancet* article was based on a talk he had given before the Section of Psychiatry, Royal Society of Medicine, on December 4, 1917.

101 "talked over": Rivers, "The Repression of War Experience."

101 "Remembering": Siegfried Sassoon, "To One Who Was with Me in the War," *Collected Poems* (London: Faber and Faber, 1984), 171–72.

102 "So long as I was an officer": W.H.R. Rivers, "Symbolism in Dreams," in Rivers, *Conflict and Dream*, 171–72.

102 "Life, with an ironic gesture": Sassoon, *Sherston's Progress*, 33.

103 "Autumn was asserting itself": Sassoon, *Sherston's Progress*, 12.

103 "When I'm asleep": Sassoon, "Sick Leave," in *Collected Poems* (London: Faber and Faber, 1984), 78.

103 "going back": Sassoon, *Sherston's Progress*, 33–34.

103 "drift on": Sassoon, *Sherston's Progress*, 21.

103 "When the windows": Sassoon, *Sherston's Progress*, 26.

103 "Love drove me to rebel": Sassoon, "Banishment," in *Collected Poems* (London: Faber and Faber, 1984), 79.

104 "I had said good-bye": Sassoon, *Sherston's Progress*, 38–39.

104 "I must never forget Rivers": Siegfried Sassoon, May 9, 1918, in *Siegfried Sassoon Diaries, 1915–1918*, 246.

104 "I was restless and overwrought": Sassoon, *Sherston's Progress*, 145.

105 "angry feeling of wanting": Sassoon, *Sherston's Progress*.

105 "Everything had fallen to pieces": Sassoon, *Sherston's Progress*, 146.

105 "And then, unexpected": Sassoon, *Sherston's Progress*, 146–47.

CHAPTER 4: AND THE GOD LEFT

109 "O Lord Asclepius": Aelius Aristedes, "Speech in Honor of Ascle-pius," *Oratio XLII*, lines 1–15, in Emma Edelstein and Ludwig Edelstein, *Asclepius: Collection and Interpretation of the Testimonies* (Baltimore: Johns Hopkins University Press, 1998; originally pub-lished 1945), 159.

110 "He stretches out his hand": Aelius Aristides, *Oratio L*, 56, in Emma J. Edelstein and Ludwig Edelstein, *Asclepius: Collection and Interpretation of the Testimonies* (Baltimore: Johns Hopkins Univer-sity Press, 1998; originally published 1945), 150.

110 "Amid the Aesculapian cult": Sir William Osler, *The Principles and Practice of Medicine*, 7th ed. (New York and London: D. Appleton, 1910), 1095.

110 What she saw was "remarkable": Arlette Leroi-Gourhan, "The Flowers Found with Shanidar IV, a Neanderthal Burial in Iraq," *Science* 190 (1975): 562.

111 "more than 50,000 years ago": Leroi-Gourhan, "The Flowers Found with Shanidar IV," 564.

111 "rang[ing] the mountainside": Ralph Solecki, an archaeologist at Columbia University, had sent soil samples to Arlette Leroi-Gourhan from the Shanidar Cave in Iraq and asked her to do an analysis of the pollen. He summarized her conclusions by stating, "Someone in the Last Ice Age had ranged the mountainside in the mournful task of collecting flowers." Ralph S. Solecki, *Shanidar: The First Flower People* (New York: Alfred A. Knopf, 1971), 247. See also Ralph Solecki, "Shanidar IV, a Neanderthal Flower Burial in Northern Iraq," *Science* 190 (1975): 880–81.

111 Some critics were maliciously tart: The most extensive discussion of evidence for and against Neanderthal burials is in a detailed review article that contains comments on the paper from scientists with a variety of viewpoints: Robert H. Gargett, "Grave Shortcomings: The Evidence for Neanderthal Burial," *Current Anthropology* 30 (1989): 157–90.

111 Flowers might have been: Jeffrey D. Sommer, "The Shanidar IV

'Flower Burial': A Re-evaluation of Neanderthal Burial Ritual," *Cambridge Archaeological Journal* 9 (1999): 127–37.

112 Scientists who studied cave structure: Harold L. Dibble, Vera Aldeias, Paul Goldberg, et al., "A Critical Look at Evidence from La Chapelle-aux-Saints Supporting an Intentional Neanderthal Burial," *Journal of Archaeological Science* 53 (2015): 649–57; Paul Goldberg, Vera Aldeias, Harold Dibble, et al., "Testing the Roc de Marsal Neanderthal 'Burial' with Geoarchaeology," *Archaeological and Anthropological Sciences* 9 (2017): 1005–15. They concluded that research "fails to provide unequivocal evidence in support of the notion that Neanderthals intentionally interred their dead, whether in any ritualistic or symbolic context or not" (Dibble, Aldeias, Goldberg, et al., "A Critical Look," 649). A recent excavation of Shanidar Cave by archaeologists from Cambridge University, however, conducted more than fifty years after the initial discovery of the Neanderthal skeletons there, concluded that at least several of the skeletons formed a "unique assemblage" and that it was likely that they had been buried in an "intentionally dug channel." The lead author of the study, Emma Pomeroy, suggested that the cave may have been "a site of memory for the repeated ritual interment of their dead" (Emma Pomeroy, interview in *Science Daily*, February 18, 2020). Emma Pomeroy, Paul Bennett, Chris Hunt, et al., "New Neanderthal Remains Associated with the 'Flower Burial' at Shanidar Cave," *Antiquity* 94 (2020): 11–26. The idea of early man buried with flowers, of conjuring sites of memory, persists as a heuristic and imaginative attraction.

112 Recent science suggests: Jan Lietava, "Medicinal Plants in a Middle Paleolithic Grave Shanidar IV?" *Journal of Ethnopharmacology* 35 (1992): 263–66; Gerhard Shipley and Kelly Kindscher, "Evidence for the Paleoethnobotany of the Neanderthal: A Review of the Literature," *Scientifica* [2016 Article ID 8927654].

112 Penny Spikins, an archaeologist: Penny Spikins, Andrew Needham, Barry Wright, et al., "Living to Fight Another Day: The Ecological and Evolutionary Significance of Neanderthal Healthcare," *Quaternary Science Reviews* 217 (2019): 98–118.

112 their 2016 article in *Nature:* Jacques Jaubert, Sophie Verheyden, Dominique Genty, et al., "Early Neanderthal Constructions Deep in Bruniquel Cave in Southwestern France," *Nature* 534 (2016): 111–14.

112 "more complex": Jaubert et al., "Early Neanderthal Constructions," 114.

114 Willow bark: Michael Desborough and David Keeling, "The Aspi-

rin Story—from Willow to Wonder Drug," *British Journal of Hae-matology* 177 (2017): 674–83; Maria Rosa Montinari, Sergio Minelli, and Raffaele De Caterina, "The First 3500 Years of Aspirin History from Its Roots," *Vascular Pharmacology* 113 (2019): 1–8.

114 in our modern pharmacopoeia: The World Health Organization estimates that approximately one in four modern drugs used in the United States are derived from plants. "Traditional Medicine," Factsheet 134 (Geneva: World Health Organization, 2013); Karen Hardy, "Paleomedicine and the Evolutionary Context of Medicinal Plant Use," *Revista Brasileira de Farmacognosia* 31 (2021): 1–15.

114 In the *Iliad:* "Cut this shaft from my thigh," it says in the *Iliad:* "And the dark blood— / wash it out of the wound with clear warm water. / And spread the soothing, healing salves across it / the powerful drugs they say you learned from Achilles." Homer, *The Iliad*, trans. Robert Fagles (New York: Penguin, 1998), 324, book 11, lines 990–993. See also: S. G. Marketos and G. J. Androutsos, "The Healing Art in the *Iliad,*" in S. A. Palpetis, ed., *Science and Technology in Homeric Epics* (New York: Springer, 2008), 275–81.

114 For thousands of years: Healing plants such as yarrow are an important part of myth and folklore, as well as a part of the healing rituals of priests and physicians. More than sixty thousand years after yarrow found its way into a Neanderthal cave, the remains of a fully clothed sixteen- to eighteen-year-old Bronze Age female were found in an oak coffin lined with ox hide. Her body, which dated to c. 1370 B.C., had been covered by a woollen blanket; a small container next to her head, made of birch bark, held cremated remains of a five- to six-year-old child. She had been buried on a summer's day, researchers concluded, because yarrow flowers had been placed in her coffin. Karin Frei, Ulla Mannering, Kristian Kristiansen, et al., "Tracing the Dynamic Life Story of a Bronze Age Female," *Scientific Reports* 5 (2015): 10431; doi 10.1038 / srep 10431 (2015). Yarrow has been a part of human existence from the earliest years and it continues to be entwined in the lore and rituals of life. The questions one asked about the presence of yarrow in a Neanderthal cave one also asks about yarrow found in a grave in Denmark sixty thousand years later: Did it mark a young death and others' mourning? Was it a nod to transience, to beauty, to the gods? Had it been a part of a religious or healing ritual? Was it just a flower to mark a summer death?

115 "No heart can think": Quoted in Margaret Grieve, *A Modern Herbal*, vol. 2 (New York: Dover, 1971; first published 1931), 632.

115 Persian doctors recommended: The history of medicinal uses of

botanicals for psychiatric conditions is a long one. See, for example: J. R. Whitwell, *Historical Notes on Psychiatry: Early Times–End of 16th Century* (London: H. K. Lewis, 1936); Stanley W. Jackson, *Melancholia and Depression: From Hippocratic Times to Modern Times* (New Haven: Yale University Press, 1986); Giuseppe Roccatagliata, *A History of Ancient Psychiatry* (New York: Greenwood Press, 1986); N. Vakili and A. Gorji, "Psychiatry and Psychology in Medieval Persia," *Journal of Clinical Psychiatry* 67 (2006): 1862–69.

115 "purge all the melancholy vapours": Robert Burton, "Herbal Alternatives," vol. 2, pt. 2, sec. 4, in *The Anatomy of Melancholy* (New York: New York Review Books, 2001; first published 1621), 216.

116 Egypt's "teeming soil": Homer, *The Odyssey*, book 4, trans. Robert Fagles (New York: Penguin, 1996), 131.

116 Dioscorides, the Greek physician: Pedanius Dioscorides, *De Materia Medica*, published A.D. 50–70. This herbal text was widely used for more than fifteen hundred years and describes the medicinal uses of approximately six hundred plants.

116 "mirth and hilarity": Dioscorides, *De Materia Medica;* Pliny the Elder, Book 25, "The Natural History of the Wild Plants."

116 "challenge[s] for the chiefest": Robert Burton, *The Anatomy of Melancholy*, "Herbal Remedies," vol. 2, pt. 2, sec. 1 (London: J. M. Dent, 1961; first published 1621), 20. More than three hundred years later, in "The Raven," Edgar Allan Poe's speaker calls for nepenthe to escape from memory and despair: "Respite—respite and nepenthe from thy memories of Lenore; / Quaff, oh quaff this kind nepenthe and forget this lost Lenore! / Quoth the Raven, 'Nevermore.'"

116 "a drug, heart's ease": Homer, *The Odyssey*, book 4, trans. Robert Fagles, 131.

117 "Stone-from-the-Meeting": The Ebers Papyrus was written c. 1500 B.C. but likely drew upon earlier texts. It is thought to have been discovered in the Theban necropolis on the west bank of the Nile; it is now at the University of Leipzig in Germany.

117 "Sixty centuries ago": Sir William Osler, *The Evolution of Modern Medicine: A Series of Lectures at Yale University for the Silliman Foundation, in April, 1913* (New Haven: Yale University Press, 1921).

117 "the first figure": Osler, *The Evolution of Modern Medicine.*

117 "for no other scientist": Isaac Asimov, *Biographical Encyclopedia of Science and Technology* (New York: Doubleday, 1972).

118 Edwin Smith Papyrus: This Egyptian medical text, dating to approximately 1600 B.C., is more grounded in scientific thinking than other ancient Egyptian medical texts, which are deeply rooted in magic and ritual. The papyrus, primarily surgical in nature,

Notes

describes forty-eight cases of injury and trauma. It is held at the New York Academy of Medicine. J. F. Nunn, *Ancient Egyptian Medicine* (London: British Museum Press, 1996).

118 "uncharted spheres": Osler, *The Evolution of Modern Medicine;* J. Walker, "The Place of Magic in the Practice of Medicine in Ancient Egypt," *Bulletin of the Australian Centre for Egyptology* 1 (1990): 85–95; Roger Forshaw, "Before Hippocrates: Healing Practices in Ancient Egypt," in *Medicine, Healing and Performance*, ed. Effie Gemi-Iordanou, Stephen Gordon, Robert Matthew, et al. (Oxford and Philadelphia: Oxbow Books, 2014), 25–41.

118 Egyptian sleep temples: Roccatagliata, *A History of Ancient Psychiatry;* K. Patton, "A Great and Strange Correction: Intentionality, Locality, and Epiphany in the Category of Dream Incubation," *History of Religions* 43 (2004): 194–223; G. T. Gotthard, "Dreams as a Constitutive Cultural Determinant—the example of Ancient Egypt," *International Journal of Dream Research* 4 (2011): 24–30; J. Assad, "Sleep in Ancient Egypt," in S. Chokroverty and M. Billiard, eds., *Sleep Medicine: A Comprehensive Guide to Its Development, Clinical Milestones, and Advances in Treatment* (New York: Springer, 2015), 13–19.

119 "Asclepius did not appear": Hippocrates, Epistulae, 15 [IX, p. 340, 1 ff. L.], in Edelstein and Edelstein, *Asclepius*, 258–59.

119 "far-flung stone": Pindar, *Pythian Ode* 3.45, in Pindar, *Olympian Odes and Pythian Odes*, vol. 1, trans. William H. Race (Cambridge, Mass.: Harvard University Press, 1997), 255–56, lines 47–56.

120 "greetings to the common hearth": Aristides, Oratio XLII, 1–15, in Edelstein and Edelstein, *Asclepius*, 159.

120 "When the harbor waves": Aristides, Oratio XLVII, 65, in Edelstein and Edelstein, *Asclepius*, 206.

120 "I myself am one": Aelius Aristides, Oratio XXXIII, 15–18, in Edelstein and Edelstein, *Asclepius*, 203. See also: John C. Stephens, "The Dreams of Aelius Aristides: A Psychological Interpretation," *International Journal of Dream Research* 5 (2012): 76–86.

120 "precious gems": Aristides, Oratio XXXIII, 15–18, 203.

120 "stern-cable of salvation": Aristides, Oratio XXXIII, 15–18, 203.

120 "I had been dead": Menander, Papyrus Didotiana, b, 1–15, in Edelstein and Edelstein, *Asclepius*, 212.

121 The Sanctuary of Asclepius: Richard Caton, *The Temple and Ritual of Asklepios at Epidauros and Athens* (London: C. J. Clay and Sons, 1900); Hedvig von Ehrenheim, "Identifying Incubation Areas in Pagan and Early Christian Times," *Proceedings of the Danish Institute*

at Athens VI, ed. Erik Hallager and Sine Riisager (Aarhus: Aarhus University Press, 2009), 237–76.

122 Temple priests drew upon: Edelstein and Edelstein, *Asclepius;* Frank J. Machovec, "The Cult of Asklipios," *American Journal of Clinical Hypnosis* 22 (1979): 85–90; James E. Bailey, "Asklepios: Ancient Hero of Medical Caring," *Annals of Internal Medicine* 124 (1996): 257–63; H. Christopoulou-Aletra, A. Togia, and C. Varlami, "The 'Smart' Asclepieion: A Total Healing Environment," *Archives of Hellenic Medicine* 27 (2010): 259–63.

123 Persians, in another time: Paul Tillich, "The Relation of Religion and Health," in Simon Doniger, ed., *Healing: Human and Divine* (New York: Association Press, 1957), 186.

123 "Unguent Asclepius": Oribasius, Synopsis and Eustathium, III, 162, in Edelstein and Edelstein, *Asclepius*, 191–192.

124 Snakes roved freely: See Edelstein and Edelstein, *Asclepius*, for extensive discussion of serpents in the cult and temples of Asclepius. Also: Sir William Osler, "Asclepius," in *The Evolution of Modern Medicine;* Albert R. Jonsen, *The New Medicine and the Old Ethics* (Cambridge, Mass.: Harvard University Press, 1990); Luciana Angeletti, Umberto Agrimi, Cristina Curia, et al., "Healing Rituals and Sacred Snakes," *The Lancet* 340 (1992): 223–25.

125 "Medicine broke its leading strings": Osler, *The Evolution of Modern Medicine*.

125 "From the brain": "The Sacred Disease," *Hippocrates*, vol. 2 (Cambridge, Mass.: Harvard University Press, 1923), 175. Medical observations attributed to Hippocrates represent the writings and practice not only of Hippocrates but of his followers. The writings of Hippocrates are disputed as to dates and actual authorship. See, for example, W.H.S. Jones, "Greek Medicine and 'Hippocrates,'" *Hippocrates*, vol. 1 (Cambridge, Mass.: Harvard University Library, 1923), ix–lxix; Robin Lane Fox, *The Invention of Medicine: From Homer to Hippocrates* (New York: Basic Books, 2020), 72–97.

126 "They say that he is sick": Purported letter from Hippocrates to the physician Crateuas; the dating and identity of the author are disputed. Cited text is from Letter 16, Hippocrates, *Pseudepigraphic Writings: Letters—Embassy—Speech from the Altar—Decree*, ed. and trans. Wesley D. Smith, *Studies in Ancient Medicine 2*, vol. 1 (Leiden: E. J. Brill, 1990), 71–73; R. J. Hankinson, "The Pseudo-Hippocratic Letters and the Greek Self-Image of Virtue, Health, and Expertise," in D. Manetti, L. Perilli, and A. Roselli, eds., *Ippocrate e gli altri* [en ligne] (Rome: Publications de l'École française de Rome, 2021).

126 Hippocrates made explicit: Hippocrates, "Decorum," *Hippocrates*, vol. 2, trans. W.H.S. Jones (Cambridge, Mass.: Harvard University Press, 1923), 279–301; Hippocrates, "The Physician," *Hippocrates*, vol. 2, 311–13.

127 "gentleman in character": Hippocrates, "The Physician," 311.

127 "grave and kind to all": Hippocrates, "The Physician."

127 "A physician who is": Hippocrates, "Decorum," 287.

127 "I swear by Apollo": Hippocrates, "The Oath," in *Hippocrates*, trans. W.H.S. Jones (Cambridge, Mass.: Harvard University Press, 1923), 299–301.

127 "sacramental seal is inviolable": R. Nolan, "The Law of the Seal of Confession," *Catholic Encyclopedia*, vol. 13 (New York: Robert Appleton, 1912).

128 The secrecy of a confession: "The secrecy of a confession is morally absolute for the confessor, and must under no circumstances be broken." The Book of Common Prayer (According to the use of the Episcopal Church) (New York: Oxford University Press, 1979), 446.

128 "Then the god stretched forth": Hippocrates, Epistulae, 15 [IX, p. 340, 1 ff. L.], in Edelstein and Edelstein, *Asclepius*.

CHAPTER 5: BEARINGS IN THE DARK

129 "Some may not have": W.H.R. Rivers, *The History of Melanesian Society*, vol. 2 (Cambridge: Cambridge University Press, 1914), 298.

130 "To sit quietly": Morag Coate, *Beyond All Reason* (London: Constable, 1964), 214.

130 "It is the physician's order": Maimonides, *M. Regimen Sanitatis*, ed. Suessmann Munter (Jerusalem: Mossad Harav Kook, 1983; first written c. 1190).

130 "uplift my abasement": Antonin Artaud, *Anthology*, trans. David Ossman (San Francisco: City Light Books, 1965), 27–28.

131 "Keep watch, dear Lord": Evening Prayer: Rite One, The Book of Common Prayer (According to the use of the Episcopal Church) (New York: Church Publishing, 1979), 71.

132 "had a low 'leper' window": Katharine Rivers, "Memories of Lewis Carroll," *McMaster University Library Research News* 3 (1976).
    And from Geoffrey Chaucer's *The Canterbury Tales*:

> *And specially from every shire's end*
> *Of England to Canterbury they travel,*
> *To seek the holy blessed martyr;*
> *Who helped them when they were sick.*

132 "cure the souls": Cited in Michael Bliss, *William Osler: A Life in Medicine* (New York: Oxford University Press, 1999), 15.

132 "wild people": Bliss, *William Osler,* 17.

132 "Drunkenness, blasphemy": Bliss, *William Osler.*

133 On the fever wards: Kate C. Mead, "A Few Vignettes of Sir William Osler," bulletin no. 9 of *International Association of Medical Museums and Journal of Technical Methods,* ed. Maude E. Abbott, Sir William Osler Memorial Number: Appreciations and Reminiscences (Montreal: Privately issued, 1926).

133 "the one great moving force": William Osler, "The Faith That Heals," *British Medical Journal* (1910): 1470–72.

133 Faith had limits: William Osler, "Medicine in the Nineteenth Century," paper presented at the John Hopkins Historical Club, January 1901, in *Aequanimitas: With Other Addresses to medical Students, Nurses and Practitioners of Medicine,* 3rd ed. (New York: McGraw Hill, 1932), 259–60.

133 "Probably when our species": John Steinbeck, *The Log from the Sea of Cortez* (New York: Penguin, 1995; first published 1951), 72.

134 "In the treatment of": Samuel Taylor Coleridge, *Specimens of the Table Talk of Samuel Taylor Coleridge* (London: Wentworth Press, 2016), 17.

134 "I will never, ever, ever": John Lipsey, MD, Johns Hopkins Hospital Department of Psychiatry.

134 the evidence of things not seen: Hebrews 11:1–2 (KJV).

134 "whose problem in the last resort": Carl Jung, "Psychotherapists or the Clergy," *Pastoral Psychology* (1956): 32.

134 "nothing whatsoever to do": Jung, "Psychotherapists or the Clergy."

134 "has heard enough": Jung, "Psychotherapists or the Clergy," 37.

134 "reconcile himself": Jung, "Psychotherapists or the Clergy."

135 It is usual for the psychotherapist: Carl Jung, *Symbols and the Interpretation of Dreams,* vol. 18 (Princeton, N.J.: Princeton University Press, 1976), 223.

135 "My method, like Freud's": Carl Jung, "Yoga and the West," in *The Collected Works of C. G. Jung,* vol. 11, ed. Gerhard Adler and R.F.C. Hull (Princeton, N.J.: Princeton University Press, 1970), 536. See Elizabeth Todd, "The Value of Confession and Forgiveness According to Jung," *Journal of Religion and Health* 24 (1985): 39–48.

135 "father-confessor": Siegfried Sassoon, *Sherston's Progress* (New York: Penguin Classics, 2013; first published 1936), 26.

135 "We have erred and strayed": Confession of Sin, Evening Prayer: Rite One, The Book of Common Prayer.

135 "Shams are over": William James, *The Varieties of Religious Experi-*

ence: A Study in Human Nature (New York: Penguin, 1982; first published 1902), 462–63.

136 make "a searching and fearless": Twelve Step Program, *Alcoholics Anonymous*, 4th ed. (New York: AA Publishing, 2001; first published 1939).

136 "most important psychotherapeutic": W.H.R. Rivers, "Psychotherapeutics," in *Encyclopedia of Religion and Ethics*, ed. James Hastings, vol. 10 (Edinburgh: T. and T. Clark, 1918), 437.

136 "I am ill because of wounds": D. H. Lawrence, "Healing," in *Complete Poems*, vol. 1, ed. V. de Sola Pinto and W. F. Roberts (New York: Penguin, 1994), 620.

137 "cannot afford to ignore": John Custance, *Wisdom, Madness and Folly: The Philosophy of a Lunatic* (New York: Pellegrini & Cudahy, 1952), 250.

137 "Can it be proved?": Coate, *Beyond All Reason*, 216.

137 "does not have to be a believer": Coate, *Beyond All Reason*, 212–13.

138 "leave their patients free": Coate, *Beyond All Reason*, 183.

138 "a real person to the patient": Coate, *Beyond All Reason*, 212.

138 "step across into": Coate, *Beyond All Reason*, 188.

138 to give his eulogy: Kay Redfield Jamison, "Eulogy for Anthony Storr (1920–2001)," memorial service at Holywell Music Room, Oxford, June 24, 2001. Reprinted in Angela Huth, ed., *Well-Remembered Friends: Eulogies on Celebrated Lives* (London: John Murray, 2004), 349–52.

138 "It's not psychopathology": Christopher Lehmann-Haupt, "Obituary for Anthony Storr," *The New York Times*, March 28, 2001.

139 "It was glorious": Anthony Storr, communication to the author.

139 "a hierarchy culminating": Anthony Storr, *Music and the Mind* (New York: Free Press, 1992), 187.

139 "source of reconciliation": Storr, *Music and the Mind*, 188.

139 "an irreplaceable, undeserved": Storr, *Music and the Mind*.

140 "has to be affected": Anthony Storr, *The Art of Psychotherapy* (London: Martin Secker & Worburg, 1979), 170.

140 "One possessed no antennae": Storr, *The Art of Psychotherapy*, 172. Here Storr is quoting from John Parry's *The Psychology of Human Communication* (London: University of London Press, 1967), 170–71.

140 "entering into another's distress": Storr, *The Art of Psychotherapy*, 170.

141 "The thing about being associated": T. H. White, *The Goshawk* (New York: New York Review Books Classics, 2007), 212.

141 "A physician of too much sensibility": John Gregory, *Lectures on the*

Duties and Qualifications of a Physician (London: Strahan and Cadell, 1772), 9. W.H.R. Rivers said likewise: The sympathy of the physician is essential in gaining the confidence of the patient, he wrote, but "unless very judiciously expressed, sympathy will have a bad effect"; for example, he argued, sympathy can encourage the continuance of psychopathology and hinder the development of self-reliance. "Psycho-therapeutics," 438.

141 "depress his spirit": Gregory, *Lectures on the Duties and Qualifications of a Physician*, 9.

141 "Afterwards he would talk": Graham Greene, *A Sort of Life* (London: Vintage, 2002; first published 1971), 79.

142 Less beneficial: Several studies document a significant decrease over time in the use of psychotherapy by psychiatrists, as well as a decrease in the use of psychotherapy by clinicians of all backgrounds, especially in treating patients who are financially at a disadvantage. Ramin Mojtabai and Mark Olfson, "National Trends in Psychotherapy by Office-Based Psychiatrists," *Archives of General Psychiatry* 65 (2008): 962–70; M. Olfson and S. C. Marcus, "National Trends in Outpatient Psychotherapy," *American Journal of Psychiatry* 167 (2010): 1456–63; Brandon A. Gaudiano and Ivan W. Miller, "The Evidence-Based Practice of Psychotherapy," *Clinical Psychology Review* 22 (2013): 813–24.

143 "Psycho-therapy is rather amazing": Robert Lowell, letter to Elizabeth Bishop, November 18, 1949, in *The Letters of Robert Lowell*, ed. Saskia Hamilton (New York: Farrar, Straus and Giroux, 2005), 150.

144 *Dictionary of Psychological Medicine:* Daniel Hack Tuke, ed., *A Dictionary of Psychological Medicine* (Philadelphia: P. Blakiston, 1892), 1034. Tuke's influence on the field of medical psychology, and his family's influence on the humane treatment of the severely mentally ill, were lasting ones. See also A. Digby, *Madness, Morality, and Medicine: A Study of the York Retreat, 1796–1914* (Cambridge and New York: Cambridge University Press, 1985); Sarah Chaney, "The Action of the Imagination: Daniel Hack Tuke and Late Victorian Psycho-therapeutics," *History of the Human Sciences* 30 (2017): 17–33.

144 Psychotherapy was restorative: Tuke, *A Dictionary of Psychological Medicine*, 1034.

144 oldest branch of medicine: W.H.R. Rivers, "Psycho-therapeutics," 433. Much of Rivers's work centered on comparative medical systems and the cultural context of healing. This focus of medical anthropology is discussed in depth by Arthur M. Kleinman at Harvard. See Arthur M. Kleinman, "Some Issues for a Comparative

Study of Medical Healing," *International Journal of Social Psychiatry* 19 (1973): 159–65.

144 "Psychotherapy is no achievement": Leopold Löwenfeld (1897), cited in Sonu Shamdasani, "'Psychotherapy': The Invention of a Word," *History of the Human Sciences* 18 (2005): 8. See also Christopher Gill, "Ancient Psychotherapy," *Journal of the History of Ideas* 46 (1985): 307–25; Chiara Thumiger, "Therapy of the Word and Other Psychotherapeutic Approaches in Ancient Greek Medicine," *Transcultural Psychiatry* 57 (2020): 741–52.

145 A British definition: D. Leigh, C.M.B. Pare, and J. Marks, eds., *A Concise Encyclopedia of Psychiatry* (Baltimore: University Park Press, 1977), 305.

145 The American Psychological Association: L. F. Campbell, J. C. Norcross, M. J. Vasques, and N. J. Kaslow, "Recognition of Psychotherapy Effectiveness: The APA Resolution," *Psychotherapy* 50 (2013): 98–101.

145 More than four hundred: T. B. Karasu, "The Specificity Versus Nonspecificity Dilemma: Toward Identifying Therapeutic Change Agents," *American Journal of Psychiatry* 143 (1986): 687–95; S. Garfield and A. Bergin, "Introduction and Historical Overview," in A. Bergin and S. Garfield, eds., *Handbook of Psychotherapy and Behaviour Change* (Chichester: Wiley, 1994), 3–18.

146 mystical and transcendent states: R. R. Griffiths, W. A. Richards, U. McCann, and R. Jesse, "Psilocybin Can Occasion Mystical-Type Experiences Having Substantial and Sustained Personal Meaning and Spiritual Significance," *Psychopharmacology* 187 (2006): 268–283; W. N. Pahnke, "Psychedelic Drugs and Mystical Experience," *International Psychiatry Clinics* 5 (1969): 149–162; R. G. Wasson, *The Wondrous Mushroom: Mycolatry in Mesoamerica* (New York: McGraw-Hill, 1980).

146 Treatment results: See, for example, Alan Davis, Frederick Barrett, Darrick May, et al., "Effects of Psilocybin-Assisted Therapy on Major Depressive Disorder: A Randomized Clinical Trial," *JAMA Psychiatry* 78 (2021): 481–89, E1–E9; David Horton, Blaise Morrison, and Judy Schmidt, "Systematized Review of Psychotherapeutic Components of Psilocybin-Assisted Psychotherapy," *American Journal of Psychotherapy* 74 (2021): 140–149; Mary Sweeney, Sandeep Nayak, Ethan Hurwitz, et al., "Comparison of Psychedelic and Near-Death or Other Non-Ordinary Experiences in Changing Attitudes about Death and Dying," *PLOS ONE* 17 (2022): e0271926; G. M. Goodwin, S. T. Aaronson, O. Alvarez, et al., "Single-Dose

Psilocybin for a Treatment-Resistant Episode of Major Depression," *New England Journal of Medicine* (2022) 387: 1637–1648.

146 use of psychedelic substances in prehistoric: Elisa Guerra-Doce, "Psychoactive Substances in Prehistoric Times: Examining the Archaeological Evidence," *Time and Mind* 8 (2015): 91–112; Michael Winkleman, "Introduction: Evidence for Entheogen Use in Prehistory and World Religions," *Journal of Psychedelic Studies* 3 (2019): 43–62.

147 *Persuasion and Healing:* Jerome D. Frank, *Persuasion and Healing: A Comparative Study of Psychotherapy* (Baltimore: Johns Hopkins Press, 1961). *Persuasion and Healing* continues to have a powerful effect on the study of psychotherapy. Kay Redfield Jamison, "Healing Through Words: Jerome Frank and Psychotherapy at Johns Hopkins: The Phipps Centennial Lectures: The Jerome Frank Lecture," *Journal of Nervous and Mental Disease* 205 (2017): 273–74.

147 "socially sanctioned": Frank, *Persuasion and Healing*, 2.

147 "a circumscribed": Frank, *Persuasion and Healing*, 2–3.

148 "knack for posing questions": Thomas Rennie, "Adolf Meyer and Psychobiology: The Man, His Methodology and Its Relation to Therapy," *American Congress on General Semantics*, vol. 2 (1943): 160.

148 "hints of excitement": Greene, *A Sort of Life*, 79.

148 To be demoralized: Jerome D. Frank, "Psychotherapy: The Restoration of Morale," *American Journal of Psychiatry* 131 (1974): 271–74; John M. de Figueiredo and Jerome Frank, "Subjective Incompetence, the Clinical Hallmark of Demoralization," *Comprehensive Psychiatry* 23 (1982): 353–63; L. Tecuta, E. Tomba, S. Grandi, and G. A. Fava, "Demoralization: A Systematic Review of Its Clinical Characterization," *Psychological Medicine* 45 (2015): 673–91.

148 "The mastery of life's direction": Paul R. McHugh and Phillip R. Slavney, *The Perspectives of Psychiatry*, 2nd ed. (Baltimore and London: Johns Hopkins University Press, 1998), 282.

148 "It is facilitated by learning": McHugh and Slavney, *The Perspectives of Psychiatry*.

149 "to organize and grow": Adolf Meyer, quoted in S. D. Lamb, *Pathologist of the Mind: Adolf Meyer and the Origins of American Psychiatry* (Baltimore: Johns Hopkins University Press, 2014), 222.

149 "Throughout the whole history": Rivers, "Psycho-therapeutics," 437.

149 behavioral techniques: Cognitive behavioral therapy (CBT) and dialectical behavior therapy (DBT) are two of the best-studied, most effective, and most widely used of the targeted psychothera-

pies. Both aim to modify specific patterns of thinking and behavior. Aaron T. Beck, *Cognitive Therapy and the Emotional Disorders* (New York: Penguin, 1979); Marsha M. Linehan, *DBT Skills Training Manual*, 2nd ed. (New York: Guilford, 2015); Christopher R. DeCou, Katherine Anne Comtois, and Sara J. Landes, "Dialectical Behavior Therapy Is Effective for the Treatment of Suicidal Behavior: A Meta-Analysis," *Behavior Therapy* 50 (2019): 60–72; Márcia Cristina Oliveira de Simoni and Murillo de Oliveira Dias, "Literature Review on Cognitive Behavioral Therapy," *British Journal of Psychology Research* 8 (2020): 39–47.

150 "depends on the patient's sense of alliance": Scott A. Baldwin, Bruce E. Wampold, and Zac E. Imel, "Untangling the Alliance-Outcome Correlation: Exploring the Relative Importance of Therapist and Patient Variability in the Alliance," *Journal of Consulting and Clinical Psychology* 75 (2007): 842–52; Bruce E. Wampold, "How Important Are the Common Factors in Psychotherapy? An Update," *World Psychiatry* 14 (2015): 270–77.

150 "The chief of these": John Gregory, *Lectures on the Duties*, 19.

150 "sensibility of heart": Gregory, *Lectures on the Duties*, 19–20.

150 "a faculty of seeing": J. C. Bucknill and D. H. Tuke, *A Manual of Psychological Medicine* (London: John Churchill, 1879).

150 Therapists require also to be: Richard D. Chessick, *How Psychotherapy Heals: The Process of Intensive Psychotherapy* (Northvale, N.J.: Jason Aronson, 1987); Steven J. Ackerman and Mark J. Hilsenroth, "A Review of Therapist Characteristics and Techniques Positively Impacting the Therapeutic Alliance," *Clinical Psychology Review* 23 (2003): 1–33.

151 "human limits and one's own limitations": Karl Jaspers, *General Psychopathology*, vol. 2 (Baltimore and London: Johns Hopkins University Press, 1997; first published 1959), 819.

151 "We do not all start": William Osler, *The Principles and Practice of Medicine* (New York: D. Appleton, 1893), 978.

151 "Diseases are like tulips": Sara Coleridge, *Memoir and Letters of Sara Coleridge*, ed. her daughter (New York: Harper & Brothers, 1874), 208.

152 "The grains of one": Willa Cather, *O Pioneers!* (New York: Vintage, 1992; first published 1913), 82.

152 "Sometimes I think": Graham Greene, *A Burnt-Out Case* (London: Penguin, 1963; first published 1960), 128.

152 Out of atrocity: Viktor Frankl, *Man's Search for Meaning* (Boston: Beacon Press, 2006; first published in German in 1946).

152 "I am unspeakably tired": Viktor Frankl, letter to Wilhelm and Ste-

pha Börner, September 1945, in *Yes to Life: In Spite of Everything* (Boston: Beacon, 2019), 111–12.

153 "Life is so infinitely meaningful": Frankl, *Yes to Life*, 112.

153 "When all this happens": Viktor Frankl, *Recollections: An Autobiography* (New York: Basic Books, 2000), 104.

154 "What can I expect from life?": "We had to teach the despairing men, that *it did not really matter what we expected from life, but rather what life expected from us.*" Frankl, *Man's Search for Meaning*, 77.

154 "Remembering is a noble": Elie Wiesel, "Hope, Despair, and Memory," Nobel Lecture, December 11, 1986, in *Nobel Lectures, Peace 1981–1990*, ed. Irwin Abrams (Singapore: World Scientific Publishing, 1997), 174–80.

154 "transform a personal": Frankl, *Man's Search for Meaning*, 112.

154 "widening and broadening": Frankl, *Man's Search for Meaning*, 110.

154 "If architects want": Frankl, *Man's Search for Meaning*, 105.

154 "a strenuous effort": Siegfried Sassoon, *Sherston's Progress* (London: Faber and Faber, 1983; first published 1936), 42.

155 "Without your wound": Thornton Wilder, *The Angel That Troubled the Waters and Other Plays* (London: Longmans, Green, 1928), 56.

155 "The most skilful physicians": *The Republic of Plato*, 3rd ed., trans. Benjamin Jowett (Oxford: Clarendon Press, 1888), 97.

155 "that gives the measure": Carl Jung, "Fundamental Questions of Psychotherapy," in *The Collected Works of C. J. Jung*, vol. 16 (Princeton, N.J.: Princeton University Press, 1966), 116.

156 Stanley Jackson: See, for example, Stanley W. Jackson, *Melancholia and Depression: From Hippocratic Times to Modern Times* (New Haven: Yale University Press, 1986); Stanley W. Jackson, *Care of the Psyche: A History of Psychological Healing* (New Haven: Yale University Press, 1999); Stanley W. Jackson, "The Wounded Healer," *Bulletin of the History of Medicine* 75 (2001): 1–36.

156 "duties of a physician": Cited in James H. Oliver, "An Ancient Poem on the Duties of a Physician," *Bulletin of the History of Medicine* 7 (1939): 315–23.

156 "No one escapes being wounded": Henri J. M. Nouwen, *The Wounded Healer: Ministry in Contemporary Society* (New York: Doubleday, 1979).

157 *The English Malady:* George Cheyne, *The English Malady: Or, a Treatise of Nervous Diseases of All Kinds, as Spleen, Vapours, Lowness of Spirits, Hypochondriacal and Hysterical Distempers* (London: G. Strahan and J. Leake, 1733).

157 "Reproach universally thrown": Cheyne, *The English Malady*, i.

157 "Of all the Miseries": Cheyne, *The English Malady*, 2–3.

157 "Horror . . . [the] perpetual Anxiety": Cheyne, *The English Malady*, 346.

157 "dropt off like autumnal Leaves": Cheyne, *The English Malady*, 328–29.

158 "It will be a great Satisfaction": Cheyne, *The English Malady*, 4.

158 "Look upon your distressed Friends": Timothy Rogers, *A Discourse Concerning Trouble of Mind, and the Disease of Melancholly* (London: Parkhurst & Cockerill, 1691), ii.

159 "Melancholly seizes on the Brain": Rogers, *A Discourse Concerning Trouble of Mind*, ii.

159 "recourse to such Doctors": Rogers, *A Discourse Concerning Trouble of Mind*, iii–iv.

159 "Tell them of others": Rogers, *A Discourse Concerning Trouble of Mind*, xxii–xxiii. Rogers suffered for much of his life from extended periods of melancholy.

CHAPTER 6: BIG SUR

160 "He was at ease with ambiguity": Kay Redfield Jamison, *An Unquiet Mind: A Memoir of Moods and Madness* (New York: Alfred A. Knopf, 1995), 88.

161 "These years were painful": G. S. Fraser, "Christmas Letter Home," *Poems of G. S. Fraser*, ed. Ian Fletcher and John Lucas (Leicester: Leicester University Press, 1981), 56.

166 "My psychiatrist saw me through": Kay Redfield Jamison, *An Unquiet Mind: A Memoir of Moods and Madness* (New York: Alfred A. Knopf, 1995), 87–88.

167 "I remember sitting in his office": Jamison, *An Unquiet Mind*, 118.

167 "Ineffably, psychotherapy heals": Jamison, *An Unquiet Mind*, 89.

168 "The sea encourages my": Douglas Dunn, "Wishful Thinking," in Norman Ackroyd and Douglas Dunn, *A Line in the Water* (London: Royal Academy, 2009), 140.

170 "The force of the great surf": John Steinbeck, *The Log from the Sea of Cortez* (New York: Penguin, 1995; first published 1951), 49.

CHAPTER 7: SOWINGS

171 "Notre-Dame de Paris": Emmanuel Macron (speech, Notre-Dame Cathedral, Paris, April 15, 2019), translated by Ioline Henter.

172 "When spring came": Willa Cather, *My Ántonia* (New York: Vintage, 2018; first published 1918), 92.

172 "Cette histoire, c'est la nôtre": President Emmanuel Macron

(speech, Notre-Dame Cathedral, Paris, April 15, 2019), translated by Ioline Henter.

172 "It is our literature": Macron (speech, Notre-Dame Cathedral, Paris, April 15, 2019), translated by Ioline Henter.

172 "the base from which we evaluate": Macron, April 15, 2019, speech.

172 our destiny: Macron (speech, Notre-Dame Cathedral, Paris, April 15, 2019), translated by Ioline Henter.

173 The bells that had rung: Allen Tempko, *Notre-Dame of Paris: The Biography of a Cathedral* (New York: Viking Press, 1955); Elizabeth Pineau, "Notre-Dame's Great Bell Tolls Once More on Anniversary of Fire," Reuters, April 15, 2020; Agnès Poirier, *Notre-Dame: The Soul of France* (London: Oneworld, 2020); Dany Sandron and Andrew Tallon, *Notre Dame Cathedral: Nine Centuries of History*, trans. Andrew Tallon and Lindsay Cook (University Park, Pa.: Penn State University Press, 2020).

173 Crown of Thorns: The Crown of Thorns relic in Notre-Dame Cathedral, not surprisingly, has an uncertain provenance: from Jerusalem in the first century A.D., to the Byzantine Emperors Chapel in Constantinople, to King Louis IX of France, who built the Saint-Chapelle in Paris to house it. It has been kept in Notre-Dame de Paris since 1806. Many of the original thorns in the relic were distributed by Louis IX and his successors and are preserved in other reliquaries.

173 "Every time, every time": President Emmanuel Macron (speech, Notre-Dame Cathedral, Paris, April 15, 2019), translated by Ioline Henter.

173 "Everything that makes France": Macron speech, April 16, 2019.

174 "passionately French": Macron speech, April 16, 2019.

174 "After this time of testing": Macron speech, April 16, 2019.

174 Proposals for new designs: Tom Ravenscroft, "Seven Alternative Spires for Notre-Dame Cathedral," *Dezeen*, April 25, 2019; Francesco Banderin, *The Art Newspaper*, August 2, 2019 (citing the French National Assembly, "New Law Regarding Notre-Dame Says Restoration Must Preserve Its 'Historic, Artistic and Architectural Interest'"); Sangeeta Singh-Kurtz, "The Notre-Dame Redesign Debate Is Over—and It Will Look Exactly the Same," *Architectural Digest*, July 15, 2020.

175 "Great edifices, like great mountains": Victor Hugo, *The Hunchback of Notre-Dame*, anonymous nineteenth-century translation used by the first Everyman edition in 1910 (New York: Alfred A. Knopf/Everyman's Library, 2012; first published in French in 1831 under the title *Notre-Dame de Paris, 1482*), 111.

176 "Nature's physician": Cited in James Wood, *Dictionary of Quotations from Ancient and Modern, English and Foreign Sources* (London: Frederick Warne and Co., 1893), 81.

176 *On the Diagnosis and Cure:* Galen, *On the Diagnosis and Cure of the Soul's Passion*, in C. J. Kühn, ed., *Claudii Galeni Opera Omnia* [*The Works of Claudius Galen*] (Leipzig: C. Cnobloch, 1821–1933; rpt. Hildesheim: Georg Olms, 1964–1965. Greek, Latin trans.).

177 "cornerstones of our humanness": Sigmund Freud, *Civilization and Its Discontents*, ed. J. Strachey, in *The Standard Edition of the Complete Psychological Works of Sigmund Freud*, vol. 21, 1927–1931 (New York: W. W. Norton, 1962).

177 "business, exercise, or recreation": Robert Burton, *The Anatomy of Melancholy* (New York: New York Review Books, 2001; first published 1621).

177 "I write of melancholy": Burton, *The Anatomy of Melancholy*, 20.

177 "unladened the abscess": Burton, *The Anatomy of Melancholy*, 21.

177 "be not idle": Burton, *The Anatomy of Melancholy*, 432.

177 "assist in cutting wood": Benjamin Rush, *Medical Inquiries and Observations Upon the Diseases of the Mind* (Philadelphia: Kimber & Richardson, 1812).

178 "a ramble and pleasure": Twenty-Third Annual Report of the Board of Visitors of the Government Hospital for the Insane, 45th Congress, Third Session, October 1878, H. Ex. Docil, 1073. See also Thomas Otto, *St. Elizabeths Hospital: A History* (Washington, D.C.: United States General Services Administration, National Capital Region, 2013); Frances McMillen and James Kane, "The Records of St. Elizabeths Hospital at the National Archives," National Archives, *Prologue Magazine* 42 (2010).

178 "an asylum indeed": President Franklin Pierce, First Annual Message to Congress, December 5, 1853.

178 "add more to the beauty": Report of the Board of Visitors of the Government Hospital for the Insane, 47th Congress, Second Session, October 1, 1882, H. Ex. Docil, 969.

178 "not unmeet": Report of the Board of Visitors, October 1, 1882.

178 "enter into moral treatment": Superintendent William Whitney Godding, quoted in *Historic American Buildings Survey: St. Elizabeths Hospital, Greenhouses (Building 20 A–H)*, HABS NO. DC-349-AY.

178 "bring to darkened minds": Godding, quoted in *Historic American Buildings Survey*.

179 "there is a comparatively greater demand": John E. Lind, "The Mental Patient and the Library," *The Washington Post*, September 30, 1928, SM8.

179 "The mind must be managed": S. B. Woodward, "Observations on the Medical Treatment of Insanity," *American Journal of Insanity* 7 (1850): 1–34.

179 "The spring would come": Willa Cather, *O Pioneers!* (New York: Vintage, 1992; first published 1913), 104.

180 "Writing is a form of therapy": Graham Greene, *Ways of Escape* (New York: Simon and Schuster, 1980), 285.

180 "How often writing": Robert Lowell, letter to Frank Bidart, September 4, 1976, in *The Letters of Robert Lowell*, ed. Saskia Hamilton (New York: Farrar, Straus and Giroux, 2005), 656.

180 "Up till now": Robert Lowell, letter to Elizabeth Bishop, January 23, 1963, in *The Letters of Robert Lowell*, 414.

180 "By creating I became well": Heinrich Heine, in K. R. Eissler, *Goethe: A Psychoanalytic Study: 1775–1786*, vol. 2 (Detroit: Wayne State University, 1963), 1182. "By creating was I able to recover / By creating I became well."

180 Work helps: This is a common belief held by psychologists, physicians, philosophers, and many writers. Sherlock Holmes, a character created by a physician, put it succinctly: "Work is the best antidote to sorrow, my dear Watson." Arthur Conan Doyle, "The Adventure of the Empty House," in *The Return of Sherlock Holmes*, *The Strand Magazine*, 1903.

180 "working till the stars": J. M. Barrie, "Courage," rectorial address delivered at the University of St. Andrews, Scotland, May 3, 1922.

181 "an impenetrable shell": Cynthia Asquith, *Portrait of Barrie* (London: James Barrie, 1954), 1.

181 "full ash-tray": Asquith, *Portrait of Barrie*, 22.

181 "a kind of benign wizardry": Asquith, *Portrait of Barrie*.

181 "fellow of infinite jest": Asquith, *Portrait of Barrie*, 4.

181 "wood and path": Philip Pullman, *Daemon Voices: On Stories and Storytelling* (New York: Alfred A. Knopf, 2018), 76.

181 "wild space . . . an unstructured space": Pullman, *Daemon Voices*, 76.

181 "contains the history": Pullman, *Daemon Voices*, 77.

181 "leads from here to there": Pullman, *Daemon Voices*.

182 "I remember an afternoon": Kay Redfield Jamison, *Nothing Was the Same: A Memoir* (New York: Alfred A. Knopf, 2009), 182.

CHAPTER 8: ISLAND AND QUEST

187 "If you don't live it": Charlie Parker, quoted in Robert George Reisner, *Bird: The Legend of Charlie Parker* (New York: Da Capo Press), 27.

188 "A little way before him": Robert Louis Stevenson, "The Isle of Voices," in *Robert Louis Stevenson: His Best Pacific Writings* (Honolulu, Hawaii: Bess Press, 2003; first published 1893), 275.

188 "To be born is to be wrecked on an island": J. M. Barrie, "Preface," in R. M. Ballantyne, *The Coral Island* (London: James Nisbet, 1913), v–viii.

188 "you are constantly making": J. M. Barrie, "Preface."

189 Look at Maui: In an earlier book about grief, I wrote about islands of one's own making. Kay Redfield Jamison, *Nothing Was the Same* (New York: Alfred A. Knopf, 2009).

189 "'Tis in ourselves": William Shakespeare, *Othello*, 1.3.313–314 (Cambridge: Cambridge University Press, 2018), 107.

191 "dark skies and dampness and rain": D. H. Lawrence, "The Man Who Loved Islands," in *Love Among the Haystacks and Other Stories* (London: Penguin, 1960; first published 1929), 98–99.

191 "crucibles of exploration": James Michener, *Hawaii* (New York: Dial Press, 2014; first published 1959), 18. Michener was eloquent in his description of why so many animal and plant species are unique to the Hawaiian Islands. As in the history of human evolution, hard conditions combined with felicitous ones to spur growth and beauty:

> Perhaps a fortunate combination of rainfall, climate, sunlight and soil accounted for this miracle. Perhaps eons of time in which diverse growing things were left alone to work out their own best destinies was the explanation. Perhaps the fact that when a grass reached here it had to stand upon its own capacities and could not be refertilized by grasses of the same kind from the parent stock, perhaps that is the explanation. But whatever the reason, the fact remains: in these islands new breeds developed, and they prospered, and they grew strong, and they multiplied. For these islands were a crucible of exploration and development. (*Hawaii*, 18)

191 "beautifully coloured": Robert Louis Stevenson, "My First Book" (1894), reprinted in Robert Louis Stevenson, *Treasure Island* (London: Penguin, 1999), 193.

191 "harbours that pleased me like sonnets": Stevenson, "My First Book."

191 "unexpected quarters": Stevenson, "My First Book."

192 "Parrot Islands": Douglas Dunn, "Parrot Islands," in *The Year's Afternoon* (London: Faber and Faber, 2000), 17.

192   "Let there be room": Dunn, "Parrot Islands."

192   "A mind on its wing": Dunn, "Parrot Islands."

193   "darken the serenitie of mans Mind": Edward Reynolds, *A Treatise on the Passions and Faculties of the Soule of Man* (London: Robert Bostock, 1640), 52.

193   "scattering and distracting": Reynolds, *A Treatise on the Passions and Faculties of the Soule of Man.*

193   "so they mutually *weaken*": Reynolds, *A Treatise on the Passions and Faculties of the Soule of Man*, 53.

193   Driving out one passion: Robert Burton, pt. 2, sect. 2, "Mind Rectified," *The Anatomy of Melancholy* (New York: New York Review Books, 2001; first published 1621), 112–14.

193   "Passion, imagination, self-will": William Hazlitt, "On the Love of Life," in *Collected Works of William Hazlitt*, vol. 1, ed. A. R. Waller and Arnold Glover (London: J. M. Dent, 1902; essay first published 1815), 3.

193   Thoreau, observed Emerson: Ralph Waldo Emerson, "Thoreau," in *Nature and Selected Essays* (New York: Penguin, 2003; first published 1862), 409.

193   "catches us and carries us off": Robert Lowell, "Hawthorne's Pegasus," in *Robert Lowell: Collected Prose*, ed. Robert Giroux (New York; Farrar, Straus and Giroux, 1987), 162.

194   "Literature is full of examples": William Osler, "The Faith That Heals," *British Medical Journal* 1 (1910): 1471.

194   "is only an active phase": Osler, "The Faith That Heals."

194   "I drew the map": Ursula K. Le Guin, *The Books of Earthsea* (New York: Saga Press, 2018), 387.

194   "All the islands were on it": Le Guin, *The Books of Earthsea.*

194   "The only way is forward": Philip Pullman, *Daemon Voices: On Stories and Storytelling* (New York: Alfred A. Knopf, 2018), 42.

195   "America's greatest and best-loved fairy tale": "The Wizard of Oz: An American Fairy Tale," an exhibit at the Library of Congress, April 21–September 23, 2000.

195   "If we walk far enough": L. Frank Baum, *The Wonderful Wizard of Oz* (New York: HarperCollins, 1987; first published 1900), 168.

195   "There was a child went forth": Walt Whitman, "There Was a Child Went Forth," *Autumn Rivulets*, in *Leaves of Grass*, ed. Sculley Bradley and Harold Blodgett (New York: W. W. Norton, 1973; first published 1856), 364–66.

195   "This is reality": Willa Cather, *My Ántonia* (London: Vintage Classics, 2018; first published 1918), 131.

195   "All those frivolities": Cather, *My Ántonia.*

196 "One by one": James Barrie, quoted in Cynthia Asquith, *Portrait of Barrie* (London: James Barrie, 1954), 220.

196 "galumphing": Lewis Carroll, *The Hunting of the Snark: An Agony in Eight Fits* (New York: Pantheon, 1966; first published 1876), 26. Carroll describes the seagoing, lace-making Beaver, who, having hunted the Snark, "went simply galumphing about." The slaying of the Jabberwock, in *Through the Looking Glass*, also led to "galumphing." Lewis Carroll, *Alice's Adventures in Wonderland* & *Through the Looking Glass* (New York: Signet, 2000; first published 1871), 138.

196 "a child who, by some divine grace": Max Beerbohm, "The Child Barrie," *Saturday Review*, January 7, 1905, 13–14.

196 "I don't know whether": J. M. Barrie, *Peter Pan: The 1911 "Peter and Wendy Edition"* (Greenwood, Wisc.: Suzeteo Enterprises, 2019), 5.

197 "Do you remember anything": T. H. White, *The Once and Future King* (New York: Ace Books, 1987; first published 1958), 285–86.

198 "Understanding courage is a timeless": General Sir Peter de la Billière, Introduction to Lord Moran's *The Anatomy of Courage* (New York: Carroll & Graf, 2007; first published 1945), xvii.

198 "is in facing danger": L. Frank Baum, *The Wonderful Wizard of Oz* (Orinda, Calif.: SeaWolf Press, 2021; first published 1900), 138.

198 "Courage is a moral quality": Lord Moran, *The Anatomy of Courage*, 67.

199 "We were primarily": Apsley Cherry-Garrard, *The Worst Journey in the World* (New York: Penguin, 2005; first published 1922), 533.

199 "Much of that": Cherry-Garrard, *The Worst Journey in the World*, 532.

201 "immense fits of depression": Cherry-Garrard, *The Worst Journey in the World*, 195.

201 "the Pole was not by any means": Cherry-Garrard, *The Worst Journey in the World*.

201 "I now see very plainly": Cherry-Garrard, *The Worst Journey in the World*, 529.

202 "I want to do something splendid": Louisa May Alcott, *Little Women* (London: Puffin Books, 2014; first published 1868), 224.

202 "I don't like to doze by the fire": Alcott, *Little Women*, 70.

203 "For this was no longer": P. L. Travers, *Mary Poppins in Cherry Tree Lane* (New York: HarperCollins Children's Books, 2016; first published 1982), 47–48.

203 "If you are looking for autobiographical facts": P. L. Travers, quoted in Stanley Kunitz and Howard Haycraft, eds., *The Junior Book of Authors*, 2nd ed. (New York: Wilson, 1951), 288.

203 "as a matter of course": "A Radical Innocence," in Pamela Lyndon

Travers, *What the Bee Knows: Reflections on Myth, Symbol and Story* (Wellingborough: Aquarian Press, 1989), 237–38.

203 "I remembered how, for a long period": "A Radical Innocence."

204 "on her own desert": "A Radical Innocence," 240.

204 "I remember his melancholy": "A Radical Innocence," 239.

204 "Where nobody explains": P. L. Travers, "Only Connect," lecture at the Library of Congress, October 31, 1967. First published in *The Quarterly Journal* (Library of Congress, 1967) and reprinted in *Only Connect: Readings on Children's Literature*, ed. Sheila Egoff, G. T. Stubbs, and L. F. Ashley (Toronto and New York: Oxford University Press, 1969), 196.

204 "one reality that underlies everything": P. L. Travers, "The Art of Fiction," no. 63, *Paris Review* 86 (1982): 217.

205 "is the pure product": W.H.R. Rivers, "The Sociological Significance of Myth," *Folklore* 23 (1912): 310.

205 "strangely shaped rocks": Rivers, "The Sociological Significance of Myth," 315.

205 "What *isn't* frightening": Travers, "Only Connect," 196.

205 "fairy godmother" of her youth: Letter from Ted Hughes to the publisher of the Mary Poppins books, undated, Mitchell Library of the State Library of New South Wales, Sydney.

205 "All the King's horses": Travers, "Only Connect," 197.

205 "You only have to open a newspaper": Travers, *What the Bee Knows*, 26.

205 "run around in our blood": Travers, *What the Bee Knows*.

205 "Life, in a sense, is myth": Travers, "Only Connect," 204.

205 "Afterwards, they make their long way": Travers, "Only Connect," 194–95.

206 "looking as though they had gone mad": P. L. Travers, *Mary Poppins* (London: HarperCollins Children's Books, 2016; first published 1934), 16.

206 "You'll never leave us, will you?": Travers, *Mary Poppins*, 22.

206 "I'll stay till the wind changes": Travers, *Mary Poppins*, 23.

207 "There was something strange": Travers, *Mary Poppins*, 21.

207 "For you, Mary Poppins": P. L. Travers, *Mary Poppins Comes Back* (London: HarperCollins Children's Books, 2016; first published 1935), 158.

207 It is right and wonderful: Feature name: Travers, ID 15773, Map of Mercury, Approval date October 19, 2018, Gazetteer of Planetary Union, Nomenclature, International Astronomical Union.

207 "All good things come to an end": Travers, *Mary Poppins Comes Back*, 215, 227.

208 "And the thing they wished": P. L. Travers, *Mary Poppins Opens the Door* (London: HarperCollins Children's Books, 2016; first published 1944), 207.

208 "is to accept everything": P. L. Travers to Jonathan Cott, July 1979, quoted in Valerie Lawson, *Mary Poppins, She Wrote* (New York: Simon & Schuster, 1999), 335.

209 "I learn by going where I have to go": Lawson, *Mary Poppins, She Wrote*, 360–61.

210 "And therein stuck a fair sword": Sir Thomas Malory, *Le Morte d'Arthur*, vol. 1 (London: Penguin Classics, 1986; first published c. 1485), 16, 19.

210 To teach is to show: Kay Redfield Jamison, *Exuberance: The Passion for Life* (New York: Alfred A. Knopf, 2004), 227–28.

211 "no bones, no crowns": Simon Armitage, *The Death of Arthur* (New York: W. W. Norton, 2012), 14.

211 "greatest English writer": Quoted in Sylvia Townsend Warner, *T. H. White: A Biography* (New York: Viking Press, 1967), 153.

211 "There lies buried in its heart": Alan Jay Lerner, *The Street Where I Live* (New York: W. W. Norton, 1978), 192.

211 "that subtle force": William Osler, "Old and New," *Bulletin of Medical and Chirurgical Faculty of Maryland* (1908–1909), May 13, 1909, 248–59.

212 "certain unwritten laws": Osler, "Old and New."

212 "And so there grew": Alfred Lord Tennyson, "The Coming of Arthur" (lines 11–13), *Idylls of the King*, 10th ed., ed. J. M. Gray (London: Penguin Classics, 1989. Originally published 1859–1885, 21.

212 "Merlyn is myself": T. H. White, "The Pleasures of Learning," lecture tour [4 lectures for American tour], 1963. Papers of T. H. White, Harry Ransom Humanities Research Center, University of Texas at Austin, 3.

212 "thirst to throw yourself": White, "The Pleasures of Learning," 54.

212 "When you know a thing": White, "The Pleasures of Learning."

212 "You have to arm yourself": White, "The Pleasures of Learning," 47.

212 "I have had to spend": White, "The Pleasures of Learning."

213 "T. H. White / 1906–1964": T. H. White is buried in the Protestant cemetery in Athens, a setting of olive and bitter orange trees and pines. His marble gravestone is flat and a broadsword is cut into the stone beneath his epitaph.

213 "chased by a mad black wind": John Warner, quoted in Sylvia Townsend Warner, *T. H. White: A Biography*, 94.

213 "I think he was 75 per cent": John Warner, quoted in Sylvia Townsend Warner, *T. H. White*, 93.

213 The actress Julie Andrews: Cited in Kurth Sprague, *T. H. White's Troubled Heart* (Rochester, N.Y.: Boydell & Brewer, 2007), xv.

213 "a great man": T. H. White diary, April 8, 1957, quoted in Sylvia Townsend Warner, *T. H. White: A Biography*, 272.

214 "He was studying Erse": Sylvia Townsend Warner, *T. H. White*, 125.

214 "The best thing for being sad": T. H. White, *The Once and Future King* (New York: Ace Books, 2011; first published 1958), 176–77.

215 "which smelt of incense and cinnamon": White, *The Once and Future King*, 24.

215 "full of salmon flies": White, *The Once and Future King*.

215 "of every possible colour": White, *The Once and Future King*, 25.

215 "propped against each other": White, *The Once and Future King*, 24.

216 "with closed eyes": White, *The Once and Future King*, 26.

217 "ravaged by all the passions": White, *The Once and Future King*, 44.

217 "Power is of the individual mind": White, *The Once and Future King*, 45.

218 "You swim along": White, *The Once and Future King*, 44.

218 "In future, you will have to go": White, *The Once and Future King*, 39.

218 "Education is experience": White, *The Once and Future King*.

218 "It is necessary": W.H.R. Rivers, "Psychology and the War," in *Instinct and the Unconscious* (Cambridge: Cambridge University Press, 1924), 257.

218 The remedies: Rivers, "Psychology and the War."

219 "came from nowhere": White, *The Once and Future King*, 158.

219 "stars of spring": White, *The Once and Future King*, 154.

219 "the sea sound": White, *The Once and Future King*, 159.

219 "which had no corners": White, *The Once and Future King*, 647.

219 "touch their nerves": Laurie Lee, "The Lying in State," in *Village Christmas and Other Notes on the English Year* (London: Penguin Classics, 2016). Although some have assumed that Laurie Lee was writing about George VI, his essay seems more obviously to be about Winston Churchill, lying in state in Westminster Hall in January 1965.

220 "without malice, vanity, suspicion": White, *The Once and Future King*, 387.

220 "Aristotelian and comprehensive tragedy": White, *The Once and Future King*, 308.

220 "The king had slept": White, *The Once and Future King*.

221 "grievous wound": "I will into the vale of Avilion to heal me of my grievous wound: and if thou hear never more of me, pray for my soul." Sir Thomas Malory, *Le Morte d'Arthur*, vol. 2 (London: Penguin Classics, 1986; first published c. 1485), 517.

221 "And that long lamentation": Wilfred Owen, "Hospital Barge," in *Wilfred Owen: The Poems*, ed. Jon Silkin (London: Penguin, 1985; poem first published 1918), 116.

221 "There was something invincible": White, *The Once and Future King*, 642.

221 "a tincture of grandness": White, *The Once and Future King*.

221 "My idea of those knights": White, *The Once and Future King*, 645.

221 "It will burn": White, *The Once and Future King*.

222 "Yet some men say": Malory, *Le Morte d'Arthur*, vol. 2, 519.

222 "The cannons of his adversary": Malory, *Le Morte d'Arthur*, vol. 2, 647.

223 "Your children shall ask": Joshua 4:21.

CHAPTER 9: THEY LOOKED TO THEIR SONGS

224 "They suffered": Paul Robeson interview with Frank B. Lenz, "When Robeson Sings," *Association Men* (July 1927), 495.

225 "You, Mr. Robeson": Citation for Honorary Doctor of Humane Letters, conferred upon Paul Robeson by Morehouse College, June 1, 1943, quoted by Paul Robeson in *Here I Stand* (Boston: Beacon Press, 1988; first published 1958), 114.

225 Bones of cave lions: Fossil deposits found under what is now Trafalgar Square date from the last interglacial, approximately 120,000 years ago. These include those of hippopotamuses, lions, pond terrapins, elephants, rhinoceroses, cave lions, and a woolly mammoth. J. W. Franks, "Interglacial Deposits at Trafalgar Square, London," *New Phytologist* 59 (1959): 145–52; Rodney Mace, *Trafalgar Square: Emblem of Empire* (London: Lawrence and Wishart, 1976); A. J. Sutcliffe, *On the Track of Ice Age Mammals* (Cambridge, Mass.: Harvard University Press, 1985); Steve Jones, "A Hippopotamus Herd in Trafalgar Square," *The Lancet* 383 (March 29, 2014): 1117–18.

225 Thousands filled the square: Joseph E. Persico, *Eleventh Month, Eleventh Day, Eleventh Hour: Armistice Day, 1918* (New York: Random House, 2005); Guy Cuthbertson, *Peace at Last: A Portrait of Armistice Day, 11 November 1918* (New Haven: Yale University Press, 2018); Alexandra Churchill, *In the Eye of the Storm: George V and the Great War* (Warwick, England: Helion & Company), 1918.

225 In the summer: On June 28, 1959, Paul Robeson spoke to a crowd of ten thousand demonstrators in Trafalgar Square participating in a Committee for Nuclear Disarmament protest.

226 "As London traffic": John Ryle, letter to the editor, *New York Review of Books*, February 22, 2018.

226 Paul Robeson was a singer: There are many sources of information about Paul Robeson's life and work, including Paul Robeson, *Here I Stand* (Boston: Beacon Press, 1988; first published 1958); Marie Seton, *Paul Robeson* (London: Dennis Dobson, 1958); Philip S. Foner, ed., *Paul Robeson Speaks: Writings, Speeches, Interviews, 1918–1974* (New York: Citadel Press, 1978); The Editors of *Freedomways, Paul Robeson: The Great Forerunner* (New York: Dodd, Mead, 1978); Charlotte Turner Bell, *Paul Robeson's Last Days in Philadelphia* (Bryn Mawr, Pa.: Dorrance, 1986); Martin Duberman, *Paul Robeson: A Biography* (New York: New Press, 1989); Lloyd L. Brown, *The Young Paul Robeson: "On My Journey Now"* (Boulder, Colo.: Westview, 1997); Sheila Tully Boyle and Andrew Bunie, *Paul Robeson: The Years of Promise and Achievement* (Amherst: University of Massachusetts Press, 2001); Paul Robeson, Jr., *The Undiscovered Paul Robeson: An Artist's Journey, 1898–1939* (New York: John Wiley, 2001); Paul Robeson, Jr., *The Undiscovered Paul Robeson: Quest for Freedom, 1939–1976* (New York: John Wiley, 2010) (henceforth, *Quest for Freedom*); Arnold H. Lubasch, *Robeson: An American Ballad* (Lanham, Md.: Rowman and Littlefield, 2012); Jeff Sparrow, *No Way But This: In Search of Paul Robeson* (Victoria, Australia: Scribe Publications, 2017).

227 "Before King dreamed": Lerone Bennett, Jr., 1998, introduction to "Paul Robeson: Wales," an exhibition created by the South Wales Miners' Library, Swansea University, Wales.

227 "lives, overwhelmingly": James Baldwin, "A Statement by James Baldwin," *The Village Voice*, March 27, 1978, 6.

227 "*know* that such a man was in the world": Baldwin, "A Statement by James Baldwin."

227 "Light / parted from": Pablo Neruda, "Ode to Paul Robeson," in *All the Odes* (New York: Farrar, Straus and Giroux, 2013), 495.

228 "cry from the depths": Music critic (unnamed), "Paul Robeson in Songs," *The New York Times*, April 20, 1925, 21.

228 "truest expression": Marie Seton, *Paul Robeson* (London: Dennis Dobson, 1958), 232.

228 Song, he said: Seton, *Paul Robeson*, 233.

228 "simply beautiful": Correspondence from Michael Hersch, Decem-

ber 21, 2021. "The very best performers," he added, "put their audience into an almost instantaneous hypnotic state which is shot through with a kind of structural awakedness . . . a rare and wonderful juxtaposition."

228 "exuded magnetism": Martin Duberman, interview with Howard "Stretch" Johnson, March 5, 1985, quoted in Martin Duberman, *Paul Robeson: A Biography* (New York: New Press, 1989), 258.

228 "as though each person": Martin Duberman, interview with Junius Scales, March 10, 1986, quoted in Duberman, *Paul Robeson: A Biography*.

228 Robeson was five: Robeson, *Here I Stand*, 7.

229 "The glory of": Robeson, *Here I Stand*, 6.

229 Born into slavery: Robeson wrote, "January is the month of emancipation. This season with its connotation of dawning freedom is close to me. My own father—not my grandfather—was a slave. He was born in 1843 in Eastern North Carolina near Rocky Mount, and escaped in 1858 over the Maryland border to Pennsylvania. He worked on farms, earned enough money and went back twice to North Carolina, to carry money to the mother he loved so dearly. So he escaped three times by the underground railroad." Paul Robeson, "Here's My Story," *Freedom*, January 1951, 1.

229 "rock-like strength": Robeson, *Here I Stand*, 9.

229 "no hint of servility": Robeson, *Here I Stand*, 11.

229 "I adored him": Robeson, *Here I Stand*, 9.

230 "I learned that Emancipation": Robeson, "Here's My Story," *Freedom*, January 1951, 1.

230 "And I've spent my life": Robeson, "Here's My Story," January 1951, 1.

230 "I honestly feel": Paul Robeson, "An Actor's Wanderings and Hopes," *The Messenger*, October 1924, 32.

230 "What would Pop think?": Robeson, "Here's My Story," *Freedom*, April 1952, 5.

230 "I often stop": Robeson, "Here's My Story," *Freedom*, April 1953, 5.

230 "Paul simply said": Brown, *The Young Paul Robeson: "On My Journey Now"* (Boulder, Colo.: Westview, 1997), 141.

231 Paul Robeson's accomplishments: See discussions in Duberman, *Paul Robeson: A Biography*; Brown, *The Young Paul Robeson*; Paul Robeson, Jr., *The Undiscovered Paul Robeson*; Boyle and Bunie, *Paul Robeson: The Years of Promise and Achievement*.

231 "the greatest defensive end": Walter Camp, quoted in Alden Whitman, "Paul Robeson Dead at 77; Singer, Actor and Activist," *The New York Times*, January 24, 1976, 30.

231 practicing French verbs: Martin Duberman, interview with Helen Rosen, April 7, 1998, American Masters Digital Archive (WNET).

231 "If he strode": Lawrence Brown, quoted in Seton, *Paul Robeson*, 59.

231 "no rest till the": "Ol' Man River," from *Show Boat* (1927), music by Jerome Kern, lyrics by Oscar Hammerstein II.

232 "because it was serious": Hal Prince, NPR interview, *All Things Considered*, April 17, 2000.

232 he had conceived the melody: Gary Giddins, liner notes for Criterion Collection release (2020) of *Show Boat* (1936 film, Universal Pictures, directed by James Whale).

232 "aching and racked": "Ol' Man River," from *Show Boat* (1927).

232 "a sorrow which": Seton, *Paul Robeson*, 44.

232 "I went in": Edna Ferber, letter to Alexander Woollcott, February 19, 1933. Alexander Woollcott Collection, Houghton Library, Harvard University.

232 "is the most interesting": Paul Robeson interview with Marguerite Tazelaar, *New York Herald Tribune*, 1935.

233 "cheered the roof off": Uta Hagen, letter to her parents, quoted in George Spector, "Hagen." Cited in Duberman, *Paul Robeson: A Biography*, 663.

233 "one of the most memorable": Burton Rascoe, "Guild's *Othello* a Triumph, Unbelievably Magnificent," *New York World-Telegram*, October 20, 1943, 16.

233 "the American theatre": V. Rogov, "Othello in the American Theatre," translated from *Literatura Iskustvo* (February 9, 1944). Cited in Duberman, *Paul Robeson: A Biography*, 277.

233 "It was deeply fascinating": Paul Robeson, "Some Reflections on *Othello* and the Nature of Our Time," *The American Scholar* 14 (Autumn 1945): 391.

234 "There is a balm": "There Is a Balm in Gilead," in *Folk Songs of the American Negro*, ed. Frederick J. Work (Nashville: Work Bros. & Hart, 1907), 31.

234 "My cradle song": Paul Robeson, "The Related Sounds of Music," written in September 1957 for a Czechoslovakian musical journal. Reprinted in English in Foner, ed., *Paul Robeson Speaks: Writings, Speeches, Interviews, 1918–1974* (New York: Brunner/Mazel, 1978), 443.

234 "there was a warmth": Robeson, *Here I Stand*, 15.

234 "the hopes of our people": Paul Robeson, interview with Frank B. Lenz, "When Robeson Sings," *Association Men* (July 1927), 495.

234 "sometimes of quiet meditation": Paul Robeson, Foreword to *Lift*

Every Voice! The Second People's Song Book (New York: Oak Publications, 1953), 3.

235   "They that walked": W.E.B. Du Bois, "The Sorrow Songs," in *The Souls of Black Folk* (Chicago: A.C. McClurg, 1903), 117.

235   "Through all the sorrow": Du Bois, "The Sorrow Songs," 122.

235   "Is there no balm": Jeremiah 8:22.

235   "sovereign remedy against despair": Robert Burton, *The Anatomy of Melancholy* (New York: New York Review Books, 2001; first published 1621), second partition, 117.

235   "tonick to the saddened soul": Burton, *The Anatomy of Melancholy*.

235   "lost in his own reverie": Reported by Howard Marshall, *Radio Review*, November 25, 1935, and described by Paul Robeson, Jr., *The Undiscovered Paul Robeson: An Artist's Journey, 1898–1939*, 242–43.

236   "emotional burning": Walter Whitworth, "Negro Spirituals and Folk Songs Admirably Presented," *The Indianapolis News*, January 21, 1926, 31.

236   "elemental, agonizingly poignant": Whitworth, "Negro Spirituals and Folk Songs Admirably Presented," *The Indianapolis News*, January 21, 1926, 31.

236   "Somewhere, sometime": Paul Robeson, in E. G. Cousins, ed., *What I Want from Life* (London: George Allen & Unwin Ltd., 1934), 74.

236   "He is without doubt": W.E.B. Du Bois, quoted in Lloyd L. Brown, Preface to Paul Robeson, *Here I Stand* (Boston: Beacon Press, 1988; first published 1958), xxvi.

237   "My art is a weapon": Paul Robeson, speech before the Union of Mine-Mill and Smelter Workers of Canada Convention, Ontario, February 1956.

237   "Why should we not sing": Lloyd George, "Mr. Lloyd George's Speech. A Letter to 'The Times,'" *The Times* (London), August 18, 1916, 3.

237   Eisteddfod: "The Right to Sing. Mr. Ll. George on War Cheerfulness. The Eisteddfod," *The Times* (London), August 18, 1916, 3.

237   "I am a citizen of the world": Paul Robeson, quoted in *Express and Star*, January 23, 1939.

237   As a child in Princeton: Paul Robeson, address at Welcome Home Rally, Rockland Palace, New York City, June 19, 1949, in Foner, ed., *Paul Robeson Speaks*, 201.

238   "There was a clear line": Paul Robeson, "Here's My Story," *Freedom*, December 1950.

238   "control his rage": Saul Fisher, a psychiatrist at Bellevue Hospital, April 1947. Quoted in Boyle and Bunie, *Paul Robeson: The Years of*

Promise and Achievement (Amherst: University of Massachusetts Press, 2001),3.

238   "We must wait": Robeson, *Here I Stand*, 74–75.

239   "It is easy": Robeson, *Here I Stand*, 76.

239   "How long?": Robeson, *Here I Stand*, 90.

239   "Every artist": Paul Robeson, speech at a rally organized by the National Joint Committee for Spanish Relief in Aid of the Spanish Refugee Children, Royal Albert Hall, London, June 24, 1937. Reprinted in Foner, *Paul Robeson Speaks*, 118–19.

240   "I gets weary": Over many years of singing "Ol' Man River," Paul Robeson changed Oscar Hammerstein II's lyrics. In one of his last public appearances, a "Salute to Paul Robeson" at Carnegie Hall in April 1973, Robeson ended with the version he had been using for years. "Though ill health has compelled my retirement," he told the audience, "you can be sure that in my heart I go on singing":

> But I keeps laughing
> Instead of crying,
> I must keep fighting
> Until I'm dying,
> And Ol' Man River
> He just keeps rolling along!

Quoted in Foner, *Paul Robeson Speaks*, 482.

240   "the purpose of art": Harry Belafonte, remarks to the Veterans of the Lincoln Brigade / Abraham Lincoln Brigade Archives, sixtieth anniversary of the Abraham Lincoln Brigade's arrival in Spain, New York City, Manhattan Community College, April 27, 1997.

240   At one point: There are several accounts of Paul Robeson "stopping the war" with his singing, including a book for children written by his granddaughter Susan Robeson, *Grandpa Stops a War: A Paul Robeson Story* (Toronto: Triangle Square, 2019).

241   "seemed inept": "Robeson to President Truman—'Government Must Act Against Lynching or the Negroes Will," *The New York Times*, September 24, 1946, 43.

241   "last refuge of freedom": Paul Robeson led a small delegation to the White House to talk about lynching with President Truman. The substance and tone of the meeting are described in Duberman, *Paul Robeson: A Biography*, 307.

241   "one of the greatest enslavers": Duberman, *Paul Robeson: A Biography*.

241   "We Charge Genocide": Paul Robeson, on behalf of the Civil Rights Congress, presented an anti-lynching petition, "We Charge Genocide," to the United Nations on December 17, 1951. It

charged that the United States was in violation of Article II of the United Nations Genocide Convention: "We maintain, therefore, that the oppressed Negro citizens of the United States, segregated, discriminated against and long the target of violence, suffer from genocide as the result of the consistent, conscious, unified policies of every branch of government." (According to the Tuskegee Institute, 3,446 African Americans were lynched between 1882 and 1968. Sources are given in the Monroe Work Today Dataset Compilation at Tuskegee Institute, which, in collaboration with seventy other institutions and data sources, determined the number of lynchings.)

241 "If there is no struggle": Frederick Douglass, "West India Emancipation," Canandaigua, New York, August 3, 1857.

242 "In 1946, at a legislative hearing": Robeson, *Here I Stand*, 38–39.

243 "What they have done to Paul": W.E.B. Du Bois, *The Daily Worker*, August 21, 1958, quoted in Duberman, *Paul Robeson*, 473, 732.

243 In 1956, Robeson: Testimony before the House Un-American Activities Committee, Eighty-Fourth Congress, Second Session, June 12, 1956, Washington, D.C., 4492–4510.

243 "Are you now a member": Testimony before the House Un-American Activities Committee, June 12, 1956.

244 The only thing wrong with Paul Robeson: W.E.B. Du Bois, quoted in "Paul Robeson. Right or Wrong? Right, Says W.E.B. Du Bois," *Negro Digest* 7 (1950): 8.

245 "Whatever has happened to Stalin": Paul Robeson testimony before the House Un-American Activities Committee, June 12, 1956.

245 "terrible fury": Seton, *Paul Robeson*, 83.

245 "This is like Mississippi": Seton, *Paul Robeson*.

246 "Negro blood": Anne Lounsbery, "Russia's Literary Genius Alexander Pushkin: The Great-Grandson of an African Slave," *The Journal of Blacks in Higher Education* (2000): 108.

246 Once, when Robeson was asked: Robeson, Jr., *The Young Paul Robeson: Quest for Freedom, 1939–1976* (New York: John Wiley, 2010), 153.

246 "fell in love with him": Robeson, Jr., *Quest for Freedom*, 88.

246 "They have never been told": Robeson, Jr., *Quest for Freedom*, 89.

246 "Maybe you'll understand": Robeson, Jr., *Quest for Freedom*, 95.

246 "I think he felt": Helen Rosen, American Masters Digital Archive (WNET), April 7, 1998.

247 In 1958, the Supreme Court: *Kent et al. v. John Foster Dulles*, 357 U.S. 116 (1958). The United States Supreme Court ruled that a passport cannot be withheld from a United States citizen because of belief or association.

247 ". . . the irretrievability of his world": Robeson, "Some Reflections on *Othello* and the Nature of Our Time."

248 "conspiracy of the government": Martin Duberman, interview with Helen Rosen, 1998.

248 "I'm a very melancholy person": Paul Robeson, quoted in *The Manchester Guardian*, November 1932.

248 unexplainably began to yell: Duberman, *Paul Robeson: A Biography*, 149. Duberman suggests that this "bout of nerves" may have marked the onset of Robeson's depressive illness.

248 The next year: Boyle and Bunie, *Paul Robeson: The Years of Promise and Achievement*, 263.

248 He came very close: Marie Seton, quoted in Duberman, *Paul Robeson: A Biography*, 163. Based on Duberman's interviews with Seton, August–September 1982.

248 "complete emotional collapse": Paul Robeson's manic and depressive episodes are described in detail in Duberman, *Paul Robeson: A Biography*; and Robeson, Jr., *Quest for Freedom*. Duberman interviewed several of Robeson's psychiatrists at length about Robeson's diagnosis and treatment. Helen Rosen (1998) discussed Robeson's breakdowns with Duberman, as well, and in an interview for a PBS program about Robeson, April 7, 1998. Joe Andrews, Robeson's dresser, described Robeson's early episode of depression in London in 1932. There is limited written information about Robeson's family history of mental illness. In 1961, his son, Paul Robeson, Jr.—in his own words, paranoid, "exhilarated," and terrified—was put into a straitjacket and hospitalized after throwing a chair through the window of his hotel room. Robeson, Jr., *Quest for Freedom*, 318–19. David Paul Robeson, Paul Robeson's grandson, died by suicide in 1998. Lubasch, *Robeson: An American Ballad* (Lanham, Md.: Roman and Littlefield, 2012), 235.

249 In 1961 Paul Robeson cut his wrists: Duberman, *Paul Robeson: A Biography*; Duberman, interview with Rosen, 1998; Robeson, Jr., *Quest for Freedom*.

249 "One could see the scars": Duberman, interview with Rosen, 1998.

249 "huddled in a fetal position": Helen Rosen, quoted in Duberman, *Paul Robeson: A Biography*, 502.

249 He was admitted: Duberman, *Paul Robeson: A Biography*; Robeson, Jr., *Quest for Freedom*.

249 One admission, which was involuntary: The admission to the Priory Hospital was in September 1961. Robeson, Jr., *Quest for Freedom*, 322.

249 "endogenous depression": Dr. John Flood, consultant psychiatrist

at the Priory Hospital in Roehampton, to Dr. Morris Perlmetter, one of Robeson's psychiatrists in New York. Cited in Duberman, *Paul Robeson: A Biography*, 502.

249 His physician: Duberman, *Paul Robeson: A Biography*, 322–23.

250 "wither away": Eslanda Robeson to Mikhail Kotov, June 22, 1962, quoted in Duberman, *Paul Robeson: A Biography*, 511.

250 "I'll never be well": Paul Robeson to Eslanda Robeson, April 9, 1963.

250 "his face blank with terror": Described by Duberman, *Paul Robeson: A Biography*, 532; and Robeson, Jr., *Quest for Freedom*, 354.

250 "I'm just putting in time": Robeson, Jr., *Quest for Freedom*, 369.

251 "I looked at him": Harry Belafonte, remarks to the Veterans of the Lincoln Brigade / Abraham Lincoln Brigade Archives, 1997.

251 "Would you introduce me": Helen Rosen, PBS interview, 1998.

251 When Lewis finally met: Duberman, *Paul Robeson: A Biography*, 540.

251 "He knew the price": Paul Robeson, Jr., spoken at his father's funeral, January 27, 1976, and quoted in Robeson, Jr., *Quest for Freedom*, 371.

252 "Going home, going home": Lyrics written by William Arms Fisher for Antonin Dvorak's "Largo" from Symphony No. 9 ("From the New World").

252 "free Negroes who refused": Paul Robeson, letter to Boris Polevoi, October 1954, *Masses & Mainstream*, quoted in Foner, *Paul Robeson Speaks*, 387.

252 "played their part in": Robeson, letter to Boris Polevoi.

252 "baying of the lynch-mob": Robeson, letter to Boris Polevoi.

252 "caress of love": Robeson, letter to Boris Polevoi.

252 "He bore on his body": Bishop J. Clinton Hoggard, eulogy for Paul Robeson, January 27, 1976, Mother A.M.E. Zion Church, New York. Printed in Charlotte Turner Bell, *Paul Robeson's Last Days in Philadelphia* (Bryn Mawr, Pa.: Dorrance, 1986), 21.

252 "Paul is medicine to me": Benjamin C. Robeson, "My Brother, Paul," in Robeson, *Here I Stand*, 113.

252 "the war with its shattering of dreams": Benjamin C. Robeson, "My Brother, Paul," 113.

253 "He hath borne our griefs": Isaiah 53:4.

253 By his suffering: Isaiah 53:5.

253 "Well done": "His lord said unto him, Well done, thou good and faithful servant." Matthew 25:21.

253 "Oh, when I come to": Lucie Eddie Campbell, *One Lord, One Faith, One Baptism: An African American Ecumenical Hymnal*, ed. James Abbington (Chicago: GIA Publications), 1933.

253 "illimitable sorrow": Paul Robeson, *Here I Stand*, 15.

253 "soared 100 feet high": "Paul Robeson Sings in St. Paul's for Benefit of South Africa" (author unnamed), *The Witness*, November 13, 1958, 3.

254 No child fidgeted: *The Witness*, November 13, 1958, 3; *The Times* (London), October 13, 1958, 5.

254 "This has been one of": *The Witness*, November 13, 1958, 3.

254 "Here in its foundations": James Elmes, *Sir Christopher Wren and His Times* (London: Chapman & Hall, 1852), 411.

254 "Get them to sing": Belafonte, remarks to the Veterans of the Lincoln Brigade, 1997.

254 "You never gave up your song": Pablo Neruda, "Ode to Paul Robeson," in *All the Odes*, 501.

255 "The major Voice": Gwendolyn Brooks, "Paul Robeson," in *The Essential Gwendolyn Brooks* (New York: Library of America, 2005; originally published in *Family Pictures*, 1970).

255 "I can never forget": Andrew Young, remarks entered into the *Congressional Record*, January 28, 1976, 1380.

255 "We know enough of history": Paul Robeson, "I Want to Be African," in *What I Want from Life*, in Foner, *Paul Robeson Speaks*, 89.

255 "to pass something on": Letter from Robert Lowell to Harriet Winslow, July 31, 1961, in *The Letters of Robert Lowell*, ed. Saskia Hamilton (New York: Farrar, Straus and Giroux, 2003), 385.

255 "Whenever faced by grave and serious decisions": Margaret Burroughs, Tribute to Paul Robeson, in Editors of *Freedomways*, eds., *Paul Robeson: The Great Forerunner* (New York: Dodd, Mead, 1978), 270.

255 Leah Zazulyer: Leah Zazulyer, "When Paul Robeson Sang to Me," *Jewish Currents* (1998): 12.

256 "To my utter amazement": Zazulyer, "When Paul Robeson Sang to Me," 183.

256 "As he sang, I forgot": Zazulyer, "When Paul Robeson Sang to Me."

256 "It was a sort of power": Frederic C. Bartlett, "Obituary—W.H.R. Rivers," *The Eagle* (St. John's College, Cambridge), 43 (1923), 12–14.

256 "stands like a giant": Cited in Jeff Sparrow, *No Way But This: In Search of Paul Robeson* (Melbourne: Scribe, 2017), 268.

256 "They knocked the leaves": Poem by Bill Brown, enclosed in a letter to Judge George W. Crockett, November 6, 1977. Quoted in Duberman, *Paul Robeson: A Biography*, 549, 763.

257 "They looked to their songs": Paul Robeson, interview with Frank B. Lenz, "When Robeson Sings," *Association Men* (July 1927), 495.

258 "By ashen roots": Alfred, Lord Tennyson, *In Memoriam*, ed. Erik Gray (New York: W. W. Norton, 2004; first published 1850), 87.

259 "We obtained in the island": W.H.R. Rivers, "The Primitive Conception of Death," *Hibbert Journal* 10 (1912): 393–407.

259 "impossible to realise": Siegfried Sassoon, November 11, 1918, *Siegfried Sassoon Diaries: 1915–1918*, ed. Rupert Hart-Davis (London: Faber and Faber, 1983), 282.

259 "with a blank mind": Siegfried Sassoon, *Siegfried's Journey: 1916–1920* (London: Faber and Faber, 1982; first published 1945), 97.

259 "outburst of mob patriotism": Sassoon, *Diaries: 1915–1918*, 282.

259 "moral authority": Sassoon, *Siegfried's Journey*, 98.

259 "It was a wretched wet night": Sassoon, *Diaries: 1915–1918*, 282.

259 "an ideal moderator": Sassoon, *Siegfried's Journey*, 98.

260 "I feel/His influence": Siegfried Sassoon, "Revisitation (W.H.R.R.)," in *Siegfried Sassoon: Collected Poems 1908–1956* (London: Faber and Faber, 1984), 205.

260 "For he was a good man": Siegfried Sassoon, June 6, 1922, in *Siegfried Sassoon Diaries: 1920–1922*, ed. Rupert Hart-Davis (London: Faber and Faber, 1981), 164. Hardy's actual wording is: "You was a good man, and did good things!" From Thomas Hardy, *The Woodlanders* (London: Penguin Classics, 1998; first published 1887).

260 "It was a day of brilliant sunshine": Sassoon, June 7, 1922, in *Siegfried Sassoon Diaries: 1920–1922*, 166–67.

262 "exists only in vigilant": Siegfried Sassoon, *Sherston's Progress* (London: Faber and Faber, 1936), 28.

262 "He had shown that he believed": Sassoon, *Sherston's Progress*, 42.

262 "a strenuous effort": Sassoon, *Sherston's Progress*.

262 "Every Toda has two funerals": W.H.R. Rivers, "The Funeral of Sinerani," *The Eagle* (St. John's College, Cambridge), 24 (1903), 337.

262 "What voice revisits me": Siegfried Sassoon, "Revisitation (W.H.R.R.)," in *Siegfried Sassoon: Collected Poems 1908–1956* (London: Faber and Faber, 1984), 205.

264 "It was ordained that you": In a letter to Robert Graves, Sassoon had quoted the French army surgeon and writer Georges Duhamel. Robert Graves, *Goodbye to All That* (London: Penguin, 2000; first published 1929), 226.

264 "can't get away from the War": Letter from T. E. Lawrence to Robert Graves, 1924 (n.d.), in *The Letters of T. E. Lawrence*, ed. David Garnett (London: Jonathan Cape, 1938), 463.

264 "by far the greatest living psychiatrist": Letter from Robert Graves

to Edmund Blunden, March 1921. Harry Ransom Center, University of Texas, Austin.

264 "still in a neurasthenic state": Robert Graves, *The Common Asphodel: Collected Essays on Poetry, 1922–1949* (New York: Haskell House, 1970), vii.

264 "therapeutic poems": Graves, *The Common Asphodel.*

265 "special powers to draw upon": Miranda Seymour, *Robert Graves: Life on the Edge* (New York: Henry Holt, 1995), 106.

265 "To T. E. Lawrence": Robert Graves, *On English Poetry* (London: Heinemann, 1922).

265 "one of my heroes": Letter from W.H.R. Rivers to Robert Graves, May 26, 1921, Morris Library, Southern Illinois University of Carbondale.

266 "I stood quite dumb": Robert Graves, "The Red Ribbon Dream," *The New Republic*, March 8, 1922, 43. See Jean Moorcroft Wilson, "Dr. W.H.R. Rivers: Siegfried Sassoon and Robert Graves, Fathering Friend," *Brain* 140 (2017): 3378–83.

266 "He was treated for shellshock": Norman Buck, Assistant Librarian of St. John's College Library, University of Cambridge, 1963. Recounted to Paul Whittle, PhD, in "W.H.R. Rivers: A Founding Father Worth Remembering," talk given to the Department of Experimental Psychology, University of Cambridge, December 6, 1997. Lieutenant William Arnold Middlebrook, East Yorkshire Regiment, was admitted to Craiglockhart War Hospital in April 1917. He was diagnosed with "neurasthenia" and treated by W.H.R. Rivers until his discharge from the hospital in June 1917.

267 "What does Keats have to teach": Letter from Wilfred Owen to his brother Harold Owen, 1916. Quoted in Jon Stallworthy, *Wilfred Owen* (London: Oxford University Press and Chatto & Windus, 1974), 131.

268 "Very dear Siegfried": Letter from Wilfred Owen to Siegfried Sassoon, October 10, 1918, in Harold Owen and John Bell, eds., *Wilfred Owen: Collected Letters* (London: Oxford University Press, 1967), 581 [letter 664].

268 "For twelve days": Letter from Wilfred Owen to his mother, Susan Owen, April 25, 1917, in *Wilfred Owen: Collected Letters*, 452 [letter 505].

268 "he is nervous about my nerves": Letter from Wilfred Owen to his mother, April 25, 1917, in *Wilfred Owen: Collected Letters.*

269 Brown's therapeutic philosophy: William Brown, "The Treatment of Cases of Shell Shock in an Advanced Neurological Centre," *The Lancet* 192 (1918): 197–200.

269 "petrification of terror": Brown, "The Treatment of Cases of Shell Shock."

269 "gospel of work": Brown, "The Treatment of Cases of Shell Shock."

269 Sassoon's doctor, W.H.R. Rivers: Staff notes from Craiglockhart War Hospital, Department of Documents, Imperial War Museum, London. Private papers of Siegfried Sassoon (catalogue no. 9059), vol. 2, MS. SS 7, Papers Relating to Dr. W.H.R. Rivers and Family, f. 301. Staff notes, 7 pages, n.d., 297–303.

269 Owen's doctor, Arthur J. Brock: Staff notes from Craiglockhart War Hospital.

270 "The minds of these patients": Arthur J. Brock, "War Psychology," in *Health and Conduct* (London: Williams and Norgate, 1923), 139–40. See also: Arthur J. Brock, "Ergotherapy in Neurasthenia," *Edinburgh Medical Journal* 6 (1911): 430–34; David Cantor, "Between Galen, Geddes and the Gael: Arthur Brock, Modernity, and Medical Humanism in Early-Twentieth-Century Scotland," *Journal of the History of Medicine* 60 (2005): 1–41.

270 "one day rank with anesthesia": Colonel Thomas W. Salmon, quoted by Eleanor Clarke Slagle in E. C. Slagle, "Occupational Therapy," *Trained Nurse and Hospital Review* 100 (1938): 375–82.

271 "I held my own": Letter from Wilfred Owen to his mother, Susan Owens, August 13, 1917, in *Wilfred Owen: Collected Letters*, 483 [letter 539].

271 Art should be more than a refuge: Arthur J. Brock, "The Re-Education of the Adult: I. The Neurasthenic in War and Peace," *Sociological Review* 10 (1918): 35.

271 "In the powerful war-poems": Arthur J. Brock, *Health and Conduct* (London: Le Play House, 1923), 171–72.

271 "Nothing like his trench life sketches": Letter from Wilfred Owen to his mother, Susan Owen, August 15, 1917, in *Wilfred Owen: Collected Letters*, 484 [letter 540].

272 "I held you as Keats": Letter from Wilfred Owen to Siegfried Sassoon, November 5, 1917, in *Wilfred Owen: Collected Letters*, 505 [letter 557].

272 "These are men whose minds": Wilfred Owen, *War Poems and Others*, ed. Dominic Hibberd (London: Chatto & Windus, 1973), 99.

273 "put the suffering of his fellow soldiers": Andrew Motion, "Wilfred Owen: The Making of a Poet," Carnegie Lecture, University of St. Andrews, Scotland, 2020.

273 "long before the outbreak of the war": Motion, "Wilfred Owen."

273 "I came out in order": Letter from Wilfred Owen to his mother,

Susan Owen, October 4 or 5, 1918, in *Wilfred Owen: Collected Letters*, 580 [letter 662].

273 "for conspicuous gallantry": Cited in *The London Gazette*, June 30, 1919.

273 "Move him into the sun": Wilfred Owen, *War Poems and Others*, 98.

274 "And you have *fixed* my Life": Letter from Wilfred Owen to Siegfried Sassoon, November 5, 1917, in *Wilfred Owen: Collected Letters*, 505 [letter 557].

274 "I go out of this year": Letter from Wilfred Owen to his mother, Susan Owen, December 31, 1917, in *Wilfred Owen: Collected Letters*, 521 [letter 578].

275 "So, soon they topped the hill": Wilfred Owen, *War Poems and Others*, 108–9.

275 "My subject is War": Wilfred Owen, *War Poems and Others*, 137.

275 his introduction to the book: *Wilfred Owen: Poems*, Introduction by Siegfried Sassoon (London: Chatto & Windus, 1920), v–vi.

275 The poem: Siegfried Sassoon, *Siegfried's Journey*, 59.

275 "Courage was mine": Wilfred Owen, "Strange Meeting," in Wilfred Owen, *War Poems and Others*, 103.

CHAPTER 11: THE ELEVENTH HOUR

276 "But death replied": Siegfried Sassoon, "The Death-Bed," in Siegfried Sassoon, *Collected Poems, 1908–1956* (London: Faber and Faber, 2002), 30–32.

277 "In all the woods": William Arthur Hill, "The Flora of the Somme Battlefield," nos. 9 & 10, *Bulletin of Miscellaneous Information*, Royal Botanic Gardens, Kew (1917), 297–300; "The Flora of the Somme Battlefield," *Nature* 100 (1918): 475–76. See also James Alexander Wearn, "The Flora of the Somme Battlefield: A Botanical Perspective on a Post-Conflict Landscape," *First World War Studies* 8 (2017): 63–77.

277 Conditions of an Armistice: "Conditions of the Armistice with Germany (November 11, 1918)," *German History in Documents and Images*, vol. 6, *Weimar Germany, 1918–1933* (Washington, D.C.: German Historical Institute, 2004); Sir Frederick Maurice, *The Armistices of 1918* (London and New York: Oxford University Press, 1943), 93–100. See also Harry R. Rudin, *Armistice 1918* (New Haven: Yale University Press, 1944).

278 "Come to me quickly": Mary Borden, *Poems of Love and War* (Brighton: Dare-Gale Press, 2015), 41. Mary Borden, poet and novelist,

was a nurse during both the First and Second World Wars. She was the first of only two American women to be awarded the Croix de Guerre (for command of the "best hospital on the Front"). She also was cited in French Army Orders for courage demonstrated during bombing on the Somme, and later awarded the Legion of Honour for bravery and wartime nursing contributions.

279 "At 11 A.M. on the morning": Alice Fitzgerald, "The War Is Over," "Memoirs of an American Nurse" (Baltimore: Maryland Historical Society, unpublished manuscript), 179. Alice Fitzgerald was head nurse at Johns Hopkins Hospital prior to the war. After the war she served as chief nurse of the American Red Cross in Europe; later she founded the International School for Public Health Nurses.

279 "Yesterday was forgotten": Fitzgerald, "The War Is Over."

280 "the war will be over": Helen Dore Boylston, *Sister: The War Diary of a Nurse* (Leeds: Kismet, 2018; first published 1925), 92. Helen Boylston served as a nurse anesthetist on the Front. After the war she remained in Europe to work for the Red Cross and then took a position as instructor in anesthesiology at Massachusetts General Hospital. Helen Dore Boylston also wrote a popular series of books for young adults about a nurse, Sue Barton. The books have sold millions of copies and are still in print.

280 "We admitted": Boylston, *Sister,* 46.

280 "The war is over": Boylston, *Sister,* 92.

280 "The scream of shells": Boylston, *Sister,* 105.

280 "We have received the news": Harvey Cushing, *From a Surgeon's Journal: 1915–1918* (Boston: Little, Brown, 1936), 495.

280 "Thus the Great War ends": Cushing, *From a Surgeon's Journal,* 497.

280 "How still it must be": Cushing, *From a Surgeon's Journal,* 498.

281 "There will be much celebrating": Cushing, *From a Surgeon's Journal,* 499.

281 "wondering what the future": Cushing, *From a Surgeon's Journal.*

281 "serious discussion of religion": Cushing, *From a Surgeon's Journal.*

281 "sheer stupidity": Walt Whitman, *Memoranda During the War* (New York: Oxford University Press, 2006; first published privately by Whitman, 1875).

281 "It is very strange": Letter from Lady Grace Osler to Mary Jacobs, December 5, 1918. Alan Mason Chesney Medical Archives, Johns Hopkins Medical Instituion.

282 "So they gave their bodies": Thucydides, "Funeral Oration of Pericles," *The Peloponnesian War,* in Alfred Eckhard Zimmern, *The Greek*

Commonwealth: Politics and Economics in Fifth-Century Athens, 5th ed. (Oxford: Oxford University Press, 1931, reprint 1977), 202.

282 "At the 11th hour": Service sheet for Remembrance Sunday, International Service of Remembrance: The Centenary of the End of the First World War, November 11, 2018, Christ Church Georgetown, Washington, D.C.

282 "They shall grow not old": Laurence Binyon, "For the Fallen," first published in *The Times* (London), September 21, 1914.

283 Thomas Cathcart Traill: Thomas Cathcart Traill began his military service in the First World War as a midshipman in the Royal Navy. He transferred to the Royal Flying Corps and remained in the Royal Air Force for the rest of his forty-year military career. During the Second World War, Traill was a staff officer in RAF Bomber Command, commanded RAF Middleton St. George, and served in North Africa. He retired in 1954 at the rank of air vice-marshal.

283 "a bugler on the cricket ground": This and other entries are from the unpublished diaries of Thomas Cathcart Traill.

284 "In the funeral procession": Thucydides, *The Peloponnesian War*, ed. Robert B. Strassler, in *The Landmark Thucydides: A Comprehensive Guide to the Peloponnesian War* (New York: Free Press, 1996), 110.

285 "Have you forgotten yet": Siegfried Sassoon, "Aftermath," in *Siegfried Sassoon: Collected Poems, 1908–1956* (London: Faber and Faber, 1984), 110.

285 John Keegan estimates: John Keegan, *The First World War* (New York: Vintage, 2000), 421–22.

285 "Their bodies had been blown": Keegan, *The First World War*, 421.

285 "Every Padre serving": David Railton, "The Origin of the Unknown Warrior's Grave," extract from *Our Empire*, November 1931, vol. 7.

286 "So I thought and thought": Railton, "The Origin of the Unknown Warrior's Grave."

286 "His Majesty is inclined": Sir Henry Wilson, speaking on behalf of George V. Quoted in Alexandra Churchill, *In the Eye of the Storm: George V and the Great War* (Warwick: Helion, 2018), 362.

288 "a singular emblem": Sir Thomas Browne, "Notes on Natural History," in *Sir Thomas Browne: The Major Works*, ed. C. A. Patrides (London: Penguin, 1977), 39.

288 "You must feed your eyes": Thucydides, *The Peloponnesian War*, 115.

289 "We have forced every sea": Thucydides, *The Peloponnesian War*, 114.

289 "So died these men": Thucydides, *The Peloponnesian War*, 115

289 "We all were made": Correspondent for *The Times* (London), November 12, 1920.

289 "For a little while": Correspondent for *The Times* (London), November 12, 1920.

289 "Lead, Kindly Light": J. H. Newman, "Lead, Kindly Light," in *The English Hymnal* (London: Oxford University Press, 1977), 373. The hymn was written in 1833 by John Henry Newman and often sung during times of tragedy: by trapped miners in England; on a lifeboat of the RMS *Titanic;* and at the Ravensbrück concentration camp. Early in 1915, British soldiers sang "Lead, Kindly Light" to accompanying artillery fire at services held before going into the trenches on the Front. The hymn, a favorite of Thomas Hardy and Mahatma Gandhi, begins:

> Lead, kindly Light, amid the encircling gloom,
> Lead thou me on;
> The night is dark, and I am far from home,
> Lead thou me on.
> Keep thou my feet; I do not ask to see
> The distant scene: one step enough for me.

290 "was the most beautiful": The King wrote in his diary, "It was a fine bright day, not cold, no wind." There were "4 Queens in the Abbey," he noted. The "whole ceremony was most moving and impressive . . . beautiful." Diary of George V, November 10–12, 1920. Royal Archives, Windsor Castle. RA GV / PRIV / GUD / 1920: 10–12 Nov.

EPILOGUE: CHESAPEAKE

291 "As for your feares": John Smith, "The Accidents that Happened in the Discovery of the Bay of Chesapeake," *The Generall Historie of Virginia, New-England and the Summer Isles* (Glasgow: J. MacLehose and Sons, 1907; first published in 1624).

292 "The young forest below": Boris Pasternak, *Doctor Zhivago*, trans. Richard Pevear and Larissa Volokhonsky (London: Vintage, 2010; first published 1957), 213.

292 "The many Rivers, Creeks, and Rivulets": Letter from the Reverend Mr. Hugh Jones to the Reverend Dr. Benjamin Woodroffe, January 23, 1698 [1699], Royal Society of London, *Philosophical Transactions*, 21, 436–42. The clergyman described the richness of the Chesapeake Bay country, its "rich and plentiful gifts": its fish of all kinds, berries, herbs and roots, deer and fowl, and the great stands of trees, chestnut, oak, cedar, black walnut, sassafras, ash, and hickory. The number of navigable rivers, creeks, and inlets made it immensely convenient, he wrote: "Noe country can compare with it."

292   The Chesapeake water: There are many navigational, historical, fictional, and natural history accounts of the Chesapeake Bay, including the writings and maps of the seventeenth-century explorer Captain John Smith: *Generall Historie of Virginia, New-England, and the Summer Isles with the Names of the Adventurers, Planters, and Governours from Their First Beginning, An: 1584 to This Present 1624* (London: Printed by John Dawson and John Haviland for Michael Sparkes, 1624); and more recently so in *The Complete Works of Captain John Smith*, 3 vols., ed. Philip Barbour (Chapel Hill: University of North Carolina Press, 1986), 2:25–488; Arthur Pierce Middleton, *Tobacco Coast: A Maritime History of Chesapeake Bay in the Colonial Era* (Baltimore: Johns Hopkins University Press and the Maryland State Archives, 1953); James A. Michener, *Chesapeake* (New York: Random House, 1978); Alice Jane Lippson and Robert L. Lippson, *Life in the Chesapeake Bay*, 3rd ed. (Baltimore: Johns Hopkins University Press, 2006); Helen C. Rountree, Wayne E. Clark, and Kent Mountford, *John Smith's Chesapeake Voyages, 1607–1609* (Charlottesville: University of Virginia Press, 2007).

293   "Heaven and earth": Captain James Smith, *Generall Historie of Virginia, New-England, and the Summer Isles*, 121–22.

293   Islands disappeared: Middleton, *Tobacco Coast*; Earl Swift, *Chesapeake Requiem* (New York: Dey Street Books, 2018).

295   throwing a summer wreath: I wrote this in the aftermath of my late husband's death. Words and necessity lured me on: "To read *In Memoriam* was to throw a summer wreath over an unclimbable fence in impassable weather. I could see life on the other side: the way over the fence would be hard, but the wreath gave me something to keep sight of, something toward which to move." Kay Redfield Jamison, *Nothing Was the Same: A Memoir* (New York: Alfred A. Knopf, 2009), 178.

Index

Page numbers in *italics* refer to illustrations.
The letter *i* following a page number denotes an illustration in the insert.

Page

15 Courtesy of the Osler Library of the History of Medicine, McGill University.

21 Courtesy of the Osler Library of the History of Medicine, McGill University.

23 (*top and bottom*) Courtesy of the Osler Library of the History of Medicine, McGill University.

26 Courtesy of the Osler Library of the History of Medicine, McGill University.

38 Image of Mary Borden from the Mary Borden Collection at the Boston University Libraries' Howard Gotlieb Archival Research Center.

46 The Chesney Archives of Johns Hopkins Medicine, Nursing, and Public Health.

57 © National Museum of the Royal Navy.

64 © National Museum of the Royal Navy.

76 Courtesy of Bethlem Museum of the Mind.

88 Copyright Siegfried Sassoon by kind permission of the Estate of George Sassoon, and Ralph Hodgson Papers, Beinecke Rare Book and Manuscript Library, Yale University.

92 © IWM Documents.9059.

100 (*left*) Copyright Siegfried Sassoon by kind permission of the Estate of George Sassoon, and Harry Ransom Center, The University of Texas at Austin.

100 (*right*) Reprinted from *The Lancet*, XCVI, W.H.R. Rivers, MD, "The Repression of War Experience," pp. 513–33, 1917.

109 © Photograph: Royal Academy of Arts, London.

121 Outline Restoration of Some of the Principal Buildings of the Hieron of Epidauros, plates by M. Cavvadias.

124 Caton, R. *The Temples and Rituals of Asklepios at Epidauros and Athens.* London: C. J. Clay and Sons, 1900.

129 From the collection of the Phoebe A. Hearst Museum of Anthropology at the University of California, Berkeley. Photo by Jim Heaphy, CC BY-SA 3.0.

131 Image of the stained-glass window of Offham Rectory, Kent. Photograph taken by Kayleigh Fitzgerald. Public domain.

153 Viktor Frankl in year 1965. Photograph by Professor Dr. Franz Vesely, CC BY-SA 3.0 de.

160 © Alain A. Moreau.

171 *Notre-Dame Cathedral in Flames;* AP Photo / Thibault Camus File.

187 Collection of the Smithsonian National Museum of African American History and Culture, ca. 1947.

200 With kind permission of Scott Polar Research Institute, University of Cambridge.

216 Courtesy of the T. H. (Terence Hanbury) White Literary File Photography Collection (Photography Collection PH-02808). Harry Ransom Center, The University of Texas at Austin.

224 Keystone Press / Alamy Stock Photo.

226 © The Valente Collection, National Portrait Gallery, Smithsonian Institution with additional permission by the family of Paul Robeson.

244 AP Photo / Bill Achatz.

258 Image courtesy of the author.

263 A. D. White Architectural Photographs, Cornell University Library.

265 *Goodbye to All That*, Penguin Random House U.K.

267 With kind permission of the Trustees of the Wilfred Owen Estate and the Bodleian Libraries, University of Oxford, MS, 12282, Photogr. 5, Item 6.

276 © IWM Q 31514.

278 © IWM Q 47886.

287 © IWM Q 31485.

291 © The Trustees of the British Museum.

PHOTO SECTION

Page

1 Courtesy of the Osler Library of the History of Medicine, McGill University.

2 (*top*) On Behalf of the Fleming Family, British Library.

2 (*bottom*) Courtesy of the Chesney Archives of Johns Hopkins Medicine, Nursing, and Public Health.

3 © National Army Museum, London, United Kingdom.

4 "La structure de la grotte de Bruniquel," Luc-Henri Fage/SSAC. Photo modified under terms of CC-BY-SA 4.0.

5 Reprinted by permission of Starregistration.net.

6 (*top*) Illustration of Scarlet Pimpernel (flowering plant) from the *Vienna Dioscurides*, circa 515.

6 (*right*) Illustration of Scarlet Pimpernel (flowering plant) from the *Vienna Dioscurides*, circa 515.

6 (*bottom*) *Nebamun Garden*, The British Museum, London. Photograph by Yann Forget.

7 (*top*) Courtesy of the Osler Library of the History of Medicine, McGill University.

7 (*bottom*) Küsnacht-Wohnhaus von C.G. Jung, Seestrasse 228, CC BY-SA 3.0 Unported.

8 © Freud Museum London.

9 (*top*) AP Photo / Thibault Camus File.

9 (*bottom*) Crown of Thorns in the circular reliquary in crystal of 1896. Notre-Dame de Paris Cathedral, CC BY-SA 3.0.

10 Copyright © 1968 by Ursula K. Le Guin. First appeared in *A Wizard of Earthsea*, published by Houghton Mifflin Harcourt in 1968. Reprinted by permission of Ginger Clark Literary, LLC.

11 Copyright 1980 and by permission of the International Wizard of Oz Club.

12 Map of Treasure Island, from the first German edition.
13 Book cover from *Mary Poppins* by P.L. Travers, published by Harcourt Children's Books (1934).
14 (*top*) British Library / Granger Historical Picture Archive—all rights reserved.
14 (*bottom*) King Arthur's Round Table at Winchester Castle—Winchester, Hampshire, England. Photo by R. S. Nourse, CC BY-SA 4.0.
15 Bettmann / Contributor.
16 © Dean and Chapter of Westminster.

PERMISSIONS ACKNOWLEDGMENTS

Grateful acknowledgment is made to the following for permission to reprint previously published materials:

Brooks Permissions: Reprinted By Consent of Brooks Permissions.

Grateful acknowledgment is made to Faber and Faber Ltd for permission to reprint an excerpt from "Parrot Islands" from *The Year's Afternoon* by Douglass Dunn. Reprinted by permission of Faber and Faber Ltd.

ROBERT LOWELL, SETTING THE RIVER ON FIRE
A Study of Genius, Mania, and Character

In this magisterial study of the relationship between illness and art, the bestselling author of *An Unquiet Mind* brings an entirely fresh understanding to the work and life of Robert Lowell (1917–1977), whose intense, complex, and personal verse left a lasting mark on the English language and changed the public discourse about private matters. In his poetry, Lowell put his manic-depressive illness (now known as bipolar disorder) into the public domain, and in the process created a new and arresting language for madness. Here Dr. Kay Redfield Jamison brings her expertise in mood disorders to bear on Lowell's story, illuminating not only the relationships between mania, depression, and creativity but also how Lowell's illness and treatment influenced his work (and often became its subject). A bold, sympathetic account of a poet who was—both despite and because of mental illness—a passionate, original observer of the human condition.

Biography

NOTHING WAS THE SAME
A Memoir

Kay Redfield Jamison, award-winning professor and writer, changed the way we think about moods and madness. Jamison uses her characteristic honesty, wit, and eloquence to look back at her relationship with her husband, Richard Wyatt, a renowned scientist who died of cancer. *Nothing Was the Same* is a penetrating psychological study of grief viewed from deep inside the experience itself.

Memoir/Psychology

EXUBERANCE
The Passion for Life

With the same grace and breadth of learning she brought to her studies of the mind's pathologies, Kay Redfield Jamison examines one of its most exalted states: exuberance. This "abounding, ebullient, effervescent emotion" manifests itself everywhere from child's play to scientific breakthrough. *Exuberance: The Passion for Life* introduces us to such notably irrepressible types as Teddy Roosevelt, John Muir, and Richard Feynman, as well as Peter Pan, dancing porcupines, and Charles Schulz's Snoopy. It explores whether exuberance can be inherited, parses its neurochemical grammar, and documents the methods people have used to stimulate it. The resulting book is an irresistible fusion of science and soul.

Psychology and Psychiatry

ALSO AVAILABLE

Night Falls Fast
An Unquiet Mind